The Joint Commission (TJC) list of abbreviations that should be spelled out.

Abbreviation	Use Instead
q.d., Q.D.	Write "daily" or "every day."
q.o.d., Q.O.D.	Write "every other day."
U	Write "unit."
IU	Write "international unit."
MS, MSO_4	Write "morphine sulfate."
$MgSO_4$	Write "magnesium sulfate."
.5 mg	Write "0.5 mg," use zero before a decimal point when the dose is less than a whole.
1.0 mg	Do not use a decimal point or zero after a whole number.

The following abbreviations could possibly be included in future Joint Commission "Do Not Use" lists. These abbreviations are as follows:

Abbreviation	Use Instead
c.c.	Use "mL" (milliliter).
μg	Use "mcg" (microgram).
>	Write "greater than."
<	Write "less than."
Drug name abbreviations	Write out the full name of the drug.
Apothecary units	Use metric units.
@	Write "at."

Other abbreviations can be found in Chapter 3, page 54.

	Metric	Standard		
Metric and Standard Measurement Conversions				
Weight	1 kilogram	2.2 lbs		
	0.45 kg	1 lb		
	30 g	1 oz		
	15 g	1/2 oz		
Volume	1 liter	32 oz	1 quart	
	500 mL	16 oz	1 pint	
	250 mL	8 oz	1 cup	
	30 mL	1 oz	2 tablespoons	
	15 mL	1/2 oz	1 tablespoon	3 teaspoons
	5 mL			1 teaspoon
	2.5 mL			1/2 teaspoon
Length	1 meter	3.28 ft	39.37 in	
	1 cm	0.39 in		

Clinical Calculations

With Applications to General and Specialty Areas

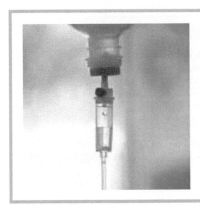
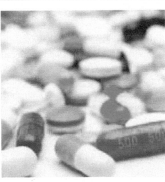
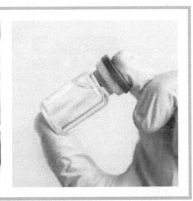

TENTH EDITION

Joyce LeFever Kee, RN, MS
Associate Professor Emerita
College of Health Sciences
Department of Nursing
University of Delaware
Newark, Delaware

Sally M. Marshall, RN, MSN
Foermerly, Nursing Service
V. A. Medical Center
Wilmington, Delaware

Kathryn Woods, RN, BSN, CRNA, DNP
American Anesthesiology of Maryland, Baltimore Practice
Greater Baltimore Medical Center
Baltimore, Maryland

Mary Catherine Forrester, RN, MSN, ACNP-BC
Vanderbilt University Hospital Trauma and Burn Center
Nashville, TN

ELSEVIER

Elsevier
3251 Riverport Lane
St. Louis, Missouri 63043

Notices

Practitioners and researchers must always rely on their own experience and knowledge in evaluating and using any information, methods, compounds or experiments described herein. Because of rapid advances in the medical sciences, in particular, independent verification of diagnoses and drug dosages should be made. To the fullest extent of the law, no responsibility is assumed by Elsevier, authors, editors or contributors for any injury and/or damage to persons or property as a matter of products liability, negligence or otherwise, or from any use or operation of any methods, products, instructions, or ideas contained in the material herein.

Previous editions copyrighted 2021, 2017, 2013, 2009, 2004, 2000, 1996, 1992, 1988

International Standard Book Number: 978-0-323-82751-5

Senior Content Strategist: Yvonne Alexopoulos
Senior Content Development Manager: Luke E. Held
Senior Content Development Specialist: Joshua S. Rapplean
Publishing Services Manager: Julie Eddy
Senior Project Manager: Abigail Bradberry
Senior Book Designer: Maggie Reid

Printed in the United States of America
Last digit is the print number: 9 8 7 6 5 4 3 2 1

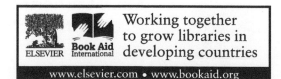

Working together
to grow libraries in
developing countries

www.elsevier.com • www.bookaid.org

To my granddaughter, Kimberly Cibroski, BSN, RN
Emergency Room, ChristianaCare, Newark, Delaware
Joyce Kee

To Bob
Sally Marshall

To my parents, Bill and Rebecca, and my husband, Mark
Katie Forrester

To my family, friends, and Roxie
Katy Woods

Preface to the Instructor

Clinical Calculations with Applications to General and Specialty Areas arose from the need to bridge the learning gap between education and practice. We believe that this bridge is needed for the student to understand the wide range of clinical calculations used in nursing practice. This book provides a comprehensive application of calculations in nursing practice and has been expanded in this tenth edition to include Next-Generation NCLEX® examination-style questions.

Clinical Calculations is unique in that it has problems not only for the general patient areas but also for the specialty units—pediatrics, critical care, pediatric critical care, labor and delivery, and community. This text is useful for nurses at all levels of nursing education who are learning for the first time how to calculate dosage problems and for beginning practitioners in specialty areas. It also can be used in nursing refresher courses, in-service programs, hospital units, home health care, and other settings of nursing practice.

The use of the latest methods, techniques, and equipment is included: unit dose dispensing system, electronic medication administration record (eMAR), computerized prescriber order system (CPOS), various methods of calculating drug doses with the use of body mass index (BMI), ideal body weight (IBW) with adjusted body weight (ABW), insulin pump, patient-controlled analgesia pumps, multi-channel infusion pumps, IV filters, and many more. This text also provides the six (6) methods for calculating drug dosages—basic formula, ratio and proportion, fractional equation, dimensional analysis, body weight, and body surface area.

This book is divided into five parts. Part I is the basic math review, written concisely for nursing students to review Roman numerals, fractions, decimals, percentages, and ratio and proportion. A post-math review test follows. The post-math test can be taken first and, if the student has a score of 90% or higher, the basic review section can be omitted. Part II covers metric and household measurement systems used in drug calculations; conversion of units; reading drug labels, drug orders, eMAR, computerized prescriber order systems, and abbreviations; and methods of calculations. We suggest that you assign Parts I and II, which cover delivery of medication, before the class. Part III covers calculation of drug and fluid dosages for oral, injectable, insulin administration, and intravenous administration. Clinical drug calculations for specialty areas are found in Part IV, which includes pediatrics, critical care for adults and children, labor and delivery, and community. Part V contains the post-test for students to test their competency in mastering oral, injectable, intravenous, and pediatric drug calculations. A passing grade is 88%. Appendix A includes guidelines for administration of medications (oral, injectable, and intravenous).

Each chapter has a content list, objectives, introduction, and numerous practice problems. The practice problems are related to clinical drug problems that are currently used in clinical settings. Illustrations of tablets, capsules, medicine cup, syringes, ampules, vials, intravenous bag and bottle, IV tubing, electronic IV devices, intramuscular injection sites, central venous sites, and many other related images are provided throughout the text.

Also included are Next-Generation NCLEX® examination-style or NGN® Prep questions, based on a Clinical Judgment Model developed by the National Council of State Boards of Nursing (NCSBN). The style of question is designed to assess critical thinking, judgment, and decision-making based on actual clinical situations.

Calculators may be used in solving dosage problems. Many institutions have calculators available. The student should work the problem without a calculator and then check the answer with a calculator.

FEATURES FOR THE TENTH EDITION

- Next-Generation NCLEX® examination-style and NGN® Prep questions have been added to relevant chapters.
- Problems using the newest drug labels are provided in most chapters.
- Six methods for calculating drug dosages have been divided into two chapters. Chapter 6 gives four methods: basic formula, ratio and proportion, fractional equations, and dimensional analysis. Chapter 7 contains two individual methods for calculating drug doses: body weight and body surface area.
- Emphasis is placed on the metric system along with the household system of measurement.
- Illustrations of intraosseous and intraspinal access are included in the Alternative Methods for Drug Administration chapter.
- Several chapters have nomograms for adults and children.
- Explanation on the unit dose dispensing system, computer-based drug administration, computerized prescriber order system, bar code medication administration, MAR, electronic medication administration record (eMAR), and automation of medication dispensing administration are provided.
- Incorporation of guidelines for safe practice and the medication administration set by the Joint Commission (TJC) and the Institute for Safe Medicine Practices (ISMP) are included.
- Explanation of the four groups of inhaled medications include: MDI inhalers with and without spacers, dry powder inhalers, and nebulizers.
- Calculations by BMI, IBW, and ABW for obese and debilitated persons are presented.
- Body Surface Area (BSA or m^2) using the square root method is included.
- Use of fingertip units for cream applications is illustrated.
- Explanations are provided for the use of the insulin pump, insulin pen injectors, and the patient-controlled analgesic pump.
- Illustrations of types of syringes, safety needle shield, various insulin and tuberculin syringes, and needleless syringes are provided.
- Illustrations of pumps are provided, including insulin, enteral infusion, and various intravenous infusion pumps (single and multi-channel, patient-controlled analgesia, and syringe).
- Coverage of direct intravenous injection (IV push or IV bolus) is provided with practice problems in Chapter 11.
- Methods and information for critical care, pediatrics, and labor and delivery calculations are presented.

ANCILLARIES

Evolve resources for instructors and students can be found online at http://evolve.elsevier.com/KeeMarshall/clinical/

The Instructor Resources are designed to help you present the material in this text and include the following:

- Test Bank—with over 500 questions.
- TEACH consists of customizable Lesson Plans and Lecture Outlines, and PowerPoint slides. It is an online resource designed to help you to reduce your lesson preparation time, give you new and creative ideas to promote student learning, and help you to make full use of the rich array of resources in the Clinical Calculations teaching package.
- Drug Label Glossary—includes all of the drug labels from the text. Instructors can search for labels by trade or generic name.
- **NEW!** NGN® Case Studies are available for instructors to assign as supplemental testing or extra NGN® preparation.

Student Resources provide students with additional tools for learning and include the following:
Elsevier's Interactive Drug Calculation Application, Version 1
- This interactive drug calculations application provides hands on, interactive practice for the user to master drug calculations. Users can select the mode (Study, Exam, or Comprehensive Exam) and then the category for study and exam modes. There are eight categories that cover the main drug calculation topics. Users are also able to select the number of problems they want to complete and their preferred drug calculation method. A calculator is available for easy access within any mode, and the application also provides history of the work done by the user.

Preface to the Student

Clinical Calculations with Applications to General and Specialty Areas, tenth edition, can be used as a self-instructional mathematics and dosage calculation review tool.

Part I, *Basic Math Review,* is a review of math concepts usually taught in middle school. Some students may need to review Part I as a refresher of basic math and then take the comprehensive math test at the end of the chapter. Others may choose to take the math test first. If your score on this test is 90% or higher, you should proceed to Part II; if your score is less than 90%, you should review Part I.

Part II, *Systems, Conversion, and Methods of Drug Calculation,* should be studied before the class on oral, injectable, insulin administration, and intravenous calculations, which are covered in Part III. In Part II you will learn the various systems of drug administration, conversion within the various systems, charting (MAR and eMAR), drug orders, abbreviations, methods of drug calculation, how to prevent medication errors, and alternative methods for drug administration. You can study Part II on your own. Chapter 6, "Methods of Calculation," gives the four methods commonly used to calculate drug dosages. You or the instructor should select one of the four methods to calculate drug dosages. Use that method in all practice problems starting in Chapter 6. This approach will improve your proficiency in the calculation of drug dosages.

Part III, *Calculations for Oral, Injectable, and Intravenous Drugs,* is usually discussed in class and during a clinical practicum. Before class, you should review the four chapters in Part III. Questions may be addressed and answered during class time. During the class or clinical practicum, you may practice drug calculations and the drawing up of drug doses in a syringe.

Part IV, *Calculations for Specialty Areas,* is usually presented when the topics are discussed in class. You should review the content in these chapters— "Pediatrics," "Critical Care," "Pediatric Critical Care," "Labor and Delivery," and "Community"— before the scheduled class. According to the requirements of your specific nursing program, this content may or may not be covered.

Part V, *Post-Test,* has 65 post-test questions you should solve to determine your competency in mastering oral, injectable, intravenous, and pediatric drug calculations. Take a look at the following features so that you may familiarize yourself with this text and maximize its value:

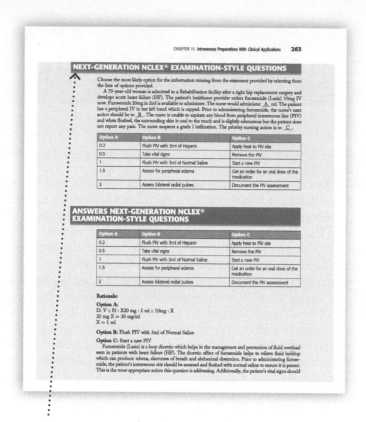

Next-Generation NCLEX® examination-style or NGN® Prep questions are designed to introduce students to new elements from the updated NCLEX® exam, assessing critical thinking, judgment, and decision-making based on actual clinical situations.

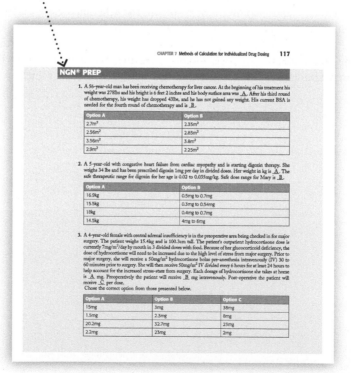

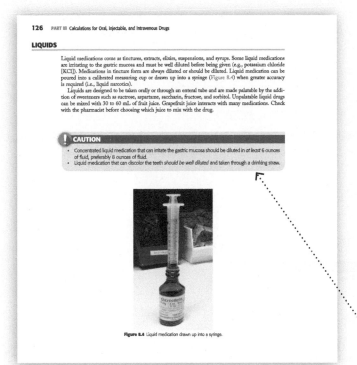

126 PART III Calculations for Oral, Injectable, and Intravenous Drugs

LIQUIDS

Liquid medications come as tinctures, extracts, elixirs, suspensions, and syrups. Some liquid medications are irritating to the gastric mucosa and must be well diluted before being given (e.g., potassium chloride [KCl]). Medications in tincture form are always diluted or should be diluted. Liquid medication can be poured into a calibrated measuring cup or drawn up into a syringe (Figure 8.4) when greater accuracy is required (i.e., liquid narcotics).

Liquids are designed to be taken orally or through an enteral tube and are made palatable by the addition of sweeteners such as sucrose, aspartame, saccharin, fructose, and sorbitol. Unpalatable liquid drugs can be mixed with 30 to 60 mL of fruit juice. Grapefruit juice interacts with many medications. Check with the pharmacist before choosing which juice to mix with the drug.

! CAUTION
- Concentrated liquid medication that can irritate the gastric mucosa should be diluted in *at least* 6 ounces of fluid, preferably 8 ounces of fluid.
- Liquid medication that can discolor the teeth *should be well diluted* and taken through a drinking straw.

Figure 8.4 Liquid medication drawn up into a syringe.

Caution boxes alert you to potential problems related to various medications and their administration.

You Must Remember boxes identify pertinent concepts that students should commit to memory.

58 PART II Systems, Conversion, and Methods of Drug Calculation

Nurse educators have resources through the Quality and Safety Education for Nurses (QSEN) Institute to assist students to learn the complexities of safe practice in drug administration.

YOU MUST REMEMBER
The person who administers the medication, usually the nurse, is responsible if an ME occurs.

Here are some examples of the types of medication errors (MEs):

1. The physician or health care provider makes a prescribing error and/or the written drug order is **NOT** legible.
2. Transcription errors occur because the medications have similar names; the decimals and zeros are not correctly written; or numbers are transposed.
3. Telephone and verbal orders are misinterpreted.
4. Interruptions occur when preparing medications.
5. Drug labels look similar (names and color), and packing obscures print on the label.
6. Trade names and generic names for drugs are used interchangeably, which causes confusion.
7. Oral dosages and intravenous dosages are different for the same drug.
8. Subcutaneous insulin is given in a tuberculin syringe and **NOT** in an insulin syringe.
9. The pharmacy delivers the wrong drug.
10. Intravenous medication is given too fast or too concentrated.
11. The amount of the drug is incorrectly calculated.
12. The drug is given intramuscularly or subcutaneously and should be given intravenously OR the drug is given intravenously and should be given intramuscularly.
13. Two incompatible drugs are given intravenously, which can cause crystallization of the drugs.
14. Two or three patients with the same names are on the same unit and their identification wristbands are hard to read. One patient receives another's medication.
15. Medication is given and not monitored, and an overdose occurs.
16. An infusion pump malfunctions or is incorrectly programmed.

Ways to prevent medication errors (MEs):

1. Ask the physician or health care provider to rewrite or clarify medication order.
2. Use only approved abbreviations from The Joint Commission (TJC) list for medication dosages. Do not use "u" for unit; it should be spelled out. Avoid use of a slash mark (/), which could be interpreted as a one (1).
3. Do not use abbreviations for medication names (e.g., MSO₄ for morphine sulfate).
4. Use leading zeros for doses less than a unit (e.g., **0.1** mg; **NOT .1** mg). Do not use a zero following a whole number (e.g., 5 mg; **NOT** 5.0 mg). The decimal point after 5 may not be noticed and would look like 50 mg.
5. Check medication orders with written order and MAR/eMAR.
6. Check the drug dose sent from the pharmacy with the MAR/eMAR.
7. Prepare medications in a clean, distraction-free environment.
8. Never administer a medication that has been prepared by another nurse.
9. Have another nurse check the dosage preparation, especially if in doubt. Recalculate drug dosage as needed.
10. Check if the patient is allergic to any specific drugs. If an allergy exists, report the type of reaction the patient experiences.
11. Check the patient's identification band with the eMAR and bar code.
12. Do not leave medication at the bedside. Stay with the patient until the medications are swallowed.

Notes emphasize important points for students as they learn material in each chapter.

Elsevier's Interactive Drug Calculation Application, Version 1

This interactive drug calculation application provides hands on, interactive practice for the user to master drug calculations. Users can select the mode (Study, Exam, or Comprehensive Exam) and then the category for study and exam modes. There are eight categories that cover the main drug calculation topics. Users are also able to select the number of problems they want to complete and their preferred drug calculation method. A calculator is available for easy access within any mode, and the application also provides history of the work done by the user.

At the end of various chapters, there are references to **Elsevier's Interactive Drug Calculation Application, Version 1** for additional practice problems and content information.

ACKNOWLEDGMENTS

Thank you to Joyce LeFever Kee for the years of collaboration and support on this text. Your encouragement of new ideas and concept in our broad field of nursing were much appreciated.

Sally M. Marshall, Author

It has been an honor and my great pleasure to work with Joyce LeFever Kee on several editions of *Clinical Calculations*. Joyce was a devoted educator and author and I thank her for her tremendous contributions in helping to educate nursing students over the years with her drug calculations and pharmacology texts. Joyce and I shared a wonderful author-editor relationship, but more importantly, we became friends over the editions and shared many stories about our travels. Joyce could tell me anything about any place in the world because she had already traveled there! I loved listening to her stories! Joyce, wishing you all the best of health and happiness in this next phase of your life, we will miss you!

Yvonne Alexopoulos, Content Strategist

The Publisher would also like to thank the following reviewers for their time and effort reviewing all the math components of this title:

Lou Ann Boose, RN, MSN
Paula Silver, BS, PHD

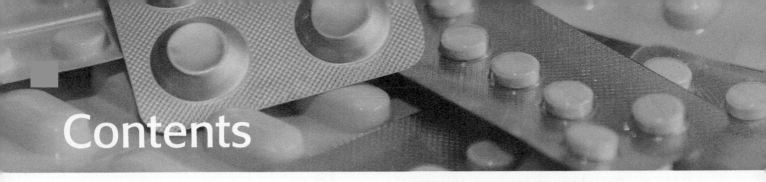

Contents

PART I

BASIC MATH REVIEW

Objectives • Express a fraction as simple, proper, or improper.
• Use the process of simplification and reduction with fractions to find the lowest common denominator.
• Add, subtract, multiply, and divide fractions.
• Express a fraction as a decimal.
• Name the value places for whole numbers and decimals.
• Use the process of rounding with decimals.
• Multiply and divide decimals.
• Change percentages to decimals, fractions, ratio and proportions.

Outline **FRACTIONS**
DECIMALS
RATIO AND PROPORTION
PERCENTAGE
POST-MATH TEST

The knowledge of basic mathematics is vital for nurses in the safe administration of medication and fluids. Medication errors are among the most common of all medical errors. Therefore, a working knowledge of mathematics is needed to calculate and accurately measure medication that will be administered to the patient.

A math test, found on pages 11 to 14, follows the basic math review. The test may be taken first, and, if a score of 90% or greater is achieved, the math review, or Part I, can be omitted. If the test score is less than 90%, the student should do the basic math review section. Some students may choose to start with Part I and then take the test.

Answers to the Practice Problems are at the end of Part I, before the Post-Math Test.

The basic math review will start with fractions and the decimal system. Ratio and proportions and percentages will be addressed. Working knowledge of arithmetic is necessary to perform the operations of addition, subtraction, multiplication, and division, which will allow the nurse to master basic math skills to solve drug dosage problems for the administration of medication.

FRACTIONS

Fractions are expressed as part(s) of a whole or part(s) of a unit. A fraction is composed of two basic numbers: a numerator (top number) represents how many parts. The denominator (bottom number) indicates the total number of parts. They are separated by a division line.

EXAMPLE Fraction: $\dfrac{3}{4}$ numerator (3 of 4 parts)
denominator (4 of 4 parts, or 4 total parts)

The value of a fraction depends mainly on the denominator. When the denominator increases, for example, from $^1/_{10}$ to $^1/_{20}$, the value of the fraction decreases, because it takes more parts to make a whole.

EXAMPLE Which fraction has the greater value: $^1/_4$ or $^1/_6$? The denominators are 4 and 6.

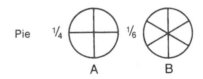

The larger value is $^1/_4$, because four parts make the whole, whereas for $^1/_6$, it takes six parts to make a whole. Therefore $^1/_6$ has the smaller value.

To make working with fractions as easy as possible, it is useful to find the lowest common denominator (LCD). The two functions used to find the LCD are simplification and reduction. Simplification means rewriting the numerator and the denominator without changing the value of the fraction to achieve the simplest and most usable fraction.

EXAMPLE To find the lowest common denominator:

Fraction: $\dfrac{30}{60} = \dfrac{3 \times 10}{3 \times 2 \times 10} =$ 1. Replace numbers with prime numbers as factors: 2, 3, 5, 7.

$\dfrac{30}{60} = \dfrac{^1\cancel{3} \times ^1\cancel{10}}{^1\cancel{3} \times 2 \times ^1\cancel{10}} = \dfrac{1}{2}$ 2. Cancel common factors above and below the division line.

3. Then re-multiply the numerator and denominator.

EXAMPLE To find the lowest common denominator when adding and subtracting, multiply the denominators to find a common value.

Fraction: $\dfrac{1}{2} + \dfrac{2}{5} =$

$$2\overline{)10} \quad \begin{array}{l}\text{quotient} \\ \text{common value}\end{array} \quad 5 \times 1 = 5 \quad \dfrac{1}{2} = \dfrac{5}{10}$$

$$5\overline{)10} \quad \begin{array}{l}\text{quotient} \\ \text{common value}\end{array} \quad 2 \times 2 = 4 \quad \dfrac{2}{5} = \dfrac{4}{10}$$

$$\dfrac{5}{10} + \dfrac{4}{10} = \dfrac{9}{10} \text{ or } \dfrac{1}{2} - \dfrac{2}{5} = \dfrac{5}{10} - \dfrac{4}{10} = \dfrac{1}{10}$$

1. Multiply denominators together to find a common value or if the denominators are too large, try using prime numbers (2, 3, 5, 7...). For this example, 10 is the common value $2 \times 5 = 10$.

2. Divide each denominator into the common value then multiply the numerator by that quotient. Take the quotient/result and multiply by the numerator to find the value of the fraction.

3. Then add or subtract.

Reduction is another means to change the numerator and denominator by the same number until they are as small as possible. If a fraction is even, divide by 2, if it is odd try 3, or if it ends in 0 try 10.

EXAMPLE Fraction: $\dfrac{10}{16} \div \dfrac{2}{2} = \dfrac{5}{8}$ and $\dfrac{21}{36} \div \dfrac{3}{3} = \dfrac{7}{12}$ or $\dfrac{30}{60} \div \dfrac{10}{10} = \dfrac{3}{6} \div \dfrac{3}{3} = \dfrac{1}{2}$

Proper, improper, and Mixed Fractions

Proper or simple fractions have numerators with numbers less than denominators, e.g., ½, ⅔, ¾, ⅘.

Improper fractions have a large numerator and a small denominator and should be simplified or

reduced, e.g., $\dfrac{4}{2} = \dfrac{2 \times \cancel{2}}{1 \times \cancel{2}} = 2$ or $\dfrac{8}{5} = 5\overline{)8} \begin{array}{l}1 \\ \underline{-5} \\ 3\end{array} = 1\dfrac{3}{5}$

A mixed number is a whole number and a fraction, e.g., $1\dfrac{3}{5}, 3\dfrac{1}{2}$. Mixed numbers can be changed to improper fractions by multiplying the denominator by the whole number and then adding the numerator, e.g., $1\dfrac{3}{5} = \dfrac{8}{5} (5 \times 1 = 5 + 3 = 8)$ and $3\dfrac{1}{2} = \dfrac{7}{2} (2 \times 3 = 6 + 1 = 7)$.

Adding Fractions

Adding fractions must be done with fractions that share the same common denominator, then, all that is necessary is the adding of the numerators.

$$\dfrac{1}{5} + \dfrac{2}{5} = \dfrac{3}{5}$$

Subtracting Fractions

Subtracting fractions must be done with fractions that share the same common denominator, again, all that is necessary is the subtracting of the numerators.

$$\dfrac{3}{5} - \dfrac{2}{5} = \dfrac{1}{5}$$

Multiplying Fractions

To multiply fractions, multiply the numerators and then the denominators. Reduce the fraction, if possible, to lowest terms.

EXAMPLES **PROBLEM 1:** $\dfrac{1}{3} \times \dfrac{3}{5} = \dfrac{\overset{1}{\cancel{3}}}{\underset{5}{\cancel{15}}} = \dfrac{1}{5}$

The answer is $^3/_{15}$, which can be reduced to $^1/_5$. The number that divides into both 3 and 15 is 3. Therefore 3 divides into 3 one time, and 3 divides into 15 five times.

PROBLEM 2: $\dfrac{1}{3} \times 6 = \dfrac{\overset{2}{\cancel{6}}}{\underset{1}{\cancel{3}}} = 2$

A whole number can also be written as that number over one ($^6/_1$). Six is divided by 3 ($6 \div 3$); 3 divides into 6 two times.

PROBLEM 3: $\dfrac{4}{5} \times 12 = \dfrac{48}{5} = 9\dfrac{3}{5}$

Dividing Fractions

To divide fractions, invert the *second fraction*, called the divisor, and then multiply.

EXAMPLES **PROBLEM 1:** $\dfrac{3}{4} \div \dfrac{3}{8}$ (divisor) $= \dfrac{\overset{1}{\cancel{3}}}{\underset{1}{\cancel{4}}} \times \dfrac{\overset{2}{\cancel{8}}}{\underset{1}{\cancel{3}}} = \dfrac{2}{1} = 2$

When dividing, invert the divisor $^3/_8$ to $^8/_3$ and multiply. To reduce the fraction to lowest terms, 3 divides into both 3s one time, and 4 divides into 4 and 8 one time and two times, respectively.

PROBLEM 2: $\dfrac{1}{6} \div \dfrac{4}{18} = \dfrac{1}{\underset{1}{\cancel{6}}} \times \dfrac{\overset{3}{\cancel{18}}}{4} = \dfrac{3}{4}$

Six and 18 are reduced, by dividing by 6, to 1 and 3.

PROBLEM 3: $3\dfrac{2}{3} \div \dfrac{5}{6} = \dfrac{11}{\underset{1}{\cancel{3}}} \times \dfrac{\overset{2}{\cancel{6}}}{5} = \dfrac{22}{5} = 4\dfrac{2}{5}$

Change $3^2/_3$ to an improper fraction and invert $^5/_6$ to $^6/_5$ and then multiply. Reduce 3 and 6 by dividing by 3, to 1 and 2.

Decimal Fractions

Change fraction to decimal. Divide the numerator by the denominator.

EXAMPLES **PROBLEM 1:** $\dfrac{3}{4} = 4\overline{)3.00}^{\,0.75}$ or 0.75

Therefore $\dfrac{3}{4}$ is the same as 0.75.

PROBLEM 2 $\dfrac{12}{8} = 8\overline{)12.0}$ or 1.5

$$\begin{array}{r} 1.5 \\ 8\overline{)12.0} \\ \underline{8} \\ 40 \\ \underline{40} \end{array}$$

PRACTICE PROBLEMS ▶ I FRACTIONS

Answers can be found on page 9.

Round off to the nearest tenth unless otherwise indicated.

1. a. Which has the greatest value: $^1/_{50}$, $^1/_{100}$, or $^1/_{150}$? _____

   b. Which has the lowest value: $^1/_{50}$, $^1/_{100}$, or $^1/_{150}$? _____

2. Reduce improper fractions to whole or mixed numbers.

   a. $^{12}/_4 =$ _____

   b. $^{20}/_5 =$ _____

   c. $^{22}/_3 =$ _____

   d. $^{32}/_6 =$ _____

3. Multiply fractions to whole number(s) or lowest fraction or decimal.

   a. $^2/_3 \times ^1/_8 =$ _____

   b. $2\,^2/_5 \times 3\,^3/_4 =$ _____

   c. $^{500}/_{350} \times 5 =$ _____

   d. $^{400,000}/_{200,000} \times 3 =$ _____

4. Divide fractions to whole number(s) or lowest fraction or decimal.

   a. $^2/_3 \div 6 =$ _____

   b. $^1/_4 \div ^1/_5 =$ _____

   c. $^1/_6 \div ^1/_8 =$ _____

   d. $^1/_{150}/^1/_{100} = (^1/_{150} \div ^1/_{100}) =$ _____

   e. $^1/_{200} \div ^1/_{300} =$ _____

   f. $9\,^3/_5 \div 4 = ^{48}/_5 \div ^4/_1 =$ _____

5. Change each fraction to a decimal.

   a. $^1/_4 =$ _____

   b. $^1/_{10} =$ _____

   c. $^2/_5 =$ _____

   d. $^{35}/_4 =$ _____

   e. $^{78}/_5 =$ _____

DECIMALS

The decimal system or metric system is a base 10 number system, 1-9, where each number or combination of numbers have a place or position that gives it value. The decimal system consists of whole numbers to the left of the decimal or zero, that start with a place value of units, tens, hundreds, thousands. Fractional numbers are to the right of the decimal point. Decimal fractions are written in tenths, hundredths, thousandths, ten-thousandths. Tenths means 0.1 or 1/10, hundredths means 0.01 or 1/100, thousandths means 0.001 or 1/1000 and ten-thousandths means 0.0001 or 1/10,000. For example, use the number 2468.8642 and assign place value.

Whole Numbers					**Decimal Fractions**			
2	4	6	8	•	8	6	4	2
Thousands	Hundreds	Tens	Units		Tenths	Hundredths	Thousandths	Ten Thousandths

With the decimal system, the answer to decimal problems can be long because decimal fractions are exact. When decimal fractions are long, they may need to be shortened to be more useful, and they are shortened by rounding.

Rounding rule: First identify the place value where the rounding will end, either the tenths, hundredths, or thousandths place. Then look at the number to the right, if that number is 5 or greater, round up by adding one to the place value. If the number to the right is less than 5, nothing is added to the place value.

EXAMPLES **PROBLEM 1:** Round 2468.8642 to the nearest hundredths. The number 4 occupies the thousandths place and is less than 5, therefore nothing is added to the hundredths place and the number is 2468.86.

PROBLEM 2: Round 2468.86 to the nearest tenth. The number 6 is greater than 5 so the number would be rounded to 2468.9.

Multiplying Decimals

To multiply decimal numbers, multiply the multiplicand by the multiplier. Count how many numbers (spaces) are to the right of the decimals in the problem. Mark off the number of decimal spaces in the answer (right to left) according to the number of decimal spaces in the problem. Answers are rounded off to the nearest **tenths.**

EXAMPLE
multiplicand　　1.34
multiplier　　　×2.3
　　　　　　　　402
　　　　　　　268
product　　　　3.082　or　3.1 (rounded off in tenths)

Answer 3.1. Because 8 is greater than 5, the "tenth" number is increased by 1.

Dividing Decimals

To divide decimal numbers, move the decimal point in the divisor to the right to make a whole number. The decimal point in the dividend is also moved to the right according to the number of decimal spaces in the divisor. Answers are rounded off to the nearest **tenths.**

EXAMPLE   Dividend ÷ Divisor = Quotient

$$2.46 \div 1.2 \text{ or } \frac{2.46}{1.2} =$$

$$\underline{2.05} = 2.1 \text{ (quotient)}$$

(divisor)   1.2)2.4 60 (dividend)

$$\underline{2\ 4}$$

60

$$\underline{60}$$

0

PRACTICE PROBLEMS ▶ II DECIMALS

Answers can be found on page 10.

Round off to the nearest tenths.

1. Multiply decimals.

   a. $6.8 \times 0.123 =$ _____

   b. $52.4 \times 9.345 =$ _____

2. Divide decimals.

   a. $69 \div 3.2 =$ _____

   b. $6.63 \div 0.23 =$ _____

   c. $100 \div 4.5 =$ _____

   d. $125 \div 0.75 =$ _____

3. Change decimals to fractions.

   a. $0.46 =$ _____

   b. $0.05 =$ _____

   c. $0.012 =$ _____

4. Which has the greatest value: 0.46, 0.05, or 0.012? Which has the smallest value? _____

RATIO AND PROPORTION

A *ratio* is the relation between two numbers and is separated by a colon, e.g., 1:2 (1 is to 2). It is another way of expressing a fraction, e.g., 1:2 =½.

Proportion is the relation between two ratios separated by a double colon (::) or equals sign (=).

To solve a ratio and proportion problem, the inside numbers *(means)* are multiplied and the outside numbers *(extremes)* are multiplied. To solve for the unknown, which is X, the X goes to the left side and is followed by an equals sign.

EXAMPLES   **PROBLEM 1:** $1:2::2:X$ (1 is to 2, as 2 is to X)

means
extremes

Multiply the extremes and the means, and solve for X.

$X = 4$ (1 X is the same as X)

Answer: 4 (1:2::2:4)

PROBLEM 2: $4:8::X:12$

$8X = 48$

$X = {}^{48}/_8 = 6$

Answer: 6 (4:8::6:12)

PROBLEM 3: A ratio and proportion problem may be set up as a fraction.

Ratio and Proportion	Fraction
$2:3::4:X$	$\dfrac{2}{3} = \dfrac{4}{X}$ (cross-multiply)
$2X = 12$	$2X = 12$
$X = {}^{12}/_2 = 6$	$X = 6$

Answer: 6. Remember to cross-multiply when the problem is set up as a fraction.

PRACTICE PROBLEMS ▶ III RATIO AND PROPORTION

Answers can be found on page 10.

Solve for X.

1. $2:10::5:X$ _____

2. $0.9:100 = X:1000$ _____

3. Change the ratio and proportion to a fraction and solve for X.
$3:5::X:10$ _____

4. It is 500 miles from Washington, DC to Boston, MA. Your car averages 22 miles per 1 gallon of gasoline. How many gallons of gasoline will be needed for the trip? _____

PERCENTAGE

Percent (%) means 100. Two percent (2%) means 2 parts of 100, and 0.9% means 0.9 part (less than 1) of 100. A percent can be expressed as a fraction, a decimal, or a ratio.

EXAMPLES

Percent		Fraction	Decimal	Ratio
60%	=	$^{60}/_{100}$	0.6	60 : 100
0.45%	=	$^{0.45}/_{100}$ or $^{45}/_{10,000}$	0.0045	0.45:100 or 45:10,000

Note: *To change a Percent to a decimal, move the decimal point two places to the left.*

PRACTICE PROBLEMS ▶ IV PERCENTAGE

Answers can be found on page 10.

Change percent to fraction, decimal, and ratio.

Percent	Fraction	Decimal	Ratio
1. 2%			
2. 0.33%			
3. 150%			
4. ½% (0.5%)			
5. 0.9%			

ANSWERS

I Fractions (Round off to the nearest tenths unless otherwise indicated.)

1. a. $^{1}/_{50}$ has the greatest value.
  b. $^{1}/_{150}$ has the lowest value.

2. a. 3
  b. 4
  c. $7^{1}/_{3}$
  d. $5^{2}/_{6}$ or $5^{1}/_{3}$

3. a. $^{2}/_{24} = ^{1}/_{12}$

  b. $^{12}/_{5} \times ^{15}/_{4} = \dfrac{180}{20} = 9$

  c. $\dfrac{\overset{10}{\cancel{500}}}{\underset{7}{\cancel{350}}} \times 5 = \dfrac{50}{7} = 7.1$

  d. $\dfrac{\overset{2}{\cancel{400,000}}}{\underset{1}{\cancel{200,000}}} \times 3 = 6$

4. a. $^{2}/_{3} \div 6 = ^{2}/_{3} \times ^{1}/_{6}$
  $= ^{2}/_{18} = ^{1}/_{9} = 0.11$

  b. $^{1}/_{4} \div ^{1}/_{5} =$
  $^{1}/_{4} \times ^{5}/_{1} = ^{5}/_{4} =$
  $1^{1}/_{4}$, or 1.25 or 1.3

  c. $\dfrac{1}{6} \div \dfrac{1}{8} = \dfrac{1}{\underset{3}{\cancel{6}}} \times \dfrac{\overset{4}{\cancel{8}}}{1} = \dfrac{4}{3} = 1.33$, or 1.3

d. $^{1}/_{150} \div ^{1}/_{100} = \dfrac{1}{\underset{3}{\cancel{150}}} \times \dfrac{\overset{2}{\cancel{100}}}{1}$
  $= ^{2}/_{3}$, or 0.666, or 0.67 or 0.7

e. $^{1}/_{200} \div ^{1}/_{300} = ^{1}/_{200} \times ^{300}/_{1} = ^{300}/_{200} = 1^{1}/_{2}$, or 1.5

f. $\dfrac{48}{5} \div \dfrac{4}{1} = \dfrac{48}{5} \times \dfrac{1}{4} = \dfrac{48}{20} = 2.4$

5. a. $\dfrac{1}{4} = 4\overline{)1.00}$ $\quad\dfrac{0.25 \text{ or } 0.3 \text{ rounded off}}{}$

  b. $\dfrac{1}{10} = 10\overline{)1.00}$ $\quad\dfrac{0.10 \text{ or } 0.1}{}$

  c. $\dfrac{2}{5} = 5\overline{)2.00}$ $\quad\dfrac{0.40 \text{ or } 0.4}{}$

  d. $\dfrac{35}{4} = 4\overline{)35.00}$ $\quad\dfrac{8.75 \text{ or } 8.8 \text{ rounded off}}{}$

  e. $\dfrac{78}{5} = 5\overline{)78.00}$ $\quad\dfrac{15.60 \text{ or } 15.6}{}$

II Decimals

1. a. 0.123
       $\times$ 6.8

        984
        738

       0.8364, or 0.8 (round off to tenths: 3 hundredths is less than 5)

   b. 489.6780, or 489.7 (7 hundredths is greater than 5)
2. a. 21.56, or 21.6 (6 hundredths is greater than 5, so the tenth is increased by one)
   b. 28.826, or 28.8 (2 hundredths is less than 5, so the tenth is not changed)

   c. $100 \div 4.5 = 4.5\overline{)100.0} = 22.2$, or 22 (rounded off to whole number)

   d. $125 \div 0.75 = 0.75\overline{)125.00} = 166.6$, or 167 (rounded off to whole number)
3. a. $^{46}/_{100} = {}^{23}/_{50}$
   b. $^{5}/_{100} = {}^{1}/_{20}$
   c. $^{12}/_{1000} = {}^{3}/_{250}$
4. 0.46 has the greatest value; 0.012 has the lowest value. Forty-six hundredths is greater than 12 thousandths.

III Ratio and Proportion

1. 2 X = 50
     X = 25
2. 100 X = 900
         X = 9
3. $^{3}/_{5} = {}^{x}/_{10} = 5$ X = 30
                   X = 6

4. 1 gal : 22 miles :: X gal : 500
         22 X = 500
           X = 22.7 gal.
   22.7 gallons of gasoline are needed.

IV Percentage

Percent	Fraction	Decimal	Ratio
1. 2	$^{2}/_{100}$	0.02	2:100
2. 0.33 or 0.3	$^{0.33}/_{100}$ or $^{33}/_{10,000}$	0.0033	0.33:100 or 33:10,000
3. 150	$^{150}/_{100}$	1.50	150:100
4. 0.5	$^{0.5}/_{100}$ or $^{5}/_{1000}$	0.005	0.5:100 or 5:1000
5. 0.9	$^{0.9}/_{100}$ or $^{9}/_{1000}$	0.009	0.9:100 or 9:1000

POST-MATH TEST

Answers can be found on pages 13 and 14.

The math test is composed of four sections: fractions, decimals, ratios and proportions, and percentages. There are 52 questions. A passing score is 47 or more correct answers (90%). A nonpass- ing score is 5 or more incorrect answers. Answers to the Post-Math Test can be found on pages 13 and 14.

Fractions

Which fraction has the larger value?

1. $1/100$ or $1/150$ _____

2. $1/3$ or $1/2$? _____

Reduce improper fractions to whole or mixed numbers.

3. $^{45}/_9 =$ _____

4. $^{74}/_3 =$ _____

Change a mixed number to an improper fraction.

5. $5^2/_3 =$ _____

Change fractions to decimals.

6. $^2/_3 =$ (reduce to tenths) $=$_____

7. $^1/_{12} =$ (reduce to tenths) $=$ _____

Multiply fractions (reduce to lowest terms or to tenths).

8. $^7/_8 \times ^4/_6 =$ _____

10. $21^3/_4 \times ^7/_8 =$ _____

9. $23/5 \times 5/_8 =$ _____

11. $4^4/_5 \times 3^2/_3 =$ _____

Divide fractions.

12. $^1/_2 \div ^1/_3 =$ _____

14. $^1/_8 \div ^1/_{12} =$ _____

13. $6^3/_4 \div 3 =$ _____

15. $20^3/_4 \div ^1/_6 =$ _____

Decimals

Round off decimal numbers to tenths.

16. 0.87 = _____

18. 0.42 = _____

17. 2.56 = _____

Change decimals to fractions.

19. 0.68 = _____

21. 0.012 = _____

20. 0.9 = _____

22. 0.33 = _____

Multiply decimals (round off to tenths or whole numbers).

23. 0.34 × 0.6 = _____

24. 2.123 × 0.45 = _____

Divide decimals.

25. 3.24 ÷ 0.3 = _____

26. 69.4 ÷ 0.23 = _____

Ratio and Proportion

Change ratios to fractions.

27. 3 : 4 = _____

29. 1 : 175 = _____

28. 65 : 90 = _____

30. 0.9 : 100 = _____

Solve ratio and proportion problems.

31. 2 : 3 :: 8: X_____

33. 0.5 : 20 :: X : 100 _____

32. 3 : 100 = X : 1000 _____

34. 5 : 25 = 10 : X _____

Change ratios and proportions to fractions and solve.

35. 1 : 2 :: 4 : X _____

37. 0.9 : 10 = X : 100 _____

36. 5 : 50 :: X : 300 _____

Percentage

Change percents to fractions.

38. 3% = _____   **39.** 27% = _____   **40.** 1.2% = _____   **41.** 5.75% = _____

Change percents to decimals (round off to tenths, hundredths, or thousandths).

42. 8% = _____   **44.** 0.9% = _____   **46.** 0.25% = _____

43. 15% = _____   **45.** 3.5% = _____   **47.** 0.45% = _____

Change percents to ratios.

48. 35% = _____   **50.** 4% = _____   **52.** 0.45% = _____

49. 12.5% = _____   **51.** 0.9% = _____

ANSWERS POST-MATH TEST

Fractions

1. $^1/_{100}$

2. ½

3. 5

4. $24^2/_3$

5. $^{17}/_3$

6. 0.66 or 0.7

7. 0.08 or 0.1

8. $\dfrac{28}{48}$ or $\dfrac{7}{12}$ or 0.58 or 0.6

9. $\dfrac{13}{\overset{}{\underset{1}{\cancel{5}}}} \times \dfrac{\overset{1}{\cancel{5}}}{8} = {}^{13}/_8 = 1^5/_8$

10. $\dfrac{87}{4} \times \dfrac{7}{8} = \dfrac{609}{32} = 19.03$ or 19.0 or 19 (rounded off)

11. $\dfrac{24}{5} \times \dfrac{11}{3} = \dfrac{264}{15} = 17.6$

12. $\frac{1}{2} \times \frac{3}{1} = \frac{3}{2} = 1\frac{1}{2}$

13. $\dfrac{\overset{9}{\cancel{27}}}{4} \times \dfrac{1}{\underset{1}{\cancel{3}}} = \dfrac{9}{4} = 2\frac{1}{4}$

14. $\dfrac{1}{\underset{2}{\cancel{8}}} \times \dfrac{\overset{3}{\cancel{12}}}{1} = \frac{3}{2} = 1\frac{1}{2}$

15. $\dfrac{83}{\underset{2}{\cancel{4}}} \times \dfrac{\overset{3}{\cancel{6}}}{1} = {}^{249}/_2 = 124.5$ or 125 whole number

Decimals

16. 0.9

17. 2.6

18. 0.4

19. $^{68}/_{100}$

20. $^9/_{10}$

21. $^{12}/_{1000}$

22. $^{33}/_{100}$

23. 0.204 or 0.2

24. 0.95535, or 0.96, or 1

25. 10.8

26. 301.739 or 301.7

Ratio and Proportion

27. $^3/_4$

28. $^{65}/_{90}$

29. $^1/_{175}$

30. $^9/_{1000}$

31. 12

32. 30

33. 2.5

34. 50

35. $\dfrac{1}{2} \times \dfrac{4}{X} =$

(cross-multiply)

$X = 8$

36. $\dfrac{\frac{1}{8}}{\underset{10}{50}} = \dfrac{X}{300}$

$10\,X = 300$

$X = 30$

37. $^{0.9}/_{10} = {^x}/_{90}$

$10\,X = 90$

$X = 9$

Percentage

38. $^3/_{100}$

39. $^{27}/_{100}$

40. $^{12}/_{1000}$

41. $^{575}/_{10,000}$

42. 0.08 or 0.1

43. 0.15

44. 0.009

45. 0.035

46. 0.0025

47. 0.0045

48. 35 : 100

49. 12.5 : 100 or 125 : 1000

50. 4 : 100

51. 0.9 : 100 or 9 : 1000

52. 0.45 : 100 or 45 : 10,000

PART II

SYSTEMS, CONVERSION, AND METHODS OF DRUG CALCULATION

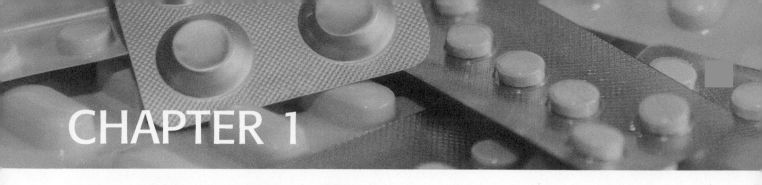

CHAPTER 1

Systems Used for Drug Administration and Temperature Conversion

Objectives
- Identify the system of measurement accepted worldwide and the system of measurement used in home settings.
- List the basic units and subunits of weight, volume, and length of the metric system.
- Explain the rules for changing grams to milligrams and milliliters to liters.
- Give abbreviations for the frequently used metric units and subunits.
- List the basic units of measurement for volume in the household system.
- Convert units of measurement within the metric system and within the household system.
- Convert Fahrenheit to Celsius and Celsius to Fahrenheit.

Outline
METRIC SYSTEM
HOUSEHOLD SYSTEM
TEMPERATURE CONVERSION

There have been three systems used for measuring drugs and solutions: metric, apothecary, and household. The metric system, or decimal system, was developed in France and is based on units of 10. It is a very precise system of measure used in medicine and science, which has been adopted worldwide, and is now known as the International System of Units (SI).

The apothecary system of measure, which dates back to the middle ages, was used for measurements of mass and volume. The pound, ounce, and grain were measurements of mass, whereas, the gallon, pint, fluid ounce, dram, and minim were used for volume. Although the larger measures of pounds, ounces, gallons, and pints are still used, the smaller measures, of grains and minums, are no longer used for medication calculation or administration. All medications are manufactured, dosed, and measured by the International Standard of Units.

Standard household measurements, teaspoon, tablespoon, and cup, are primarily used in the home setting. Standard household measure can be converted to metric only if standard measuring devices are used, not tableware. Tableware cups and spoons vary in size and are not accurate for measuring. Standard measuring spoons and measuring cups are preferred. Medication for children should only use metric measuring devices, standard measuring devices should be discouraged because of the danger of inaccuracy.

Roman numerals were at one time used for prescribing and dosing of medication. Roman numerals are no longer used for medication prescribing but can be seen in labeling such as the I-IV designation on controlled substances. Roman numerals are not used for computation and cannot be broken down into fractions and like the apothecary system have been superceded by advances in mathematics.

METRIC SYSTEM

The metric system is a decimal system based on multiples of 10 and decimal fractions of 10. There are three basic units of measurement. These basic units are as follows:

Gram (g): unit for weight
Liter (L): unit for volume or capacity
Meter (m): unit for linear measurement or length

Prefixes are used with the basic units to describe whether the units are larger or smaller than the basic unit. The prefixes indicate the size of the unit in multiples of 10. The prefixes for basic units are as follows:

Prefix for Larger Unit		**Prefix for Smaller Unit**	
Kilo	1000 (one thousand)	Deci	0.1 (one-tenth)
Hecto	100 (one hundred)	Centi	0.01 (one-hundredth)
Deka	10 (ten)	Milli	0.001 (one-thousandth)
		Micro	0.000001 (one-millionth)
		Nano	0.000000001 (one-billionth)

Abbreviations of metric units that are frequently written in drug orders are listed in Table 1.1. Lower-case letters are usually used for abbreviations rather than capital letters.

The metric units of weight, volume, and length are given in Table 1.2. Meanings of the prefixes are stated next to the units of weight. Note that the larger units are 1000, 100, and 10 times the basic units (in bold type) and the smaller units differ by factors of 0.1, 0.01, 0.001, 0.000001, and 0.000000001. The size of a basic unit can be changed by multiplying or dividing by 10. Micrograms and nanograms are the exceptions: one (1) milligram = 1000 micrograms, and one (1) microgram = 1000 nanograms. Micrograms and nanograms are changed by 1000 instead of by 10.

Conversion Within the Metric System

Drug administration often requires conversion within the metric system to prepare the correct dosage. Two basic methods are given for changing larger to smaller units and smaller to larger units.

TABLE 1.1 Metric Units and Abbreviations

	Names	Abbreviations
Weight	Kilogram	kg
	Gram	g
	Milligram	mg
	Microgram	mcg
	Nanogram	ng
Volume	Kiloliter	kL
	Liter	L
	Deciliter	dL
	Milliliter	mL
	Microliter	mcL
Length	Kilometer	km
	Meter	m
	Centimeter	cm
	Millimeter	mm

TABLE 1.2 Units of Measurement in the Metric System With Their Prefixes

Weight per Gram	Meaning
*1 kilogram (kg) = 1000 grams	One thousand
1 hectogram (hg) = 100 grams	One hundred
1 dekagram (dag) = 10 grams	Ten
*1 gram (g) = 1 gram	**One**
1 decigram (dg) = 0.1 gram ($^1/_{10}$)	One-tenth
1 centigram (cg) = 0.01 gram ($^1/_{100}$)	One-hundredth
*1 milligram (mg) = 0.001 gram ($^1/_{1000}$)	One-thousandth
*1 microgram (mcg) = 0.000001 gram ($^1/_{1,000,000,000}$)	One-millionth
*1 nanogram (ng) = 0.000000001 gram ($^1/_{1,000,000,000}$)	One-billionth

Volume per Liter	Length per Meter
*1 kiloliter (kL) = 1000 liters	*1 kilometer (km) = 1000 meters
1 hectoliter (hL) = 100 liters	1 hectometer (hm) = 100 meters
1 dekaliter (daL) = 10 liters	1 dekameter (dam) = 10 meters
*1 liter (L) = 1 liter	**1 meter (m) = 1 meter**
1 deciliter (dL) = 0.1 liter	1 decimeter (dm) = 0.1 meter
1 centiliter (cL) = 0.01 liter	*1 centimeter (cm) = 0.01 meter
*1 milliliter (mL) = 0.001 liter	*1 millimeter (mm) = 0.001 meter
1 microliter (mcL) = 0.000001 liter	

*Commonly used units of measurements.

Larger Units to Smaller Units

To change from a *larger* unit to a *smaller* unit, multiply by 10 for each unit decreased, or move the decimal point one space to the right for each unit changed.

When changing three units from larger to smaller, such as from gram to milligram (a change of three units), multiply by 10 three times (or by 1000), or move the decimal point three spaces to the right.

Change 1 gram (g) to milligrams (mg):

a. $1 \times 10 \times 10 \times 10 = 1000$ mg

b. $1 \text{ g} \times 1000 = 1000$ mg

or

c. 1 g = 1.000 mg (1000 mg)

When changing two units, such as kilogram to dekagram (a change of two units from larger to smaller), multiply by 10 twice (or by 100), or move the decimal point two spaces to the right.

Change 2 kilograms (kg) to dekagrams (dag):

a. $2 \times 10 \times 10 = 200$ dag

b. $2 \text{ kg} \times 100 = 200$ dag

or

c. 2 kg = 2.00 dag (200 dag)

When changing one unit, such as liter to deciliter (a change of one unit from larger to smaller), multiply by 10, or move the decimal point one space to the right.

Change 3 liters (L) to deciliters (dL):

a. $3 \times 10 = 30$ dL

b. $L \times 10 = 30$ dL

or

c. 3 L = 3.0 dL (30 dL)

A micro unit is one thousandth of a milli unit, and a nano unit is one thousandth of a micro unit. To change from a milli unit to a micro unit, multiply by 1000, or move the decimal place three spaces to the right. Changing micro units to nano units involves the same procedure, multiplying by 1000 or moving the decimal place three spaces to the right.

EXAMPLES   **PROBLEM 1:**   Change 2 grams (g) to milligrams (mg).

$$2 \text{ g} \times 1000 = 2000 \text{ mg}$$

or

$$2 \text{ g} = 2.000 \text{ mg (2000 mg)}$$

PROBLEM 2:   Change 10 milligrams (mg) to micrograms (mcg).

$$10 \text{ mg} \times 1000 = 10,000 \text{ mcg}$$

or

$$10 \text{ mg} = 10.000 \text{ mcg (10,000 mcg)}$$

PROBLEM 3:   Change 4 liters (L) to milliliters (mL).

$$4 \text{ L} \times 1000 = 4000 \text{ mL}$$

or

$$4 \text{ L} = 4.000 \text{ mL (4000 mL)}$$

PROBLEM 4:   Change 2 kilometers (km) to hectometers (hm).

$$2 \text{ km} \times 10 = 20 \text{ hm}$$

or

$$2 \text{ km} = 2.0 \text{ hm (20 hm)}$$

Smaller Units to Larger Units

To change from a *smaller* unit to a *larger* unit, divide by 10 for each unit increased, or move the decimal point one space to the left for each unit changed.

When changing three units from smaller to larger, divide by 1000, or move the decimal point three spaces to the left.
Change 1500 milliliters (mL) to liters (L):
a. $1500 \text{ mL} \div 1000 = 1.5 \text{ L}$
      or
b. $1500 \text{ mL} = 1\,500. \text{ L (1.5 L)}$

When changing two units from smaller to larger, divide by 100, or move the decimal point two spaces to the left.
Change 400 centimeters (cm) to meters (m):
a. $400 \text{ cm} \div 100 = 4 \text{ m}$
      or
b. $400 \text{ cm} = 4\,00. \text{ m (4 m)}$

When changing one unit from smaller to larger, divide by 10, or move the decimal point one space to the left.

Change 150 decigrams (dg) to grams (g):

a. 150 dg ÷ 10 = 15 g

or

b. 150 dg = 15 0̬ g (15 g)

EXAMPLES   **PROBLEM 1:** Change 8 grams (g) to kilograms (kg).

8 g ÷ 1000 = 0.008 kg

or

8 g = 008̬ kg (0.008 kg)

PROBLEM 2: Change 1500 milligrams (mg) to decigrams (dg).

1500 mg ÷ 100 = 15 dg

or

1500 mg = 15 00̬ dg (15 dg)

PROBLEM 3: Change 750 micrograms (mcg) to milligrams (mg).

750 mcg ÷ 1000 = 0.75 mg

or

750 mcg = 750̬ mg (0.75 mg)

PROBLEM 4: Change 2400 milliliters (mL) to liters (L).

2400 mL ÷ 1000 = 2.4 L

or

2400 mL = 2 400̬ L (2.4 L)

PRACTICE PROBLEMS ▶ **1 METRIC SYSTEM (CONVERSION WITHIN THE METRIC SYSTEM)**

Answers can be found on page 24.

1. Conversion from larger units to smaller units: *Multiply* by 10 for each unit changed (multiply by 10, 100, 1000), or move the decimal point one space to the *right* for each unit changed (move one, two, or three spaces).

   a. 7.5 grams to milligrams _____

   b. 10 milligrams to micrograms _____

   c. 35 kilograms to grams _____

   d. 2.5 liters to milliliters _____

   e. 1.25 liters to milliliters _____

   f. 20 centiliters to milliliters _____

   g. 18 decigrams to milligrams _____

   h. 0.5 kilograms to grams _____

2. Conversion from smaller units to larger units: *Divide* by 10 for each unit changed (divide by 10, 100, 1000), or move the decimal point one space to the *left* for each unit changed (move one, two, or three spaces).

   a. 500 milligrams to grams _____

   b. 7500 micrograms to milligrams _____

   c. 250 grams to kilograms _____

   d. 4000 milliliters to liters _____

   e. 325 milligrams to grams _____

   f. 100 milliliters to deciliters _____

   g. 2800 milliliters to liters _____

   h. 75 millimeters to centimeters _____

HOUSEHOLD SYSTEM

The use of household measurement is common in the home because that is what is readily available for cooking and baking. The household system of measurement is considered less accurate than the metric system because it lacks standardization. However, newer measuring cups and spoons have both household and metric measure. A teaspoon (t) is considered 5 mL and 15 mL is considered one tablespoon (T). One cup is 250 mL and 500 mL is a pint. Since oral intake at home is measured in household measure, it is useful to know the conversions.

The community health nurse may use and teach the household units of measurements to patients and caregivers.

Table 1.3 gives the commonly used units of measurement in the household system. You might want to memorize the equivalents in Table 1.3 or refer to the table as needed.

TABLE 1.3 Units of Measurement in the Household System

1 teaspoon (t)	= 5 mL	1 measuring cup	= 8 ounces (oz)
1 tablespoon (T)	= 3 teaspoons (t)	2 cups	= 1 pint
1 ounce (oz)	= 2 tablespoons (T)	4 cups	= 1 quart

Conversion Within the Household System

For changing larger units to smaller units and smaller units to larger units within the household system, the same methods that applied to the apothecary system can be used. With household measurements, a fluid ounce is usually indicated as an ounce.

Larger Units to Smaller Units

To change a ***larger*** unit to a ***smaller*** unit, multiply the constant value found in Table 1.3 by the number of the larger unit.

EXAMPLES **PROBLEM 1:** 1/2 cup juice glass = _____ ounces (oz).

1 cup = 8 oz (8 is the constant value)

1/2 c × 8 oz = 4 oz

PROBLEM 2: 3 tablespoons (T) = _____ teaspoons (t).

1 T = 3 t (3 is the constant value)

3 × 3 = 9t

PROBLEM 3: 5 ounces (oz) = _____ tablespoons (T).

1 oz = 2 T (2 is the constant value)

5 × 2 = 10 T

PROBLEM 4: 1/2 ounce (oz) = _____ tablespoon (T)

1 oz = 2 T (2 is the constant value)

1/2 × 2 = 1T

Smaller Units to Larger Units

To change a *smaller* unit to a *larger* unit, divide the constant value found in Table 1.3 into the number of the larger unit.

NOTE

The constant values are the numbers of the smaller units in Table 1.3.

EXAMPLES **PROBLEM 1:**

9 teaspoons (t) = _____ tablespoons (T).

1 T = 3 t (3 is the constant value)

9 ÷ 3 = 3 T

PROBLEM 3:

4 tablespoons (T) = _____ ounces (oz).

1 oz = 2 T (2 is the constant value)

4 ÷ 2 = 2 oz

PROBLEM 2:

24 ounces (oz) = _____ cups (c).

1 c = 8 oz (8 is the constant value)

24 ÷ 8 = 3 c

PRACTICE PROBLEMS ▶ II HOUSEHOLD SYSTEM (CONVERSION WITHIN THE HOUSEHOLD)

Answers can be found on page 24.

1. Give the equivalents, changing larger units to smaller units.

   a. 2 glasses = _____ oz

   b. 3 ounces = _____ T

   c. 4 Tablespoons = _____ t

   d. 1½ c (cups) = _____ oz

   e. ½ Tablespoon = _____ t

2. Give the equivalents, changing smaller units to larger units.

a. 9 teaspoons = _____ T

b. 6 tablespoons = _____ oz

c. 6 teaspoons = _____ oz

d. 12 ounces = _____ cups

e. 24 ounces = _____ cups

TEMPERATURE CONVERSION

Temperature is commonly measured by two scales, Celsius and Fahrenheit (Figure 1.1). Celsius (C), or centigrade, describes temperature with 0° C as the freezing point of water and 100° C as the boiling point of water. The Celsius scale is widely used around the world. Medical devices and scientific equipment often use the Celsius scale because it is a base-10 system like the metric system. The Fahrenheit (F) scale describes temperature with the freezing point of water as 32° F and the boiling point of water as 212° F. The Fahrenheit scale is primarily used in the United States and its territories.

To convert from Fahrenheit to Celsius the formula is:

$[C] = ([°F] - 32) \times 5/9$

To convert from Celsius to Fahrenheit the formula is:

$[F] = ([°C] \times 9/5) + 32$

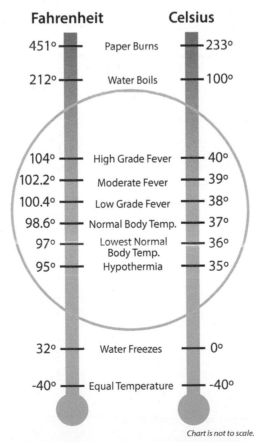

Figure 1.1 Comparison of Fahrenheit and Celsius.

PRACTICE PROBLEMS ▶ III TEMPERATURE CONVERSION

Answers can be found below.

a. Change 98.8° F to Celsius _____

b. Change 101° F to Celsius _____

c. Change 103° F to Celsius _____

d. Change 22° C to Fahrenheit _____

e. Change 30° C to Fahrenheit _____

ANSWERS

I Metric System

1. a. 7.5 g to mg
$7.5 \text{ g} \times 1000 = 7500 \text{ mg}$
or
$7.\underset{\frown}{500} \text{ mg (7500 mg)}$

b. 35,000 g
c. 2500 mL
d. 1250 mL
e. 200 mL
f. 1 dL
g. 1800 mg
h. 500 g

2. a. 500 mg to g
$500 \div 1000 = 0.5 \text{ g}$
or
$500 \text{ mg} = \underset{\frown}{500}. \text{ g (0.5 g)}$

b. 7.5 mg
c. 0.25 kg
d. 4 L
e. 0.325 g
f. 1 dL
g. 2.8 L
h. 7.5 cm

II Household System

1. a. 2 glasses = _____ oz
$2 \times 8 = 16 \text{ oz}$
b. 6 T
c. 12 t
d. 12 oz
e. 1½ t

2. a. 9 teaspoons = _____T
$9 \div 3 = 3T$
b. 3 oz
c. 1 oz
d. 1V2 cups
e. 3 cups

III Temperature Conversion

a. $°C = ([98.8° \text{ F}] - 32) \times 5/9$
$°C = 66.8 \times 5/9$
$= 334/9$
$°C = 37.1$

b. $°C = ([101° \text{ F}] - 32) \times 5/9$
$°C = 69 \times 5/9$
$= 345/9$
$°C = 38.3$

c. $°C = ([103 \text{ °F}] - 32) \times 5/9$
$°C = 71 \times 5/9$
$= 355/9$
$°C = 39.4$

d. $°F = ([22° \text{ C}] \times 9/5) + 32$
$= 198/5 + 32$
$= 39.6 + 32$
$°F = 71.6$

e. $°F = ([30° \text{ C}] \times 9/5) + 32$
$= 270/5 \ 1 \ 32$
$= 54 \ 1 \ 32$
$°F = 86$

SUMMARY PRACTICE PROBLEMS

Answers can be found below.

Make conversions within the two systems.

1. Metric system

   a. 30 mg = _____ mcg

   b. 3 g = _____ mg

   c. 6 L = _____ mL

   d. 1.5 kg = _____ g

   e. 10,000 mcg = _____ mg

   f. 500 mg = _____ g

   g. 2500 mL = _____ L

   h. 125 g = _____ kg

   i. 120 mm = _____ cm

   j. 5 m = _____ cm

2. Household system

   a. 12 t = _____ T

   b. 5 cups = _____ oz

   c. 3 T = _____ t

   d. 2 cups = _____ oz

   e. 24 oz = _____ c (cups)

   f. 4 oz = _____ T

ANSWERS SUMMARY PRACTICE PROBLEMS

1. a. 30,000 mcg
   b. 3000 mg
   c. 6000 mL
   d. 1500 g
   e. 10 mg
   f. 0.5 g
   g. 2.5 L
   h. 0.125 kg
   i. 12 cm
   j. 500 cm

2. a. 4 T
   b. 40 oz
   c. 9 t
   d. 16 oz
   e. 3 c (cups)
   f. 8 T

CHAPTER 2

Conversion Within the Metric and Household Systems

Objectives • Name the metric equivalents that are commonly used in health care.
• Name the metric equivalents for length, weight, and volume.
• Convert length, weight, and volume between metric and household measurements.
• Explain units, milliequivalents, and percents.

Outline **UNITS, MILLIEQUIVALENTS, AND PERCENTS**
METRIC AND HOUSEHOLD EQUIVALENTS
CONVERSION IN METRIC AND HOUSEHOLD SYSTEMS BY WEIGHT
CONVERSION IN METRIC AND HOUSEHOLD SYSTEMS BY LIQUID VOLUME
CONVERSION IN METRIC AND HOUSEHOLD SYSTEMS BY LENGTH

Health care primarily uses the metric system to measure for length, volume, and weight. Sometimes it is necessary to convert measurements from the common household system (cups, ounces, tablespoons, pounds, inches, etc.) to the metric system. Unlike the household system, the metric system has three fundamental units (grams, liters, and meters) which can be multiplied or divided by factors of 10. The metric system has prefixes based upon multiples of 10, which can make conversion with the system much easier.

Medications, such as drugs and intravenous fluids, are predominately ordered in metric units (grams, milligrams, liters, and milliliters). Standard household measurements are never used. Household measurements are commonly used in liquid measure, height, and weight. It is still necessary for the nurse to memorize the few common household and metric equivalents to easily convert between the two systems.

UNITS, MILLIEQUIVALENTS, AND PERCENTS

Units, milliequivalents, and percents are measurements and are used to indicate the strength or potency of certain drugs. When a drug is developed, its strength is based on chemical assay or biological assay. Chemical assay denotes strength by weight, e.g., milligrams. Biological assays are used for drugs in which the chemical composition is difficult to determine. Biological assays assess potency by determining the effect that one unit of the drug can have on a laboratory animal. Units mainly measure the potency of hormones, vitamins, anticoagulants, and some antibiotics. Drugs that were once standardized by units and were later synthesized to their chemical composition may still retain units as an indication of potency, e.g., insulin.

Milliequivalents measure the strength of an ion concentration. Ions are given primarily for electrolyte replacement. They are measured in milliequivalents (mEq), one of which is $1/1000$ of the equivalent weight of an ion. Potassium chloride (KCl) is a common electrolyte replacement and is ordered in milliequivalents.

Percents, the concentrations of weight dissolved in a volume, are always expressed as units of mass per units of volume. Common concentrations are g/mL, g/L, and mg/mL. These concentrations, expressed as percentages, are based on the definition of a 1% solution as 1 g of a drug in 100 mL of solution. Dextrose 50% in a 50-mL pre-filled syringe is a concentration of 50 g of dextrose in 100 mL of water. Calcium gluconate 10% in a 30-mL bottle is a concentration of 10 g of calcium gluconate in 100 mL of solution. Proportions can also express concentrations. A solution that is 1:100 has the same concentration as a 1% solution. Epinephrine 1:1000 means that 1 g of epinephrine was dissolved in a 1000-mL solution.

Units, milliequivalents, and percents cannot be directly converted into the metric system of measure.

METRIC AND HOUSEHOLD EQUIVALENTS

Knowing how to convert drug doses between the systems of measurement is essential in the clinical setting. In discharge teaching for individuals receiving liquid medication converting metric to household measurement may be important. Table 2.1 gives the metric and household equivalents by weight, volume, and length.

TABLE 2.1 Approximate Metric and Household Equivalents

	Metric System	Household System
Weight	1 kg = 1000 g	2.2 lbs
	30 g	1 oz
	15 g	0.5 oz
Volume	1 L = 1000 mL	1 qt = 32 fl oz
	0.5 L = 500 mL	1 pt = 16 fl oz
	0.25 L = 250 mL	1 c or 8 oz
	0.18 L = 180 mL	6 oz
	30 mL	2 l or 6 t or l oz
	15 mL	1 T or 0.5 oz
	4-5 mL	1 t
	1 mL	15-16 gtt (drops)
Length	1 meter	3.2808 feet
	0.3048 m	1 foot
	0.0254 m	1 inch
	2.54 cm	1 inch

CONVERSION IN METRIC AND HOUSEHOLD SYSTEMS BY WEIGHT

 MEMORIZE

Metric and Household Equivalents
1 Kilogram (kg) = 2.2 pounds (lbs)
30 grams (g) = 1 ounce (oz)

To convert kg to lbs, multiply the number of kg by 2.2 lbs/kg, the constant value.

EXAMPLE Change 45 kilograms to pounds. $45 \, kg \times 2.2 \, lbs/kg = 99 \, lbs$

To convert lbs to kg, divide the number of lbs by 2.2 lbs/kg, the constant value.

EXAMPLE Change 150 pounds to kilograms. $\dfrac{150 \, lbs}{2.2 \, lbs/kg} = 68.18 \, kg$

To convert g to oz, divide the number of g by 30 g/oz, the constant value.

EXAMPLE Change 90 grams to ounces. $\dfrac{90 \, g}{30 \, g/oz} = 3 \, oz$

To convert oz to g, multiply the number of ounces by 30 g/oz, the constant value.

EXAMPLE Change 6 ounces to grams. $6 \, oz \times 30 \, g/oz = 180 \, g$

PRACTICE PROBLEMS ▶ I CONVERSION BY WEIGHT

Answers can be found on page 30.

1. 195 lbs = _____ kg   **3.** 120 g = _____ oz   **5.** 60 kg = _____ lbs

2. 184 lbs = _____ kg   **4.** 5 oz = _____ g   **6.** 14 kg = _____ lbs

CONVERSION IN METRIC AND HOUSEHOLD SYSTEMS BY LIQUID VOLUME

 MEMORIZE

Metric and Household Equivalents
1 liter (L) = 32 ounces (oz)
30 milliliter (mL) = 1 ounce

To convert liters to ounces, multiply the number of liters by 32 oz/L, the constant value.

EXAMPLE Change 3 liters to ounces. $3 \, L \times 32 \, oz/L = 96 \, oz$

To convert ounces to liters, divide the number of ounces by 32 oz/L, the constant value.

EXAMPLE Change 64 oz to liters. $\dfrac{64 \, oz}{32 \, oz/L} = 2 \, L \text{ (liters)}$

To convert ounces to milliliters, multiply the number of ounces by 30 mL/oz, the constant value.

EXAMPLE   Change 5 oz to mL.   5 o̶z̶ × 30 mL/o̶z̶ = 150 mL

To convert milliliters to ounces, divide the number of milliliters by 30 mL/oz, the constant value.

EXAMPLE   Change 120 mL to ounces. $\dfrac{120 \text{ m̶L̶}}{30 \text{ m̶L̶/oz}} = 4\,oz$

PRACTICE PROBLEMS ▶ II CONVERSION BY LIQUID VOLUME

Answers can be found on page 30.

Liters and Ounces (Round to the nearest tenths.)

1. 2.5 L = _____ oz
2. 0.25 L = _____ oz
3. 40 oz = _____ L
4. 24 oz = _____ L

Ounces and Milliliters

1. 4 oz (fl oz) = _____ mL
2. 6½ oz = _____ mL
3. ½ oz = _____ mL
4. 5 mL = _____ oz
5. 150 mL = _____ oz
6. 15 mL = _____ oz

CONVERSION IN METRIC AND HOUSEHOLD SYSTEMS BY LENGTH

 MEMORIZE

Metric and Household Equivalents
0.3048 meter = 1 foot
2.54 centimeters = 1 inch

To convert feet to meters, multiply the number of feet by 0.3048 m/ft, the constant value.

EXAMPLE   Change 5 feet to meters.   5 f̶t̶ × 0.3048 m/f̶t̶ = 1.52 m

To convert meters to feet, divide the number of meters by 0.3048 m/ft, the constant value.

EXAMPLE   Change 2 meters to feet. $\dfrac{2 \text{ m̶}}{0.3048 \text{ m̶/ft}} = 6.56\text{ ft}$

To convert inches to centimeters, multiply the number of inches by 2.54 cm/in, the constant value.

EXAMPLE   Change 4 inches to centimeters.   4 i̶n̶ × 2.54 cm/i̶n̶ = 10.16 cm

To convert centimeters to inches, divide the number of centimeters by 2.54 cm/in, the constant value.

EXAMPLE   Change 60 centimeters to inches. $\dfrac{60 \text{ c̶m̶}}{2.54 \text{ c̶m̶/in}} = 23.6\text{ inches}$

PRACTICE PROBLEMS ▶ III CONVERSION BY LENGTH

Answers can be found below.

Feet to meters	Meters to feet	Inches to centimeters	Centimeters to inches
1. 6 ft __ m	**4.** 1.88 m __ ft	**7.** 2.5 in __ cm	**10.** 3.8 cm __ in
2. 5 ft __ m	**5.** 1.575 m __ ft	**8.** 5 in __ cm	**11.** 2.6 cm __ in
3. 4 ft __ m	**6.** 0.864 m __ ft	**9.** 10 in __ cm	**12.** 4.2 cm __ in

ANSWERS

I Conversion by Weight

1. $\dfrac{195\ lbs}{2.2\ kg/lbs} = 88.6\ kg$ **3.** $\dfrac{120\ g}{30\ g/oz} = 4\ oz$ **5.** $60\ kg \times 2.2\ lbs/kg = 132\ lbs$

2. $\dfrac{184\ lbs}{2.2\ kg/lbs} = 83.6\ kg$ **4.** $5\ oz \times 30\ g/oz = 150\ g$ **6.** $14\ kg \times 2.2\ lbs/kg = 30.8\ lbs$

II Conversion by Liquid Volume

Liters and Ounces

1. $2.5\ L \times 32\ oz/L = 80\ oz$
2. $0.25\ L \times 32\ oz/L = 8\ oz$

3. $40\ oz \div 32\ oz/L = 1.25\ L$ or $1.3\ L$
4. $24\ oz \div 32\ oz/L = 0.75\ L$ or $0.8\ L$

Ounces and Milliliters

1. $4\ oz \times 30\ mL/oz = 120\ mL$
2. $6.5\ oz \times 30\ mL/oz = 195\ mL$
3. $0.5\ oz \times 30\ mL/oz = 15\ mL$

4. $45\ mL \div 30\ mL/oz = 1\frac{1}{2}\ oz$ or $1.5\ oz$
5. $150\ mL \div 30\ mL/oz = 5\ oz$
6. $15\ mL \div 30\ mL/oz = \frac{1}{2}\ oz$ or $0.5\ oz$

III Conversion by Length

1. $6\ ft \times 0.3048\ m/ft = 1.82$ or $1.8\ m$
2. $5\ ft \times 0.3048\ m/ft = 1.52$ or $1.5\ m$
3. $4\ ft \times 0.3048\ m/ft = 1.22$ or $1.2\ m$

4. $\dfrac{1.88\ m}{0.3048\ m/ft} = 6.18$ or $6.2\ ft$

5. $\dfrac{1.575\ m}{0.3048\ m/ft} = 5.16$ or $5.2\ ft$

6. $\dfrac{0.864\ m}{0.3048\ m/ft} = 2.83$ or $2.8\ ft$

7. $2.5\ in \times 2.54\ cm/in = 6.35$ or $6.4\ cm$
8. $5\ in \times 2.54\ cm/in = 12.7$ or $13\ cm$
9. $10\ in \times 2.54\ cm/in = 25.4\ cm$

10. $\dfrac{3.8\ cm}{2.54\ cm/in} = 1.49$ or $1.5\ in$

11. $\dfrac{2.6\ cm}{2.54\ cm/in} = 1.02$ or $1\ in$

12. $\dfrac{4.2\ cm}{2.54\ cm/in} = 1.65$ or $1.7\ in$

SUMMARY PRACTICE PROBLEMS

Answers can be found on page 32.

May refer to Table 2.1

Weight: Metric and Household Conversion

a. To convert kg to pounds, multiply/divide by _____.

b. To convert pounds to kg, multiply/divide by _____.

1. 60 kg to _____ lbs
2. 75 kg to _____ lbs
3. 1.75 kg to _____ lbs
4. 12 kg to _____ lbs
5. 373 lbs to _____ kg
6. 196 lbs to _____ kg
7. 2.7 lbs to _____ kg
8. 22 lbs to _____ kg

a. To convert grams to ounces, multiply/divide by _____.

b. To convert ounces to grams, multiply/divide by _____.

1. 40 g to _____ oz
2. 100 g to _____ oz
3. 75 g to _____ oz
4. 200 g to _____ oz
5. 6 oz to _____ g
6. 10 oz to _____ g
7. 2 oz to _____ g
8. 4 oz to _____ g

Volume: Metric and Household Conversion

a. To convert liters to ounces, multiply/divide by_____.

b. To convert ounces to liters, multiply/ divide by_____.

1. 3 L =_____oz
2. 48 oz =_____L
3. 64 oz =_____L
4. 0.5 L =_____oz
5. 8 oz =_____L
6. 24 oz =_____L

a. To convert ounces to milliliters, multiply/divide by_____.

b. To convert milliliters to ounces, multiply/divide by_____.

1. 1.5 oz =_____mL
2. 15 mL =_____oz
3. 60 mL =_____oz
4. 75 mL =_____oz
5. 3 oz =_____mL
6. 8 oz =_____mL

Length: Metric and Household Conversion

a. To convert meters to feet, multiply/divide by _____.

b. To convert feet to meters, multiply/divide by_____.

1. 10 m to _____ ft
2. 1.2 m to _____ ft
3. 2 m to _____ ft
4. 6.2 m to _____ ft
5. 15 ft to _____ m
6. 1.5 ft to _____ m
7. 20 ft to _____ m
8. 50 ft to _____ m

a. To convert centimeters to inches, multiply/divide by_____.

b. To convert inches to centimeters, multiply/divide by_____.

1. 7 in to _____ cm
2. 3 in to _____ cm
3. 40 in to _____ cm
4. 52 in to _____ cm
5. 75 cm to _____ in
6. 2 cm to _____ in
7. 36 cm to _____ in
8. 40 cm to _____ in

ANSWERS SUMMARY PRACTICE PROBLEMS

Weight

a. multiply 2.2 kg/lbs
b. divide 2.2 kg/lbs
1. 60 kg × 2.2 kg/lbs = 132 lbs
2. 75 kg × 2.2 kg/lbs = 165 lbs
3. 1.75 kg × 2.2 kg/lbs = 3.85 lbs
4. 12 kg × 2.2 kg/lbs = 26.4 lbs
5. $\dfrac{373 \text{ lbs}}{2.2 \text{ lbs} / kg} = 169.5\text{kg}$
6. $\dfrac{196 \text{ lbs}}{2.2 \text{ lbs}/kg} = 89 \text{ kg}$
7. $\dfrac{2.7 \text{ lbs}}{2.2 \text{ lbs} / kg} = 1.2\text{kg}$
8. $\dfrac{22 \text{ lbs}}{2.2 \text{ lbs} / kg} = 10 \text{ kg}$

a. divide 30 g/oz
b. multiply 30 g/oz
1. $\dfrac{40 \text{ g}}{30 \text{ g} / oz} = 1.3 \text{ oz}$
2. $\dfrac{100 \text{ g}}{30 \text{ g} / oz} = 3.3 \text{ oz}$
3. $\dfrac{75 \text{ g}}{30 \text{ g} / oz} = 2.5 \text{ oz}$
4. $\dfrac{200 \text{ g}}{30 \text{ g} / oz} = 6.7 \text{ oz}$
5. 6 oz × 30 g/oz = 180 g
6. 10 oz × 30 g/oz = 300 g
7. 2 oz × 30 g/oz = 60 g
8. 4 oz × 30 g/oz = 120 g

Volume

a. multiply, 32 oz/L
b. divide, 32 oz/L
1. 3 L × 32 oz/L = 96 oz
2. $\dfrac{48 \text{ oz}}{32 \text{ oz} /L} = 1.5 \text{ L}$
3. $\dfrac{64 \text{ oz}}{32 \text{ oz} /L} = 2 \text{ L}$
4. 0.5 L × 32 oz/L = 16 oz
5. $\dfrac{8 \text{ oz}}{32 \text{ oz} /L} = 0.25 \text{ L}$
6. $\dfrac{24 \text{ oz}}{32 \text{ oz} /L} = 0.75 \text{ L}$

a. multiply, 30 mL/oz
b. divide, 30 mL/oz
1. 1.5 oz × 30 mL/oz = 45 mL
2. $\dfrac{15 \text{ mL}}{30 \text{ mL} /oz} = 0.5 \text{ oz}$
3. $\dfrac{60 \text{ mL}}{30 \text{ mL} /oz} = 2 \text{ oz}$
4. $\dfrac{75 \text{ mL}}{30 \text{ mL} /oz} = 2.5 \text{ oz}$
5. 3 oz × 30 mL/oz = 90 mL
6. 8 oz × 30 mL/oz = 240 mL

Length

a. divide by 0.3048 m/ft
b. multiply by 0.3048 m/ft
1. 10 m × 0.3048 m/ft = 3.048 or 3.05 ft
2. 1.2 m × 0.3048 m/ft = 0.365 or 0.37 ft
3. 2 m × 0.3048 m/ft = 0.609 or 0.61 ft
4. 6.2 m × 0.3048 m/ft = 1.889 or 1.89 ft
5. $\dfrac{15 \text{ ft}}{0.3048 \text{ m} / ft} = 49.2 \text{ m}$
6. $\dfrac{1.5 \text{ ft}}{0.3048 \text{ m} / ft} = 4.92 \text{ m}$
7. $\dfrac{20 \text{ ft}}{0.3048 \text{ m} / ft} = 65.6 \text{ m}$
8. $\dfrac{50 \text{ ft}}{0.03048 \text{ m} / ft} = 164 \text{ m}$

a. divide 2.54 inches/cm
b. multiply 2.54 inches/cm
1. 7 in × 2.54 in/cm = 17.78 or 17.8 cm
2. 3 in × 2.54 in/cm = 7.62 or 7.6 cm
3. 40 in × 2.54 in/cm = 101.6 cm
4. 52 in × 2.54 in/cm = 132 cm
5. $\dfrac{75 \text{ cm}}{2.54 \text{ in}/ cm} = 29.5 \text{ in}$
6. $\dfrac{2 \text{ cm}}{2.54 \text{ in}/ cm} = 0.78 \text{ in}$
7. $\dfrac{36 \text{ cm}}{2.54 \text{ in}/ cm} = 91.4 \text{ in}$
8. $\dfrac{40 \text{ cm}}{2.54 \text{ in}/ cm} = 15.7 \text{ in}$

APPLICATION: INTAKE PRACTICE PROBLEMS

Answers can be found below.

1. Patient intake for lunch included a carton of milk (8 oz), cup of coffee (6 oz), small glass of apple juice (4 oz), and gelatin (4 oz). How many milliliters (mL) did the patient consume for lunch? _____ mL
2. Add 8-hour intake: IV/30 mL/hr, 230 mL in IV medications. PO intake: juice (4 oz), tea (6 oz), water (3 oz), gelatin (4 oz), ginger ale (5 oz), and milk (8 oz). What was the patient's intake (IV and PO) in 8 hours? _____ mL
3. Add 8-hour intake: IV/ 60 mL/hr; 250 mL in IV medications. PO intake: juice 4 oz, water 3 oz, gelatin 2 oz, and broth 4 oz. What was the patient's intake (IV and PO) in 8 hours? _____ mL

ANSWERS APPLICATION: INTAKE PRACTICE PROBLEMS

1. Milk = 240 mL
    Coffee = 180 mL
    Apple juice = 120 mL
    Gelatin = 120 mL
    ──────────
    660 mL

The patient's intake for lunch is 660 mL.

2. IV: 30 mL × 8 hr = 240 mL
    IV medications = 230 mL
    Juice (4 oz × 30 mL) = 120 mL
    Tea = 180 mL
    Water = 90 mL
    Gelatin = 120 mL
    Ginger ale = 150 mL
    Milk = 240 mL
    ──────────
    1370 mL

The patient's intake in 8 hours (IV and PO) is 1370 mL.

3. IV: 60 mL/hr × 8 hr = 480 mL
    IV medications = 250 mL
    Juice = 120 mL
    Water = 90 mL
    Gelatin = 60 mL
    Broth = 120 mL
    ──────────
    1120 mL

The patient's intake in 8 hours (IV and PO) is 1120 mL.

For additional practice problems, refer to the Conversions and Equivalents section of the Elsevier's Interactive Drug Calculation Application, version 1 on Evolve.

NGN® PREP

1. A post-partum new mother is breast feeding her newborn. To ensure her milk supply, she should consume at least 2 liters of fluid/day. This amount in household measure would be __A__ or __B__.

Option A	Option B
64oz	8 - 8 oz cups
32oz	10 - 8oz cups
16oz	16 - 8 oz cups

2. A newborn infant at his first well baby visit weighs 6 ½ lbs. His birth weight was 8lbs. The infant's current weight in kg is __A__ and his weight loss in kg is __B__.

Option A	Option B
3.64kg	0.82kg
2.95kg	0.68kg
3.24kg	0.49kg

3. Patient admitted to Emergency Department with two lacerations of the right lower leg from a construction accident. The lateral proximal laceration is 3 inches long and the distal posterior laceration is 6 inches long. The length of the proximal wound in centimeters is __A__ and the length of the distal laceration is __B__.

Option A	Option B
8.5cm	15.2cm
6.5cm	10.2cm
5.5cm	14cm
7.6cm	12.5cm

4. Mr. Smith is receiving a bladder irrigation thru a 3-way foley catheter after a transurethral resection of the prostate to control for bleeding. The irrigation was run at 100ml/hr for 4 hours then reduced to 75ml/hr for the next 4 hours. Patient's total output, irrigation and urine, was 1940ml. The total amount of irrigating solution was __A__ and the total amount of urine was __B__.

Option A	Option B
800mL	1240mL
900mL	1140mL
1000mL	940mL
700mL	1040mL

ANSWERS - NGN® PREP

1. **Option A:** 2L × 32 oz/L = 64oz
   Option B: 64oz ÷ 8oz cups = 8 cups
2. **Option A:** 6.5lbs ÷ 2.2lbs/kg = 2.95kg
   Option B: 8 lbs ÷ 2.2lbs/kg = 3.63kg
   3.63kg − 2.95kg = 0.68kg
3. **Option A:** 3 inches × 2.54cm/inch = 7.6cm
   Option B: 6 inches × 2.54cm/inch = 15.2cm
4. **Option A:** Irrigation solution 100mL/hr × 4hr = 400mL
   75mL/hr × 4hr = 300mL
   Total irrigation solution 400mL + 300mL = 700 mL
   Option B: Total output 1940ml − 700ml = 1240 urine output

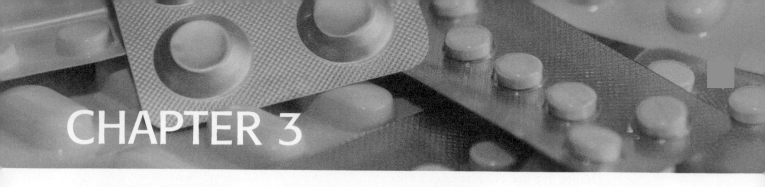

CHAPTER 3

Interpretation of Drug Labels, Drug Orders, Bar Codes, MAR and eMAR, Automation of Medication Dispensing Administration, and Abbreviations

Objectives
- Identify brand names, generic names, drug forms, dosages, expiration dates, and lot numbers on drug labels.
- Explain difference between military and traditional time.
- Give examples of drugs with "look-alike" drug names.
- Name the components of a drug order.
- Explain the computer-based medication administration system.
- Explain the use of the bar code for unit dose drug.
- Identify drug information for charting.
- Provide meanings of abbreviations: drug form, drug measurement, and routes and times of drug administration.

Outline
INTERPRETATION OF DRUG LABELS
DRUG DIFFERENTIATION
UNIT-DOSE DISPENSING SYSTEM (UDDS)
COMPUTERIZED DRUG ADMINISTRATION
MEDICATION DISTRIBUTION
DOCUMENTATION OF MEDICATION ADMINISTRATION
ABBREVIATIONS

INTERPRETATION OF DRUG LABELS

Pharmaceutical companies label drugs with their brand name of the drug in large letters and the generic name in smaller letters. The form of the drug (tablet, capsule, liquid, or powder) and dosage are printed on the drug label.

Many of the calculation problems in this book use drug labels. By using drug labels, the student can practice solving drug problems that are applicable to clinical practice. The student should know what information is on a drug label and how this information is used in drug calculations. All drug labels provide eight basic items of data: (1) brand (trade) name, (2) generic name, (3) dosage, (4) form of the drug, (5) expiration date, (6) lot number, (7) name of the manufacturer, and (8) drug information and directions.

EXAMPLE DRUG LABEL

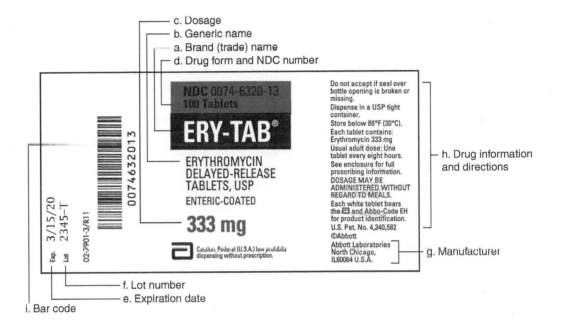

a. The brand (trade) name is the commercial name given by the pharmaceutical company (manufacturer of the drug). It is printed in large, bold letters.
b. The generic name is the chemical name given to the drug, regardless of the drug manufacturer. It is printed in smaller letters, usually under the brand name. Drugs are usually referred to by their generic name.
c. The dosage strength is the drug dose per drug form (tablet, capsule, liquid) as stated on the label.
d. The National Drug Code number (NDC) is the universal product identifier required by the U.S. Food and Drug Administration. The numbers identify the manufacturer, distributor, strength, dosage, formulation (tablets, capsules, liquids), and package size.
e. The expiration date refers to the length of time the drug can be used before it loses its potency. Drugs should not be administered after the expiration date. The nurse must check the expiration date of all drugs that he or she administers.
f. The lot number identifies the drug batch in which the medication was produced. Occasionally, a drug is recalled according to the lot number.
g. The manufacturer is the pharmaceutical company that produces the brand-name drug.
h. Specific drug-related information and directions. This information along with more detail can be found in the package insert.
i. The bar code contains all drug identifiers, such as control lot, batch number, NDC number, and expiration date. This is on all prescription and nonprescription medications.

Examples of drug labels are given, and practice problems for reading drug labels follow the examples.

EXAMPLE **ORAL DRUG (SOLID FORM)**

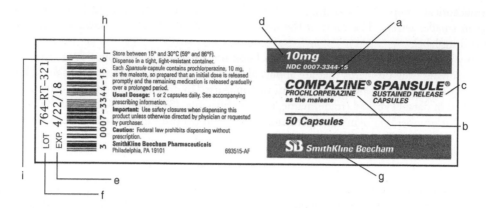

a. Brand (trade) name is Compazine.
b. Generic name is prochlorperazine.
c. Drug form is a sustained-release capsule (SR capsule).
d. Dosage is 10 mg per capsule.
e. Expiration date is 4/22/18 (after this date, the drug should be discarded).
f. Lot number is 764-RT-321.
g. Manufacturer name is SmithKline Beecham Pharmaceuticals.
h. Drug information includes dosages, storage, and safety measures.
i. Bar code.

EXAMPLE **ORAL DRUG (LIQUID FORM)**

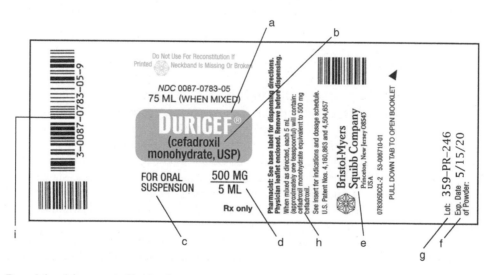

a. Brand (trade) name is Duricef.
b. Generic name is cefadroxil monohydrate.
c. Drug form is oral suspension.
d. Dosage is 500 mg per 5 mL.
e. Manufacturer is Bristol-Myers Squibb Company.
f. Expiration date is 5/15/20.
g. Lot number is 359-PR-246.
h. See package insert for more information.
i. Bar code.

EXAMPLE INJECTABLE DRUG

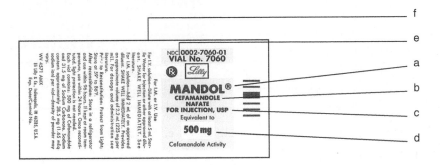

a. Brand name is Mandol.

b. Generic name is cefamandole nafate.

c. Drug form is drug powder that must be reconstituted in sterile water for use.

d. Dosage is 500 mg drug powder.

e. Drug container is vial.

f. Directions for drug reconstitution. For IV use: Add 5 mL of sterile water into the vial. Shake the vial well to completely dissolve the drug powder. For IM use: Add 2 mL of sterile water into the vial and shake thoroughly. The total volume of sterile water in the vial will equal 2.2 mL. The powder will increase the total volume by 0.2 mL.

Refer to Chapter 9 for more information on medication reconstitution.

PRACTICE PROBLEMS ▶ I INTERPRETATION OF DRUG LABELS

Answers can be found on pages 55 and 56.

1.

Store below 86°F (30°C).	NDC 0049-5340-66	4238
Dispense in tight, light-resistant containers (USP).	100 Capsules	MADE IN USA
DOSAGE AND USE See accompanying prescribing information.	**Sinequan®** (doxepin HCl)	
*Each capsule contains doxepin hydrochloride equivalent to 10 mg doxepin.	**10 mg***	
CAUTION: Federal law prohibits dispensing without prescription.	Distributed by **Pfizer** Roerig Division of Pfizer Inc, NY, NY 10017	

a. Brand (trade) name _____

b. Generic name _____

c. Drug form _____

d. Dosage _____

e. Manufacturer _____

2.

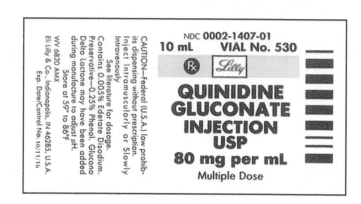

Directions for mixing: Tap bottle until all powder flows freely. Add approximately 1/3 total amount of water for reconstitution (total=33 mL); shake vigorously to wet powder. Add remaining water; again shake vigorously. Each 5 mL (1 teaspoonful) will contain amoxicillin trihydrate equivalent to 200 mg amoxicillin.
Net contents: Equivalent to 2.0 grams amoxicillin.
Store dry powder at or below 25°C (77°F).
Keep tightly closed.
Shake well before using.
Refrigeration preferable but not required.
Discard suspension after 14 days.

200mg/5mL
NDC 0029-6048-54

AMOXIL®
AMOXICILLIN
FOR ORAL
SUSPENSION

50mL (when reconstituted)

SmithKline Beecham Pharmaceuticals
Philadelphia, PA 19101

SB SmithKline Beecham

9069-B-B-B/B

LOT T54325
EXP. 11/15/16

Dosage: Administer every 12 hours.
See accompanying prescribing information.   R only

a. Brand (trade) name _____   e. Lot number _____

b. Generic name _____   f. Expiration date _____

c. Drug form _____   g. Manufacturer _____

d. Dosage _____

3.

NDC 0002-1407-01
10 mL   **VIAL No. 530**
Rx   *Lilly*

QUINIDINE GLUCONATE INJECTION USP
80 mg per mL
Multiple Dose

CAUTION—Federal (U.S.A.) law prohibits dispensing without prescription.
Inject Intramuscularly or Slowly Intravenously
See literature for dosage.
Contains 0.005% Edetate Disodium.
Preservative—0.25% Phenol. Glucono Delta Lactone may have been added during manufacture to adjust pH.
Store at 59° to 86°F.
WV 6820 AMX
Eli Lilly & Co., Indianapolis, IN 46285, U.S.A.
Exp. Date/Control No. 10/11/16

a. Brand (trade) name _____   d. Type of drug container _____

b. Generic name _____   e. Dosage _____

c. Drug form _____   f. Methods of administration _____

4.

Batch:
Expires: 3/15/20

RECOMMENDED STORAGE:
STORE BELOW 86°F (30°C).
PROTECT FROM LIGHT.
PROTECT FROM MOISTURE.
Each tablet contains **30 mg** nifedipine.
Tablets should be swallowed whole, not bitten or divided.
DOSAGE: See accompanying prescribing information.
Dispense in tight, light resistant containers (U.S.P.).

884120   NDC 0026-8841-51

ADALAT® CC

(nifedipine)
Extended Release Tablets
30 mg
100 Tablets
Caution: Federal (USA) law prohibits dispensing without prescription.

Bayer

Bayer Corporation
Pharmaceutical Division
400 Morgan Lane
West Haven, CT 06516

N 3 0026-8841-51 4

5695
©1995 Bayer Corporation
Printed in USA

PL500044

a. Brand (trade) name _____

b. Generic name _____

c. Drug form _____

d. Dosage _____

e. Expiration date _____

5.

NDC 0006-7782-30
2.5 mL INJECTION
AquaMEPHYTON®
(PHYTONADIONE)
Aqueous Colloidal Solution
10 mg per mL
Dist. by:
MERCK & CO., INC.
West Point, PA 19486, USA

MULTIPLE DOSE VIAL
FOR ROUTE OF
ADMINISTRATION AND DOSAGE:
SEE ACCOMPANYING CIRCULAR
Store in a dark place.
CAUTION: Federal (USA)
law prohibits dispensing
without prescription.
2.5 mL | No. 7782 9073108

a. Brand name _____

b. Generic name _____

c. Drug form _____

d. How many mL in vial _____

e. Dosage 1 mL = _____ mg

f. Manufacturer _____

g. Drug label suggests storing _____

Military (International) Time versus Traditional Time

Understanding the difference between military time and traditional time is essential in the health care field because almost all nursing settings use military time for documentation, medication administration, and for scheduling routine care and treatments. Military time uses a 24-hour clock, preventing potential documentation and medication errors as each time occurs only once a day. Military time requires 4 digits, the first two representing the hour and the second two digits representing the minutes. Unlike traditional time, military time does not separate the hours and minutes with a colon. Also, AM and PM are omitted because a 12-hour clock is not used in military time. Example: 5:43 AM = 0543. Example: 11:07 PM = 2307.

Use Figure 3.1 to solve conversion problems.

PRACTICE PROBLEMS ▶ II MILITARY TIME AND TRADITIONAL TIME CONVERSIONS

Answers can be found on page 56.

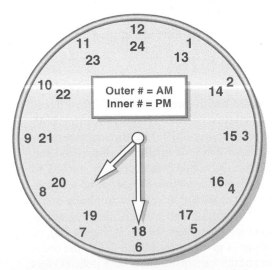

Figure 3.1 24-hour clock. In military time, midnight is considered 2400; however, midnight is referred to and written as 0000 in the medical field.

Convert traditional times to military time.
1. 9:30 AM =
2. 10:05 PM =
3. 4:55 PM =

Convert military times to traditional time.
4. 0245 =
5. 1515 =
6. 0001 =

DRUG DIFFERENTIATION

Some drugs with similar names, such as quinine and quinidine, have different chemical drug structures. Extreme care must be exercised when administering drugs that "look alike" or have similar spellings.

EXAMPLES **PERCOCET**

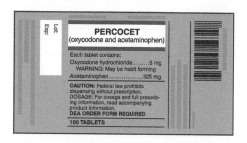

PERCODAN

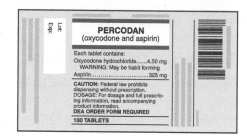

Percocet contains oxycodone and acetaminophen, whereas Percodan contains oxycodone and aspirin. A patient may be allergic to aspirin or should not take aspirin; therefore it is important that the patient be given Percocet. *Read the drug labels carefully and check.patient for an allergy band.*

EXAMPLES **HYDROXYZINE AND HYDRALAZINE**

Hydroxyzine is an antianxiety drug, and hydralazine is an antihypertensive drug.

EXAMPLES **QUINIDINE AND QUININE**

Quinidine sulfate is an antidysrhythmic drug, and quinine sulfate is an antimalarial drug.

Drug Orders

Medication orders may be prescribed and written by a licensed health care provider (HCP) with prescriptive authority, which includes physicians (MD), osteopathic physicians (DO), naturopathic physicians (ND), dentists (DDS), podiatrists (DPM), nurse practitioners (NP), and physician assistants (PA). Drug prescriptions in private practice or in clinics are written on a small prescription pad and are filled by a pharmacist at a drugstore or hospital (Figure 3.2). Some facilities have moved to computerized prescriptions. The physician enters the patient's drug order into a prescription template on a computer. The prescription then can be printed out for the patient or sent electronically over a secure network directly to the patient's chosen pharmacy. For hospitalized patients, the drug orders may be written on a doctor's order sheet and signed by the prescribing licensed HCP (Figure 3.3), or a computerized drug order system may be used. If the order is given by telephone (TO), the order must be cosigned by the physician within 24 hours. Most health care institutions have policies concerning verbal or telephone drug orders. The nurse must know and follow the institution's policy.

Robert B. Faber, M.D.
678 Apple Street
Wilmington, Delaware 19810

(123) 456-7891

Name _____ Age _____

Address _____ Date _____

R$_x$

Generic permitted _____

Label _____   _____ M.D.

Safety cap _____

Refill _____ times

Figure 3.2 Prescription pad medication order.

CITY HOSPITAL Dover, Delaware		PATIENT'S NAME Room #
Date	Time	Patient's Orders
12/2/16	0900	Zoloft 75mg po daily

Figure 3.3 Doctor's order sheet.

The basic components of a drug order are (1) date and time the order was written, (2) drug name, (3) drug dosage, (4) route of administration, (5) frequency of administration, and (6) physician's or HCP's signature. It is the nurse's responsibility to follow the physician's or HCP's order, but if any one of these components is missing, the drug order is incomplete and cannot be carried out. If the order is illegible, is missing a component, or calls for an inappropriate drug or dosage, clarification from the provider who wrote the order must be obtained before the order is carried out. It is the nurse's responsibility to know what medication he or she is giving and why the patient is receiving it.

Examples of drug orders and their interpretations are as follows:

6/3/16   0900   Digoxin 0.25 mg, po, daily
                    (give 0.25 mg of digoxin by mouth daily)

                       Ibuprofen 400 mg, po, q4h, PRN for pain
                    (give 400 mg of ibuprofen by mouth every 4 hours as needed)

                       Cefadyl 500 mg, IM, q6h
                    (give 500 mg of Cefadyl intramuscularly every 6 hours)

                       Prednisone 5 mg, po, q8h × 5 days
                    (give 5 mg of prednisone by mouth every 8 hours for 5 days)

PRACTICE PROBLEMS ▶ III INTERPRETATION OF DRUG ORDERS

Answers can be found on page 56.

Interpret these drug orders. For abbreviations that you do not know, see the section on abbreviations later in this chapter.

1. Procrit 40,000 units, SC, weekly

_____

2. Furosemide 40 mg, IV, bid

_____

3. Meperidine 50 mg, IM, q3-4h, PRN

_____

4. Prednisone 10 mg, po, tid × 5 days

_____

List what is missing in the following drug orders.

5. Codeine 30 mg, po, PRN for pain _____

6. Digoxin 0.25 mg, daily _____

7. TheoDur 200 mg _____

8. Penicillin V K 200,000 units, for days _____

TABLE 3.1 Types of Drug Orders

Types/Description	Examples
Standing orders: A standing order may be typed or written on the patient's order sheet. It may be an order that is given for a number of days, or it may be a routine order that is part of an order set that applies to all patients who have had the same type of procedure. Standing orders may include PRN orders.	Erythromycin 250 mg, po, q6h, 5 days Demerol 50 mg, IM, q3-4h, PRN, pain Colace 100 mg, po, hs, PRN
One-time (single) orders: One-time orders are given once, usually at a specified time. One-time orders can include STAT orders.	Preoperative orders: Meperidine 75 mg, IM, 0730 Atropine SO$_4$ 0.4 mg, IM, 0730
PRN orders: PRN orders are given at the patient's request and at the nurse's discretion concerning safety and need. Narcotics are time-framed and renewed every 48-72 hours.	Acetaminophen 1000 mg IV q6h PRN × 24 hr for fevers > 38° C Ondansetron HCl (Zofran), 4 mg, q4-8h, PRN for nausea
STAT orders: A STAT order is for a one-time dose of drug to be given immediately.	Regular insulin 10 units, subQ, STAT

There are four types of drug orders: (1) standing order, (2) one-time (single) order, (3) PRN (whenever necessary) order, and (4) STAT (immediate) order (Table 3.1). Many of the drugs ordered for nonhospitalized patients are normally standing orders that can be renewed (refilled) for 6 to 12 months. Narcotic orders are *not* automatically refilled; if the narcotic use is extended, the physician writes another prescription or calls the pharmacy.

UNIT-DOSE DISPENSING SYSTEM (UDDS)

The unit-dose dispensing system (UDDS) was developed to decrease medication errors, reduce the waste of medication, and improve the efficiency of the nurse when administering medications. In unit-dose dispensing, the pharmacy can provide individual doses in packets or containers for each patient. The pharmacy buys the drug in bulk and repackages the medication in individual dose packets labeled with the drug name, dosage, and usually a barcode. This method of distribution has almost replaced the ward stock system. In the ward stock system, bulk drug supplies were delivered to the medication room in each patient area. The nurse would then prepare the patients dose from large multi-dose containers or multiple dose vials. The medication would be labeled and then given to the patient.

Unit-dose dispensing has eliminated the need for many drug calculations that were essential with the ward stock system. Drug manufacturers are working to develop single doses for all medications, but extra packaging is costly. Additionally, not all medications that are prescribed for a patient are dosed in the exact amount manufactured. Therefore, the nurse must master manual calculations and have working knowledge of the process and formulas needed for medications to be given safely.

COMPUTERIZED DRUG ADMINISTRATION

While many health care facilities still use paper documentation, most facilities have moved to an electronic health care record, which includes medication ordering. This system is designed to reduce medication errors. Paper (handwritten) charting involves the prescriber writing an order on an order page. The nurse then transcribes the order onto a paper medication administration record (MAR). Handwritten orders pose many problems such as illegible handwriting and transcription errors. Computerized ordering and delivery systems enhance communication between pharmacists and nurses, decrease medication errors, and help prevent delays in delivery of therapy.

Computerized Prescriber Order System

Computerized order entry is the process of a health care provider (HCP) entering medication orders or other instructions electronically. The HCP can search for and select medications from a scrolling list (Figure 3.4). Once the medication is selected, the next screen displays all the possible doses, routes, and schedules (Figure 3.5). Once the HCP selects the components of the order, he or she can view the screen and make changes. If the information is correct, the HCP signs the order, which is then delivered to the pharmacy, where the order is processed.

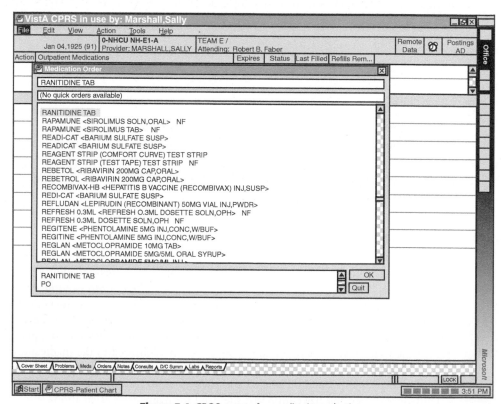

Figure 3.4 CPOS screen for medication selection.

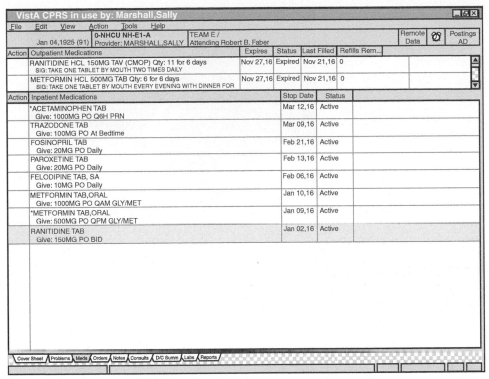

Figure 3.5 CPOS medication selection screen.

Bar Code Medication Administration

Bar code medication administration (BCMA) systems are electronic scanning systems that intercept medication errors at the point of administration. The system requires that the client wear a wristband with a unique barcode assigned specifically to that client. All medications also have a barcode. The nurse then scans the barcode on both the patient and the medication to verify that it is the correct patient, medication, dose, time, and route (Figures 3.6 and 3.7).

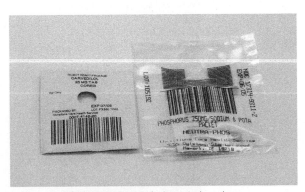

Figure 3.6 Bar code for unit drug dose.

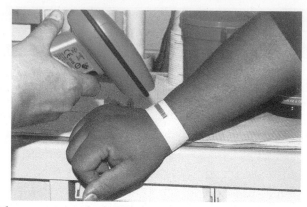

Figure 3.7 Bar-code reader. It is used to scan the patient's wristband.

MEDICATION DISTRIBUTION

There are a variety of ways that medications are stored and dispensed, and they vary from facility to facility. The two most common forms of medication distribution are discussed in the following sections.

Unit-Dose Cabinet

Unit-dose cabinets (Figure 3.8) are located in patient areas and have individualized drawers that are labeled with the patient's name, room number, and bed number. Each drawer is filled with 24 hours of medication as prescribed by the HCP and filled and verified by the pharmacist. When the nurse administers medication, the patient's drawer is accessed, and the appropriate drug is withdrawn.

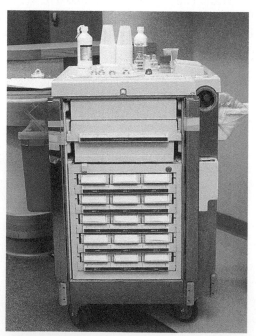

Figure 3.8 Unit-dose cabinet. (From Clayton BD, Willihnganz M: *Basic pharmacology for nurses,* ed 17, St Louis, 2017, Mosby.)

Automated Dispensing Cabinets (ADCs)

An automated dispensing cabinet is a computerized drug storage system that allows medications to be stored and dispensed in a patient care area. ADCs are supplied daily by the pharmacy with stock and patient specific medications. This system eliminates the nurse from having to wait for the medication to come from a centralized pharmacy. ADCs permit the nurse to access the machine by using either a user ID, personal password, or fingerprint scan. It tracks user access and dispensed medications. The most common systems are the AcuDose Rx, Omnicell Omni Rx, and the Pyxis MedStation (Figure 3.9).

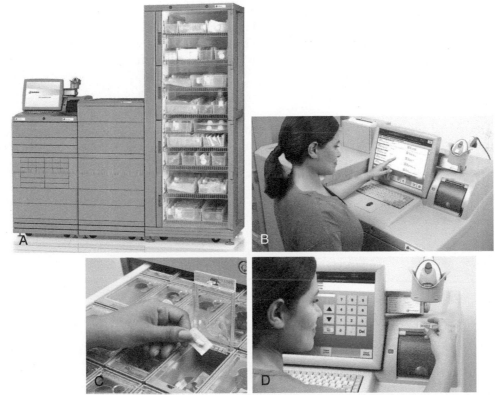

Figure 3.9 A, Pyxis MedStation. **B,** The nurse enters personal security codes or scans a fingerprint to gain access to confidential patient information. The nurse then selects the patient's name and the appropriate medication. **C,** The appropriate drawer(s) are opened and the nurse takes the needed medication. **D,** The nurse scans the medication. If the medication selected is not the correct drug or the correct dosage, the scan will cause the computer to issue a warning stating the reason. (From Becton, Dickinson, and Company, Franklin Lakes, NJ.)

DOCUMENTATION OF MEDICATION ADMINISTRATION

Documentation of medication administration should be completed immediately after medications are administered. Failure to do so may result in (1) forgetting to chart/document, or (2) administration of drugs by another nurse who thought the drugs were not given. Documentation of medication administration is either done in the paper chart or electronically.

MAR

The MAR is the medication administration record. Handwritten MARs include basic patient information including the patient's name, medical record number, date of birth, patient location, weight, allergies, sex, and date of admission. Handwritten MARs (Figure 3.10) have a list of the patient's medications that have been transcribed from the health care provider's medication orders. After giving the medication, the nurse records his or her initials next to the time the medication was administered.

eMAR

The eMAR (Figure 3.11) is the electronic medication administration record. It is a paperless system that displays the medications to be given on the computer screen. The nurse uses his or her own specific code to log onto the system, and when the drug is scanned (via the barcode), it will be documented as given.

HOPE HOSPITAL		Patient's Name	John Smith

HOPE HOSPITAL Medication Administration Record (MAR)		Patient's Name *John Smith* *123-24-8449* Age: *78* Room# *6033*
Nurse's signature/Title	Initial	
Joyce L. Kee, RN	JK	
Sally Marshall, RN	SM	Allergies: *Penicillin*
Jane Jones, LPN	JJ	

DATE ORDER	STOP DATE	Medication Dose – Route – Frequency	TIME	Date, Initial, HT Rate, BP											
				5/16		5/17		5/18		5/19					
5/16		Digoxin 0.25 mg po daily Hold if HR < 60	0800	JK	92	JK	86	JK	88	SM	84				
5/16	5/20 @0000	Prednisone 5 mg po q8h × 5 days	0800	JK		JK		JK		SM					
			1600	SM		JJ		SM		JK					
			0000	JJ		SM		JJ		JJ					
5/16		Atenolol 50 mg po daily Hold if SBP < 100	0800	JK	152/110	JK	146/90	JK	148/72	SM	145/75				

One-Time/PRN/STAT Medications				
Date	Medication/Dose Route/Frequency	Time/ Initial	Reason	Result
5/18	Ibuprofen 400 mg po q4h PRN	0930 SM	Left knee pain 5 of 10	1030 knee pain has improved 1 of 10

Figure 3.10 Medication administration record (MAR).

FRIDAY 10/12/16 - 0700   thru   SATURDAY 10/13/16 - 0659   ST ANNE HOSPITAL

Meyer, Lois M.   Unit#:   MEDICATION ADMINISTRATION RECORD
WESOF W303-2   Admitted: 10/12/16   Acct#:   Page: 1
Age: 87   Sex: F   Ht: 152.40 cm   Wt: 49.8 kg   Attending Dr: Benjamin Simmons, MD
Primary Dx: Chest pain   Run Date/Time: 10/12/16 - 2237
                                                                                          DOB: 12/28/1928

ALLERGIES: Drug: PCN, ERYTHROMYCIN, IV DYE
                     Other: NO ALLERGIES RECORDED
                     Pharmacy: IODINE (INCLUDES RADIOPAQUE AGENTS W/IODINE). MACROLIDE ANTIBIOTICS, PENICILLINS

Init	IV Flushes: Routine		0700-1459	1500-2259	2300-0659
	Sodium Chloride 0.9% **IV** Flush peripheral IV lines with 5 mls 0.9 NS q 8 hours and central lines per protocol.		Time _____ Init _____ # Flushed_____	Time _____ Init _____ # Flushed_____	Time _____ Init _____ # Flushed_____

Init	SCHED MEDS	DOSE		0700-1459	1500-2259	2300-0659
	DOCUSATE SODIUM (DOCUSATE SODIUM) START: 10/12 D/C: 11/11/16 AT 2244	**100 MG**	PO Q12 RX 002306792			
	PRAVACHOL (PRAVASTATIN SODIUM) Give at: BEDTIME START: 10/12 D/C: 11/11/16 AT 2244	**80 MG**	PO RX 002306793			
	METOPROLOL TARTRATE (METOPROLOL TARTRATE) HOLD FOR SBP<110 OR HR<55 Check apical rate and BP before drug admin. START: 10/12 D/C: 11/11/16 AT 2244	**50 MG**	PO Q12 RX 002306794			
	ACCUPRIL (QUINAPRIL HCL) HOLD FOR SBP<120 START: 10/12 D/C: 11/11/16 AT 2244	**40 MG**	PO Q12 RX 002306795			
	NITROGLYCERIN 2% (NITROGLYCERIN 2%) HOLD FOR SBP<100 START: 10/12 D/C: 11/11/16 AT 2244	**1 INCH**	TP Q6 RX 002306796			0000 0600
	ALPRAZOLAM (ALPRAZOLAM) START: 10/12 D/C: 10/14/16 AT 1601	**0.25 MG**	PO Q8 RX 002306791			0000

Init	PRN MEDS	DOSE		0700-1459	1500-2259	2300-0659
	NITROSTAT 25 TABS/BOTTLE (NITROGLYCERIN) Chest discomfort. May repeat q 5 min x 3. If no relief after 3 doses. Stat ECG & call Physician. START: 10/12 D/C: 11/11/16 at 1833	**0.4 MG**	SL STAT RX 002306718 PRN			

Figure 3.11 Electronic medication administration record (eMAR).

Note all medication hold parameters before administering any medication.

ABBREVIATIONS

Drug Measurements and Drug Forms

Many abbreviations, symbols, acronyms, and dose designations in health care developed over time from the need to communicate and document care. The nurse must learn these and properly interpret them when administering drug therapy. Here are lists of acceptable abbreviations used in three categories: (1) drug measurements and drug forms, (2) routes of drug administration, and (3) times of administration. Not all abbreviations are used in every institution. The nurse should follow the institution's policies for documentation and communication.

Abbreviation	Meaning
cap	capsule
elix	elixir

g, gm, G, GM	gram
gtt	drops
kg	kilogram
l, L	liter
m^2	square meter
mcg	microgram
mEq	milliequivalent
mg	milligram
mL, ml	milliliter
m, min	minim
oz	ounce
pt	pint
qt	quart
SR	sustained release
supp	suppository
susp	suspension
T.O.	telephone order
T, tbsp	tablespoon
t, tsp	teaspoon
V.O.	verbal order

Routes of Drug Administration

Abbreviation	Meaning
ID	intradermal
IM	intramuscular
IV	intravenous
IVPB	intravenous piggyback
KVO	keep vein open
Ⓛ	left
NGT	nasogastric tube
PO, po, os	by mouth
R, Ⓡ	right
Subcut	subcutaneous
SL, sl, subl	sublingual
TKO	to keep open
Vag	vaginal

Times of Administration

Abbreviation	Meaning
AC, ac	before meals
ad lib	as desired
B.i.d., b.i.d., bid	twice a day
c̄	with
NPO	nothing by mouth
PC, pc	after meals
PRN, p.r.n.	whenever necessary, as needed
q	every
qAM	every morning

qh	every hour
q2h	every 2 hours
q4h	every 4 hours
q6h	every 6 hours
q8h	every 8 hours
Qi.d., q.i.d., qid	four times a day
s̄	without
SOS	once if necessary; if there is a need
STAT	immediately
T.i.d., t.i.d., tid	three times a day

"Do Not Use" Abbreviations

Misconstrued and misinterpreted abbreviations can result in harmful outcomes. Two organizations, The Joint Commission (TJC), formerly known as The Joint Commission on Accreditation of Healthcare Organizations, and the Institute for Safe Medication Practices (ISMP), whose purpose is to improve quality of care and promote patient safety, have issued "Do Not Use" lists of error-prone abbreviations, symbols, acronyms, and dose designations with suggestions for alternatives to avoid mistakes and patient harm. The nurse must be alert and recognize drug orders with abbreviations or symbols that could cause potential problems.

The following is a combined list from TJC and ISMP of abbreviations and symbols that have been frequently misinterpreted and that have caused harmful errors.

The "Do Not Use" Abbreviation List

Abbreviation	Meaning	Use Instead
A.D., ad	Right ear	Right ear
&	and	and
A.S., as	Left ear	Left ear
@	at	at
A.U., au	Both ears	Both ears
cc	cubic centimeter	mL (milliliter)
D/C	Discharge or discontinue	Discharge or discontinue
Drug name abbreviations		Write out the full name of the drug
hs	At bedtime	Bedtime
HS	Half-strength	Half-strength or at bedtime
i/d	One daily	1 daily
IJ	Injection	Injection
IN	Intranasal	Intranasal or NAS
IU	International unit	International unit
< and >	Less than and greater than	Less than and greater than
o.d. or OD	Once daily	Daily
O.D., od	Right eye	Right eye
OJ	Orange juice	Orange juice
O.S., os	Left eye	Left eye
O.U., ou	Both eyes	Both eyes
Per os	By mouth, orally	PO, by mouth, or orally
q.d. or QD	Every day	Daily
qhs or qHS	Nightly at bedtime	Nightly
qn	Nightly or at bedtime	Nightly or at bedtime
q.o.d. or QOD	Every other day	Every other day
qld	Daily	Daily
q6PM	Every evening at 6 PM	6 PM daily

Abbreviation	Meaning	Use Instead
/ (slash mark)	Separates doses or means per	per
ss	Sliding scale or 1/2	Sliding scale
SSI	Sliding scale insulin	Sliding scale insulin
SSRI	Sliding scale regular insulin	Sliding scale insulin
tiw or TIW	Three times a week	Three times weekly
U or u	Unit	Unit
UD	ut dictum or as directed	As directed
Ug	microgram	mcg (microgram)

Please refer to TJC website at *www.jointcommission.org* and to the Institute for Safe Medication Practices at *www.ismp.org* for more detailed safety information.

PRACTICE PROBLEMS ▶ IV ABBREVIATIONS

Answers can be found on page 56.

If you have more than three incorrect answers, review the abbreviations and meanings. Then quiz yourself again.

1. cap _____
2. SR _____
3. fl oz _____
4. g, G, gm, GM _____
5. gtt _____
6. L _____
7. mL _____
8. mcg _____
9. mg _____
10. oz _____
11. T, tbsp _____
12. t, tsp _____
13. IM _____
14. IV _____
15. KVO or TKO _____
16. subcut _____
17. c̄ _____
18. A.C., ac _____
19. NPO _____
20. PC, pc _____
21. q4h _____
22. Qi.d., q.i.d., qid _____
23. T.i.d., t.i.d., tid _____
24. B.i.d., b.i.d., bid _____
25. STAT _____

ANSWERS

I Interpretation of Drug Labels

1. a. Sinequan
   b. doxepin
   c. capsule
   d. 10 mg per capsule
   e. Pfizer/Roerig

2. a. Amoxil
   b. amoxicillin
   c. liquid for oral suspension when reconstituted
   d. 200 mg/5 mL
   e. Lot #T54325
   f. Expiration date: 11/15/16
   g. SmithKline Beecham

3. a. quinidine gluconate
   b. quinidine gluconate (same as brand name)

c. liquid for injection
d. vial (multiple-dose vial), total amount is 10 mL per vial
e. 80 mg per mL
f. IM or IV

4. a. Adalat
   b. nifedipine
   c. extended-release tablet
   d. 30 mg per tablet
   e. 3/15/20
5. a. Aquamephyton
   b. phytonadione

c. Aqueous colloidal solution, injectable
d. 2.5 mL
e. 10 mg
f. Merck & Co.
g. In a dark place

II Military Time and Traditional Time Conversions

1. 0930
2. 2205

3. 1655
4. 2:45 AM

5. 3:15 PM
6. 12:01 AM

III Interpretation of Drug Orders

1. Give 40,000 units of Procrit subcutaneously, once a week
2. Give 40 mg of furosemide intravenously, two times per day
3. Give 50 mg of meperidine intramuscularly every 3 to 4 hours as needed for pain
4. Give 10 mg of prednisone by mouth three times a day for 5 days
5. frequency of administration
6. route of administration
7. route and frequency of administration
8. route and frequency of administration and stop date

IV Abbreviations

1. capsule
2. sustained release
3. fluid ounce
4. gram
5. drop
6. liter
7. milliliter
8. microgram
9. milligram

10. ounce
11. tablespoon
12. teaspoon
13. intramuscular
14. intravenous
15. keep vein open
16. subcutaneous
17. with

18. before meals
19. nothing by mouth
20. after meals
21. every 4 hours
22. four times a day
23. three times a day
24. two times a day
25. immediately

CHAPTER 4

Prevention of Medication Errors

Objectives
- Know the organizations that are monitoring medication errors.
- Identify high-alert drugs.
- Discuss some of the causes of medication errors (MEs).
- Explain ways that medication errors can be prevented.
- Describe the Rights in drug administration.

Outline **PREVENTING MEDICATION ERRORS**
THE RIGHTS IN DRUG ADMINISTRATION

PREVENTING MEDICATION ERRORS

The purpose of drug therapy is to improve the patient's quality of life while minimizing the risk. An adverse drug event/reaction (ADE/ADR) is an incident that causes physical, mental, or functional harm associated with a medication. One type of adverse drug event/reaction is a medication error (ME). According to the National Coordinating Council for Medication Error Reporting and Prevention, a ME is defined as "any preventable event that may cause or lead to inappropriate medication use or patient harm while the medication is in control of the health care professional, patient, or consumer." Although medication errors are considered preventable, over 100,000 MEs were reported by hospitals nationwide in 2011, according to a study conducted by the Institute for Safe Medication Practices (ISMP). As a result of these medication errors, at least 7,000 deaths occurred per year at a cost of $2 billion. However, the reporting of MEs is voluntary, not mandatory. So the actual figures of MEs are probably much higher. Of the MEs reported in 2011, about half are intercepted, and of those, 86% were intercepted by nurses.

There are currently over 40 health care groups—private, governmental, and professional—that are working together to report, understand, and prevent medication errors. Examples include: the ISMP, the Food and Drug Administration (FDA), the United States Pharmacopeia (USP), and The Joint Commission (TJC).

There are many strategies that have been implemented by various organizations to prevent medication errors. Some examples include:
- The FDA rules state that a bar code and the national drug code, which identifies the drug strength and its dosage form, are required for all human drug and blood products. Bar coding is discussed in Chapter 3.
- The FDA implemented the "black box" warning, which appears on the package insert, to alert health care providers that a drug may have significant risk of serious or life-threatening adverse effects.
- The ISMP has identified lists of high-alert drugs that should be carefully monitored to prevent adverse drug reactions. Examples of high alert drugs include: potassium chloride, insulin, heparin, opiates, and anti-cancer agents.

Nurse educators have resources through the Quality and Safety Education for Nurses (QSEN) Institute to assist students to learn the complexities of safe practice in drug administration.

 YOU MUST REMEMBER

The person who administers the medication, usually the nurse, is responsible if an ME occurs.

Here are some examples of the types of medication errors (MEs):

1. The physician or health care provider makes a prescribing error and/or the written drug order is **NOT** legible.
2. Transcription errors occur because the medications have similar names; the decimals and zeros are not correctly written; or numbers are transposed.
3. Telephone and verbal orders are misinterpreted.
4. Interruptions occur when preparing medications.
5. Drug labels look similar (names and color), and packing obscures print on the label.
6. Trade names and generic names for drugs are used interchangeably, which causes confusion.
7. Oral dosages and intravenous dosages are different for the same drug.
8. Subcutaneous insulin is given in a tuberculin syringe and **NOT** in an insulin syringe.
9. The pharmacy delivers the wrong drug.
10. Intravenous medication is given too fast or too concentrated.
11. The amount of the drug is incorrectly calculated.
12. The drug is given intramuscularly or subcutaneously and should be given intravenously OR the drug is given intravenously and should be given intramuscularly.
13. Two incompatible drugs are given intravenously, which can cause crystallization of the drugs.
14. Two or three patients with the same names are on the same unit and their identification wristbands are hard to read. One patient receives another's medication.
15. Medication is given and not monitored, and an overdose occurs.
16. An infusion pump malfunctions or is incorrectly programmed.

Ways to prevent medication errors (MEs):

1. Ask the physician or health care provider to rewrite or clarify medication order.
2. Use only approved abbreviations from The Joint Commission (TJC) list for medication dosages. Do not use "u" for unit; it should be spelled out. Avoid use of a slash mark (/), which could be interpreted as a one (1).
3. Do not use abbreviations for medication names (e.g., MSO_4 for morphine sulfate).
4. Use leading zeros for doses less than a unit (e.g., **0.1** mg; **NOT .1** mg). Do not use a zero following a whole number (e.g., 5 mg; **NOT** 5.0 mg). The decimal point after 5 may not be noticed and would look like 50 mg.
5. Check medication orders with written order and MAR/eMAR.
6. Check the drug dose sent from the pharmacy with the MAR/eMAR.
7. Prepare medications in a clean, distraction-free environment.
8. Never administer a medication that has been prepared by another nurse.
9. Have another nurse check the dosage preparation, especially if in doubt. Recalculate drug dosage as needed.
10. Check if the patient is allergic to any specific drugs. If an allergy exists, report the type of reaction the patient experiences.
11. Check the patient's identification band with the eMAR and bar code.
12. Do not leave medication at the bedside. Stay with the patient until the medications are swallowed.

13. Know whether the medication the patient is to receive would be contraindicated because of the patient's health (liver disease and Tylenol [acetaminophen]) or because of a possible drug interaction with another drug the patient is taking.
14. Assess physical parameters (e.g., apical pulse, respiration, BP, INR, and electrolyte values) before administering the medication that could affect these parameters.
15. Monitor the effects of the administered drug, the rate of IV flow, and the patient's response to the medication.
16. Check when to administer medication for a patient whose status is nothing by mouth (NPO). When in doubt, check with the health care provider (HCP) or nurse manager.
17. Record medications that are given immediately after their administration.
18. Report MEs immediately to the HCP.
19. Educate the patient and family about the drug and its action.
20. Know the compatibility of drugs that are being given. Report any contraindications.

Nurses often work in busy environments with constant distractions. When giving medications, it is important to concentrate fully on the task and know the usual drug dosage of the medication you are giving. If your facility does not have a current drug reference book that is easily accessible, then a drug reference text should be obtained. If a nurse is unsure about a drug order or dosage, then consultation is required with the pharmacy, physician, HCP, or nurse manager before administering the medication. Keeping the patient safe is the nurse's responsibility. The nurse is the licensed practitioner who administers the medication and monitors the medication's response. Nurses are the final line of defense. Be a patient advocate, and always ask if you are unsure.

THE RIGHTS IN DRUG ADMINISTRATION

To provide safe drug administration, the nurse should practice the "10 Rights": the right patient, the right drug, the right dose, the right time, the right route, the right documentation, the right to refuse the medication, the right assessment, the right education (patient), and the right evaluation (Box 4.1).

Right Patient

The patient's identification band should always be checked before a medication is given. The nurse should do the following:
- Verify the patient's identity by checking his or her identification bracelet/wristband.
- Ask the patient his or her name and birth date. Do not call the patient by name. Some individuals answer to any name. The patient may have difficulty in hearing.
- Check the name on the patient's medication label.
- Check if the patient has allergies (check chart and ask the patient).

Right Drug

To avoid error, the nurse should do the following:
- Check the drug label three times: (1) first contact with the drug bottle or drug pack, (2) before pouring/preparing the drug, and (3) after preparation of the drug.
- Check that the drug order is complete and legible. If it is not, contact the physician, HCP, or charge nurse.
- Know the drug action.
- Check the expiration date. Discard an outdated drug or return the drug to the pharmacy.
- If the patient questions the drug, recheck the drug and drug dose. If in doubt, seek another HCP's advice, i.e., pharmacist, physician, licensed HCP. Some generic drugs differ in shape or color.

Right Dose

Stock drugs and unit doses are the two methods frequently used for drug distribution. Not all health care institutions use the unit-dose method (drugs prepared by dose in the pharmacy or by the pharmaceutical company). If the institution uses the unit-dose method, drugs in bottles should *not* be administered without the consent of the physician or pharmacist. The nurse should:

- Be able to calculate drug dose using the ratio and proportion, basic formula, fractional equation, or dimensional analysis methods.
- Know how to calculate drug dose by body weight (kg) or by body surface (BSA; m^2). Doses of potent drugs (e.g., anticancer agents) and doses for children are frequently determined by body weight or BSA.
- Know the recommended dosage range for the drug. Check the *Physicians' Desk. Reference,* the *American Hospital Formulary Service (AHFS) Drug Information,* nursing drug reference books, computerized drug reference programs, or other drug references. If the nurse believes that the dose is incorrect or is not within the therapeutic drug range, he or she should notify the charge nurse, physician, or pharmacist and should document all communications.
- Recalculate the drug dose if in doubt, or have a colleague recheck the dose and calculation.
- Question drug doses that appear incorrect.
- Have a colleague check the drug dose of potent or specified drugs, such as insulin, digoxin, narcotics, and anticancer agents. This procedure is required by some facilities.

Right Time

The drug dose should be given at a specified time to maintain a therapeutic drug serum level. Too-frequent dosing can cause drug toxicity, and missed doses can nullify the drug action and its effect. The nurse should:

- Administer the drug at the specified time(s). Usually, drugs can be given 30 minutes before or after the time prescribed.
- Omit or delay a drug dose according to specific circumstance, e.g., laboratory or diagnostic tests may be necessary. Notify the appropriate personnel of the reason.
- Administer drugs that are affected by food (e.g., tetracycline) 1 hour before or 2 hours after meals.
- Administer drugs that can irritate the gastric mucosa (e.g., potassium or aspirin) with food.
- Give some medications promptly or at a specified time (e.g., STAT drugs for pain or nausea drugs).
- Know that drugs with a long half-life ($t_{1/2}$) (e.g., 20 to 36 hours) are usually given once per day. Drugs with a short half-life, e.g., 1 to 6 hours, are given several times a day.
- Administer antibiotics at even intervals (e.g., q8h: 8 AM, 4 PM, midnight), rather than tid (8 AM, noon, 4 PM); q6h (6, 12, 6, 12), rather than qid (8-12-4-8) to maintain therapeutic drug serum level. If the patient is to receive a diuretic twice a day, q12h, 8 AM and 8 PM, the evening dose may be given at 4 PM (e.g., bid) because of the diuretic effect. If dose is given in the evening, it could cause urination late at night.

Right Route

The right route is necessary for the appropriate absorption of the medication. The more common routes of absorption are: (1) oral (by mouth, po) tablet, capsule, pill, liquid, or suspension; (2) sublingual (under the tongue for venous absorption, *not* to be swallowed); (3) buccal (between gum and cheek, *not* to be swallowed); (4) topical (applied to the skin); (5) inhalation (aerosol sprays); (6) instillation (in nose, eye, ear, rectum, or vagina); and (7) four parenteral routes: intradermal, subcutaneous, intramuscular, and intravenous. The nurse should:

- Know the drug route. If in doubt, check with the pharmacy. Ointment for the eye should have "ophthalmic" written on the tube. Drugs given sublingually (e.g., nitroglycerin tablet) should *not* be swallowed, because the effect of the drug would be lost.

- Administer injectables (subcutaneous and intramuscular) at appropriate sites (see Chapter 9).
- Use aseptic technique when administering drugs. Sterile technique is required with parenteral routes.
- Document the injection site used on the patient's paper chart (MAR) or eMAR.

Right Documentation

Document on the MAR or eMAR (computer), the time the drug was administered and the nurse's initials. To avoid overdosing or underdosing of drug, administration of medication should be recorded immediately.

- Put your initials on the MAR sheet or eMAR at the proper space immediately after administering the drug. With eMAR, click the mark as given, and the system will automatically sign the medication off with your initials.
- Refused drug: Circle your initials and document on the nurse's notes or on the MAR or eMAR.
- Omitted drug: Circle your initials and document on the nurse's notes or the MAR/eMAR. Document why the drug was omitted, such as the patient was NPO because of a laboratory or diagnostic test. The charge nurse or HCP should be notified.
- Delay in administering drug should be documented on the nurse's notes, MAR sheet, or eMAR. If the drug is to be administered once a day and is delayed, document the time the drug is given. Medications can be retimed on eMAR.
- High-alert medications must be cosigned whenever a dose changes or a new IV bag is hung. Check with your institution.

Right to Refuse Medication

The patient has a right to refuse medication. However,

- Explain to the patient the therapeutic effect of the drug. This will often diminish the patient's refusal.
- Document the medication and time the patient refused the drug and the reason for the patient's refusal.
- Notify the physician, HCP, and/or charge nurse that the patient refused the drug and why.
- If the refusal is due to the mental status of the patient, it should be reported.

Right Assessment

- Assess whether the ordered medication is safe to administer.
- Assess the patient's vital signs (VS) to determine medication safety. For example, a patient may be ordered Dilaudid 0.5 mg, IV. The patient's VS are BP 95/60, pulse 60, and respirations 8. After assessing VS, the Dilaudid IV would be determined to be unsafe to administer.
- Know that opioids can decrease blood pressure, pulse, and respirations.
- Assess the effects of the medication being administered.

Right Education

- Educate the patient about the purpose(s) for the ordered medications.
- Answer patient's questions about the medication he or she is taking. The patient will most likely comply in taking the medication if the patient understands the purpose and effects of the drug(s).
- Educate the patient about the possible effects of the medication, including side effects, especially with potent drugs.

Right Evaluation

- Evaluate the effects of the medication, particularly whether it was effective or not.
- Record on the MAR or eMAR the positive or negative effects of the medication(s).
- Report to the health care provider (HCP) if the medication was ineffective.
- Evaluate whether the medication is causing adverse reactions. Report immediately any adverse reactions.

BOX 4.1 CHECKLIST FOR THE "10 RIGHTS" IN DRUG ADMINISTRATION

Right Patient

- Check patient's identification bracelet.
- Ask the patient his or her name and birth date.
- Check the name on the patient's medication label.

Right Drug

- Check that the drug order is complete and legible.
- Check the drug label three times.
- Check the expiration date.
- Know the drug action.

Right Dose

- Calculate the drug dosage.
- Know the recommended dosage range for the drug.
- Recalculate the drug dosage with another nurse if in doubt.

Right Time

- Administer drug at the specified time(s).
- Document any delay or omitted drug dose.
- Administer drugs that irritate gastric mucosa with food.
- Administer drugs that cannot be administered with food 1 hour before or 2 hours after meals.
- Administer antibiotics at even intervals (q6h or q8h).

Right Route

- Know the route for administration of the drug.
- Use aseptic techniques when administering a drug.
- Document the injection site on the MAR/eMAR.

Right Documentation

- Place nurse's initials on the MAR sheet or eMAR.
- Document the reason for a patient **not** taking the drug.
- Indicate on the MAR sheet or eMAR whether the drug dose was delayed and the time it was given.

Right to Refuse Medication

- Document the time and date the patient refused the drug and the refusal reason.
- Notify the charge nurse and physician that the patient refused the drug.
- Explain the purpose and therapeutic effect of the drug to the patient.
- Record if the refusal could be due to the patient's mental status.

BOX 4.1 CHECKLIST FOR THE "10 RIGHTS" IN DRUG ADMINISTRATION-Cont'd

Right Assessment

- Assess if the ordered medication is safe to administer.
- Assess the patient's vital signs and determine whether they are safe for the drug.
- Know that opioids can decrease vital signs.
- Assess the effects of the medication(s) being administered.

Right Education

- Educate the patient about the purpose(s) for the medication.
- Answer the patient's questions about the medication he or she is receiving.
- Educate the patient about possible side effects of the medication.

Right Evaluation

- Evaluate the effects of the medication.
- Record on the MAR or eMAR the effects of the medication(s).
- Report to the HCP if the medication was ineffective.
- Evaluate whether the medication caused adverse reactions.

NEXT-GENERATION NCLEX® EXAMINATION-STYLE QUESTIONS

A 64 year-old patient is admitted to the hospital for diverticulitis. Her course has been complicated by the development of an abdominal abscess which does require further surgical debridement. She has a gastric feeding tube but is nothing by mouth (NPO) except for medications and is scheduled for surgery at 1600. The abdominal wound dressing is getting changed and packed every 12 hours with a moist sterile dressing and was last changed at 0900. She did not require a dose of hydromorphone during the previous dressing change. Her medication administration record (MAR) states:

oxycodone 5mg po q6h prn for pain
hydromorphone 0.5mg IV q12h with dressing changes
extended- release morphine 15mg po TID (0800, 1600, 2400)

Her blood pressure is 157/74mmHg, heart rate is 107 beats per minute, Sao2 on room air is 98% and respiratory rate is 18 breaths per minute. At 1200, the patient asks if she can have a dose of pain medication.

Choose the most likely options for the missing information from the selection below:

The nurse understands that she cannot give the hydromorphone since it is _A_. Extended release morphine cannot be given because _B_. Oxycodone is the available option since it is a prn medication choice and can be _C_.

Option A	Option B	Option C
For dressing change only	It is the wrong route	Crushed and given per feeding tube
Break through pain	Must be crushed for the feeding tube	Given whole by mouth
Incorrect form for a feeding tube	Not the right time to administer	Can be given intravenously
Not the right time to administer	It is a prn medication	Can be given at the right time

ANSWERS-NEXT-GENERATION NCLEX®
EXAMINATION-STYLE QUESTIONS

Option A	Option B	Option C
For dressing change only	It is the wrong route	**Crushed and given per feeding tube**
For breakthrough	**Must be crushed for the feeding tube**	Given whole by mouth
Incorrect form for a feeding tube	For breakthrough pain	Can be given intravenously
Not the right time to administer	It is a prn medication	Can be given at the right time

Rationale:

Option A: Hydromorphone is ordered for dressing change only and cannot be used for breakthrough pain. This is an intravenous form of the drug which is ineffective if given per tube and it is not the time to administer. Administering this medication for this situation would be a drug error.

Option B: Extended release morphine can be given by mouth but should never be crushed and given per tube because more drug will be released when crushed and may lead to a drug overdose. The extended release morphine is ordered for 3 times a day and is not given whenever necessary. Giving this medication would be a drug error.

Option C: Oxycodone can be given whenever necessary, can be crushed and given per tube and is ordered for breakthrough pain. The oral formulation cannot be given intravenously.

CHAPTER 5

Alternative Methods for Drug Administration

Objectives
- Explain the correct method of applying a transdermal patch.
- Describe the administration of nasal and ophthalmic medications.
- Explain the different techniques for administering ear drops to adults and children.
- Recognize when intraosseous or intraspinal access should be utilized in the clinical setting.

Outline
TRANSDERMAL PATCH
TYPES OF INHALERS AND NEBULIZERS
NASAL SPRAY AND DROPS
EYE DROPS AND OINTMENT
EAR DROPS
PHARYNGEAL SPRAY, MOUTHWASH, AND LOZENGE
TOPICAL PREPARATIONS: LOTION, CREAM, AND OINTMENT
RECTAL SUPPOSITORY
VAGINAL SUPPOSITORY, CREAM, AND OINTMENT
INTRAOSSEOUS ACCESS
INTRASPINAL ACCESS

The properties of a medication significantly influence its route of administration, which determines how it will be absorbed into the body. The two major routes of administration are enteral and parenteral. The parenteral route directly delivers the medication into the patient's systemic circulation (e.g., intravenous, intramuscular, intraosseous, and subcutaneous). Drugs taken orally or sublingually are using an enteral route of administration. Other methods of administration may be less common but are still important alternatives for medication delivery. Some other forms of medication administration include transdermal, inhalation, pharyngeal, topical, rectal, vaginal, nasal, eye, or ear drops, and intraspinal. The general nursing procedure for any drug administration is to wash hands, apply clean gloves, then proceed to administer the medication.

TRANSDERMAL PATCH

Purpose

The transdermal patch contains medication (Figure 5.1) that's delivered via a patch that's applied to the skin for slow, systemic absorption, usually over 24 hours. Use of the transdermal route avoids the gastrointestinal problems associated with some oral medications and provides a more consistent drug level in the patient's blood.

Method

Transdermal Patch
1. Wear gloves to remove existing patch if present, then cleanse and dry the area of skin where the new patch will be applied. Commonly used areas are the chest, abdomen, arms, or thighs. Avoid areas that have hair.
2. Label the patch with date, time, and nurse's initials.
3. Remove the transparent cover (inside) of the patch. Do not touch the inside of the patch.
4. Apply the adhesive side of the patch (inside) to the chosen area with the dull plastic side up.
5. Document location of transdermal patch on medication administration record or chart.

Note: There are some transdermal patches that absorb over 3 days (e.g., duragesic), some over 7 days (e.g., Catapres), and some over 1 month (e.g., contraceptive agents).

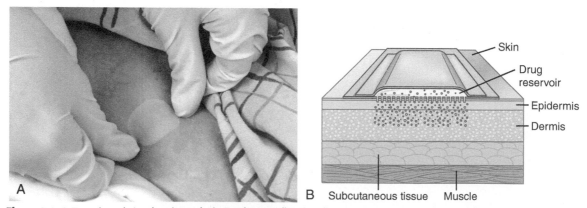

Figure 5.1 A, Transdermal nitroglycerin patch. (In Snyder JS, Collins SR, Lilley LL [2020]. *Pharmacology and the nursing process,* 9th ed., St. Louis: Mosby. From Rick Brady, Riva, MD.) **B,** Interior of the transdermal patch.

TYPES OF INHALERS AND NEBULIZERS

Purpose

The drug inhaler delivers a prescribed dose to be absorbed rapidly by the mucosal lining of the respiratory tract. The drug categories for respiratory inhalation are bronchodilators, which dilate bronchial tubes; glucocorticoids, which are anti-inflammatory agents; and mucolytics, which liquefy bronchial secretions.

Types

Inhalers can be divided into four groups: metered-dose inhalers (MDIs), MDIs with spacers, dry powder inhalers, and nebulizers. Standard MDIs use a pressurized gas that expels the medication. The user must press the canister downward to initiate the release of the medication and inhale fully at the same time, for the dose to be delivered to the lungs. For some, it can be challenging to coordinate the use of the MDI (spraying the medication) and inhaling simultaneously. Breath-activated MDIs are another type, in which the dose is triggered by inhaling through the mouthpiece; requiring less coordination from the user.

Spacer devices can be used with MDIs, acting as a reservoir to hold the medication until it is inhaled. These devices have a one-way valve that prevents the aerosol from escaping. Due to the spacer's reservoir function, coordination by the user is not necessary.

Dry powder inhalers contain small amounts of medications that have to be strongly inhaled if the powder is to get into the lungs. This method is difficult for children younger than 6 years.

Nebulizers are devices that convert medication into a fine mist. The medication is usually prescribed in a prefilled dosette, which is placed in a nebulizer connected to a small compressor that aerosolizes the medication. The medication is inhaled via mouthpiece or face mask. Nebulizers are the choice for the weak, elderly, small children, and infants because no coordination is needed for this type of delivery.

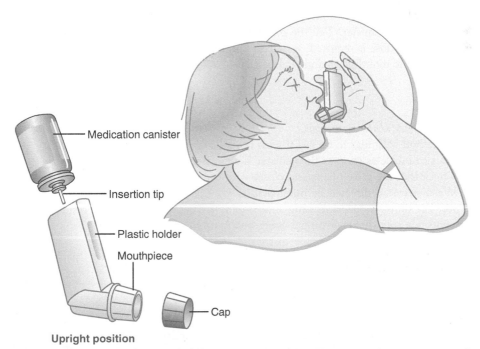

Medication canister

Insertion tip

Plastic holder

Mouthpiece

Cap

Upright position

Figure 5.2 Technique for using the aerosol inhaler. (From McCuistion LE, DiMaggio K, Winton MB, Yeager JJ [2018]. *Pharmacology: A patient-centered nursing process approach,* 9th ed., Philadelphia: Saunders.)

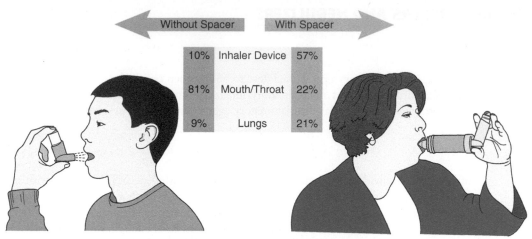

Figure 5.3 Distribution of medication with and without a spacer.

Method

Metered-Dose Inhaler
1. Insert the medication canister into the plastic holder. If the inhaler has not been used recently or if it is being used for the first time, test spray before administering the metered dose.
2. Shake the inhaler well before using. Remove the cap from the mouthpiece.
3. Instruct the patient to breathe out through the mouth, expelling air. Place the mouthpiece into the patient's mouth, holding the inhaler upright (Figure 5.2).
4. Instruct the patient to keep his or her lips securely around the mouthpiece and inhale. While the patient is inhaling, push the top of the medication canister once.
5. Instruct the patient to hold his or her breath for a few seconds. Remove the mouthpiece and take your finger off the canister. Tell the patient to exhale slowly.
6. If a second dose is required, wait 1 to 2 minutes, and repeat steps 3 to 5.
7. Cleanse the mouthpiece and replace cap.

Method

Metered-Dose Inhaler with Spacer
This method is similar to an MDI with the following additions; see Figure 5.3.
1. Start to inhale as soon as the canister is depressed.
2. Check that the valve opens and closes with each breath.
3. Wash spacer as directed by manufacturer.
Note: For steroid inhalers, rinsing and gargling are necessary to remove residual steroid medication, thus preventing a sore throat or fungal overgrowth and infection.

NASAL SPRAY AND DROPS

Purpose

Most drugs in nasal spray and drop containers are intended to relieve nasal congestion typically caused by upper respiratory tract infections by shrinking swollen nasal membranes. Types of drugs given by this method are vasoconstrictors and glucocorticoids.

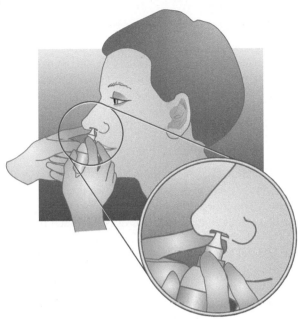

Figure 5.4 Administering nasal spray. (From McCuistion LE, DiMaggio K, Winton MB, Yeager JJ [2018]. *Pharmacology: A patient-centered nursing process approach,* 9th ed., Philadelphia: Saunders.)

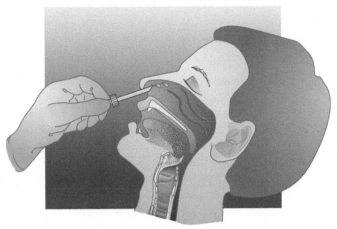

Figure 5.5 Administering nasal drops. (From McCuistion LE, DiMaggio K, Winton MB, Yeager JJ [2018]. *Pharmacology: A patient-centered nursing process approach,* 9th ed., Philadelphia: Saunders.)

Method

Nasal Spray
1. Instruct the patient to sit with his or her head tilted slightly back or slightly forward, according to the directions on the spray container.
2. Insert the tip of the container into one nostril and occlude the other nostril (Figure 5.4).
3. Instruct the patient to inhale as you squeeze the drug spray container. Repeat with the same nostril or other nostril if ordered.
4. Encourage the patient to keep his or her head tilted back for several minutes to promote absorption of the medication. The nose should not be blown until the head is upright.
5. Drink plenty of fluids after using a steroid nasal spray to avoid microbial overgrowth.

Method

Nasal Drops
1. Instruct the patient to sit with his or her head tilted back.
2. Insert the dropper into the nostril without touching the nasal membranes (Figure 5.5).
3. Instill the number of drops prescribed.
4. Instruct the patient to keep his or her head tilted back for 5 minutes and to breathe through the mouth.
5. Cleanse the dropper.
6. For the medication to reach the frontal and maxillary sinuses, the patient should slowly alternate turning his or her head from side to side while in the supine position. For the medication to reach the ethmoidal and sphenoidal sinuses, the patient will need to lean forward, bringing his or her head toward the knees.

EYE DROPS AND OINTMENT

Purpose

Eye medications are prescribed for various eye disorders, such as glaucoma, infection, and allergies, as well as eye examinations and eye surgery.

Method

Eye Drops
1. Instruct the patient to lie or sit with his or her head tilted back.
2. Instruct the patient to look up toward the ceiling and away from the dropper. Pull down the lower lid of the affected eye (Figure 5.6). Place the number of drops prescribed into the lower conjunctival sac. This prevents the drug from dropping onto the cornea. To prevent contamination DO NOT touch the end of the dropper on the eye or eyelashes.
3. Press gently on the medial nasolacrimal canthus (side closer to the nose) with a tissue to prevent systemic drug absorption.
4. If the other eye is affected, repeat the procedure in the other eye.
5. Instruct patient to blink once or twice and then to keep his or her eyes closed for several minutes. Use a tissue to blot away excess drainage from the eye.
6. When administering two or more different types of eye drops, wait 5 minutes between medications.

Method

Eye Ointment
1. Instruct the patient to lie or sit with his or her head tilted back.
2. Pull down the lower lid to expose the conjunctival sac of the affected eye (Figure 5.7).
3. Squeeze a strip of ointment about ¼-inch long (unless otherwise indicated) onto the conjunctival sac. Medication placed directly onto the cornea can cause discomfort or damage.
4. If the other eye is affected, repeat the procedure.
5. Instruct the patient to close his or her eyes for 2 to 3 minutes. Educate the patient to expect blurred vision for a short time after the application of the ointment.

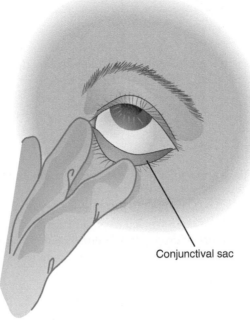

Conjunctival sac

Figure 5.6 To administer eye drops, gently pull down the skin below the eye to expose the conjunctival sac. (From McCuistion LE, DiMaggio K, Winton MB, Yeager JJ [2018]. *Pharmacology: A patient-centered nursing process approach,* 9th ed., Philadelphia: Saunders.)

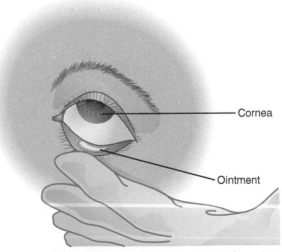

Cornea

Ointment

Figure 5.7 To administer eye ointment, squeeze a ¼-inch-long strip of ointment onto the conjunctival sac. (From McCuistion LE, DiMaggio K, Winton MB, Yeager JJ [2018]. *Pharmacology: A patient-centered nursing process approach,* 9th ed., Philadelphia: Saunders.)

EAR DROPS

Purpose

Ear medication is frequently prescribed to soften and loosen the cerumen (wax) in the ear canal, for anesthetic effect, to immobilize foreign objects (e.g., insects) in the ear canal, and to treat infections such as fungal infections.

Method

Ear Drops
1. Instruct the patient to lie on the unaffected side or to sit upright with his or her head tilted toward the unaffected side.
2. Straighten the external ear canal (Figure 5.8) as follows: *Adult:* Pull the auricle of the ear up and back. *Child:* Pull the auricle of the ear down and back until age 3.
3. Instill the prescribed number of drops. Avoid contaminating the dropper.
4. Instruct the patient to remain in this position for 2 to 5 minutes to prevent the medication from leaking out of the ear.

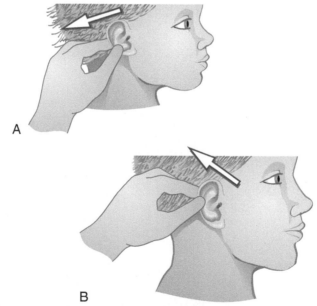

Figure 5.8 To administer ear drops, straighten the external ear canal by **(A)** pulling down and back on the auricle in children until age 3, and **(B)** pulling up and back on the auricle in adults. (From McCuistion LE, DiMaggio K, Winton MB, Yeager JJ [2018]. *Pharmacology: A patient-centered nursing process approach,* 9th ed., Philadelphia: Saunders.)

PHARYNGEAL SPRAY, MOUTHWASH, AND LOZENGE

Purpose

Sprays, mouthwashes, and lozenges can be prescribed to reduce throat irritation and for antiseptic and anesthetic effects. These methods are prescribed for a local effect on the throat and *not* for infections use.

Method

Pharyngeal Spray
1. Instruct the patient to sit upright.
2. Place a tongue blade over the patient's tongue to improve visualization of the mouth and to prevent the tongue from becoming numb if an anesthetic is being administered.
3. Hold the spray pump nozzle outside the patient's mouth, and direct the spray to the back of the throat.

Method

Pharyngeal Mouthwash
1. Instruct the patient to sit upright.
2. Instruct the patient to swish the solution around the mouth, but *not* to swallow the solution, and then to spit it into an emesis basin or sink.

Method

Pharyngeal Lozenge
1. Instruct the patient to sit upright.
2. Instruct the patient to place the lozenge into his or her mouth and suck until it is fully dissolved. The lozenge should *not* be chewed or swallowed whole.

TOPICAL PREPARATIONS: LOTION, CREAM, AND OINTMENT

Purpose

Topical lotions, creams, and ointments are used to protect skin areas, prevent skin dryness, treat itching of skin areas, and relieve pain.

Method

Topical Lotion
1. Cleanse skin area with soap and water. Allow time for the area to air-dry, or gently pat it dry.
2. Shake the lotion container. Rub the lotion thoroughly into the skin unless otherwise indicated.

Method A

Topical Cream or Ointment
1. Cleanse the skin area. Allow time for the area to air-dry, or gently pat it dry.
2. Use a sterile tongue blade or gauze to apply the cream or ointment to the affected skin area. Use long, smooth strokes. A piece of sterile gauze may be placed over the medicated area after the application to prevent the soiling of clothing.

Method B

Topical Cream or Ointment
1. Cleanse the skin area. Allow time for the area to air-dry, or gently pat it dry.
2. Squeeze a line of ointment from the tube onto your gloved finger from the tip to the first skin crease; this is known as a fingertip unit (FTU) (Figure 5.9).
   One FTU weighs about 0.5 g.
3. Use the guidelines shown in Figure 5.10 to determine the number of FTUs to apply to various body areas.
4. Apply the medication to the affected area.

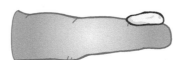

Figure 5.9 Fingertip unit: ointment squeezed from the tip of the finger to the first skin crease.

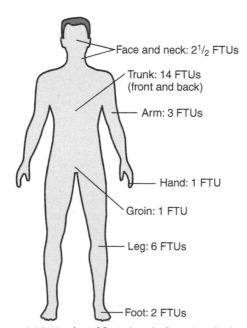

Figure 5.10 Number of fingertip units for various body areas.

RECTAL SUPPOSITORY

Purpose

Rectal medications are used to relieve vomiting when the client is unable to take oral medication, to relieve pain or anxiety, to promote defecation, and to administer drugs that could be destroyed by digestive enzymes.

Method

Rectal Suppository
1. Place the patient on his or her left side in the modified left lateral recumbent position.
2. Expose the anus by lifting the upper portion of the buttock. Check that the anus/rectum is not full of stool.
3. Lightly lubricate the suppository with water-soluble lubricant, and insert the narrow (pointed) end of the suppository into the anus, past the anal sphincter and into the rectum, approximately 3 inches or 7 to 8 centimeters (Figure 5.11).
4. Instruct the patient to remain in a supine or left lateral recumbent position for 5 to 10 minutes.

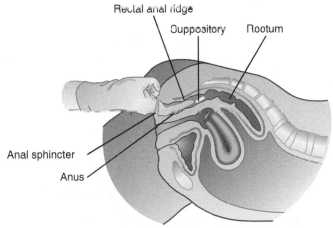

Figure 5.11 Inserting a rectal suppository. (From McCuistion LE, DiMaggio K, Winton MB, Yeager JJ [2018]. *Pharmacology: A patient-centered nursing process approach,* 9th ed., Philadelphia: Saunders.)

VAGINAL SUPPOSITORY, CREAM, AND OINTMENT

Purpose

Vaginal medications are used to treat vaginal infections or inflammation.

Method

Vaginal Suppository, Cream, and Ointment
1. Place patient into a lithotomy position (knees bent with feet on the table or bed).
2. Place the vaginal suppository at the tip of the applicator.
   or
   Connect the top of the vaginal cream or ointment tube with the tip of the applicator. Squeeze the tube to fill the applicator.
3. Lubricate the applicator with water-soluble lubricant if necessary.
4. Insert applicator downward first, then upward and backward 3 to 4 inches or 8 to 10 centimeters (Figure 5.12).
5. Instruct patient to remain lying down for at least 5 to 15 minutes after the application. The patient may use a light pad in her underwear to prevent the soiling of clothing. Bedtime is the suggested time for vaginal drug administration.
6. Instruct the patient to avoid using tampons after insertion of the vaginal medication.

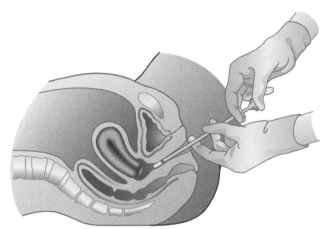

Figure 5.12 Inserting a vaginal suppository. (From McCuistion LE, DiMaggio K, Winton MB, Yeager JJ [2018]. *Pharmacology: A patient-centered nursing process approach,* 9th ed., Philadelphia: Saunders.)

INTRAOSSEOUS ACCESS

Purpose

Intraosseous (IO) access is used for patients in emergent, urgent, and medically necessary situations when intravenous access is difficult or unobtainable. In the clinical setting, IO access is commonly used in trauma, pediatric, and cardiac arrest patients to administer medications, fluid, and blood products. IO vascular access has been recognized as a reliable method of intravenous administration and incorporated into the resuscitation guidelines for both Advanced Cardiac Life Support (ACLS) and Pediatric Advanced Life Support (PALS).

IO access is established by placing an appropriately sized IO needle directly though the bone's cortex into the soft marrow interior of the medullary space. The IO needle can be inserted manually but, more commonly, the assistance of a spring-loaded device or a battery powered drill or driver is used to penetrate the patient's highly vascular medullary cavity. The IO route is able to provide immediate access into the patient's venous system for medication administration and blood draws. IO access sites have a greater resistance to flow when compared to IV lines, therefore a pressure bag may be needed when infusing IV fluids via gravity. Additionally, intravenous infusion pumps should be used to assist with administering IV fluids to pediatric patients.

The proximal and distal ends of long bones have been identified as the ideal location to establish IO access. IO needles/catheters are typically inserted in the proximal and distal tibia, proximal humerus, and sternum (Figure 5.13). The distal femur is a common insertion site in the pediatric patient population. When caring for a patient with IO access it's important to monitor the site for potential complications, such as extravasation, that could compromise the limb's circulation.

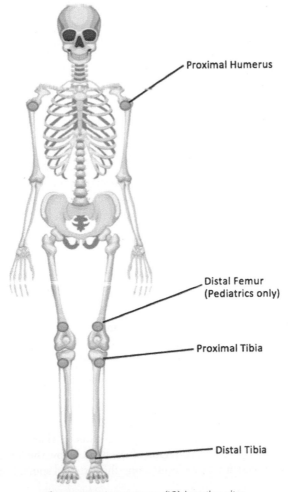

Figure 5.13 Intraosseous (IO) insertion sites.

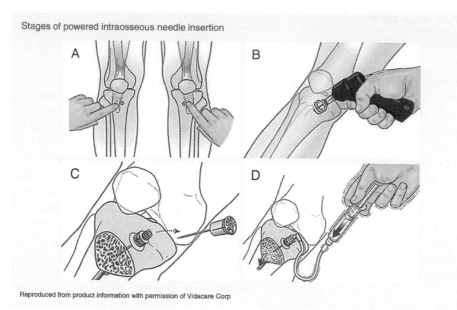

Stages of powered intraosseous needle insertion

A B C D

Reproduced from product information with permission of Vidacare Corp

Figure 5.14 Intraosseous vascular access placement. **A,** Insertion site identified and palpated. **B,** IO needle placed with battery powered drill device. **C,** Medullary space accessed and stylet removed. **D,** Tubing extension set attached to catheter hub and flushed with normal saline.

Figure 5.14 demonstrates IO placement in the proximal tibia using a battery powered IO drill. IO devices only provide temporary IV access with a dwell time of 24 to 48 hours, after which an alternative route of access should be obtained. To remove the IO device, attach an empty 6 or 10 mL luer lock syringe to the hub of the IO catheter at the skin. While maintaining a 90-degree angle to the site, use the syringe to remove the IO device by rotating it clockwise and gently pulling the catheter out. Specialty training is needed to correctly identify landmarks, safely insert and remove IO devices, and properly manage the IO access site.

Method

1. Monitor according to organizational policy, procedures, and practice guidelines.
2. Document response to therapy, i.e., vital signs improvement, urine output, site pain.
3. Maintain IO device placement, care, and maintenance.

INTRASPINAL ACCESS

Purpose

Intraspinal access devices are catheters and infusion pumps used for the delivery of narcotics, anesthetic agents, or antispasmodic medications to relieve pain or to control severe muscle spasms. The two access areas for intraspinal medication are the epidural space and the intrathecal space of the spine (Figure 5.15). Accessing these areas is accomplished through a sterile procedure and is performed by trained providers such as anesthesia providers. The anesthesia provider sterilely inserts a needle into the subarachnoid (intrathecal) space of the spine, where cerebrospinal fluid (CSF) is contained, between the pia mater and the arachnoid mater for intrathecal or spinal access. Local anesthetics and/or opioids are injected into this space as a single dose or continuously by a catheter that's threaded through the needle. Spinal access is only performed in the lumbar region of the back, below the termination of the spinal cord, unlike epidurals that can be placed at varying levels along the vertebral spine. For the epidural, a needle is sterilely placed between the dura mater and the ligamentum of flavum where a catheter is threaded into the space and secured. Once the catheter is secured, medication, typically local anesthetics and/or opioids, are administered through the catheter via infusion pumps known as epidural patient-controlled analgesia (EPCA) pumps. Epidurals are placed frequently for pain management in the labor and delivery setting, and both intrathecal and epidural procedures are used for surgical pain management.

Small implantable pumps can be surgically placed under the skin of the abdomen to deliver medication through an intrathecal catheter for chronic conditions (Figure 5.16). Medications such as baclofen, morphine, or ziconotide may be delivered in this manner to minimize the side effects often associated with the higher doses used in oral or intravenous delivery of these drugs. The goal of a drug pump is to better control symptoms and to reduce oral medications, thus reducing their associated side effects.

Method

1. Monitor according to the institution's policy, procedures, and practice guidelines.
2. Document responses to therapy (e.g., pain scale, sedation level, head or neck pain).
3. Maintain infusions according to physician orders and established policy and procedures.
4. Identify and label intraspinal access devices and administration sets to differentiate from other infusion administration systems.

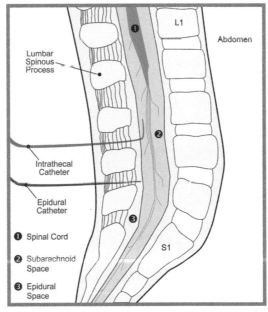

Figure 5.15 Intrathecal and epidural insertion sites.

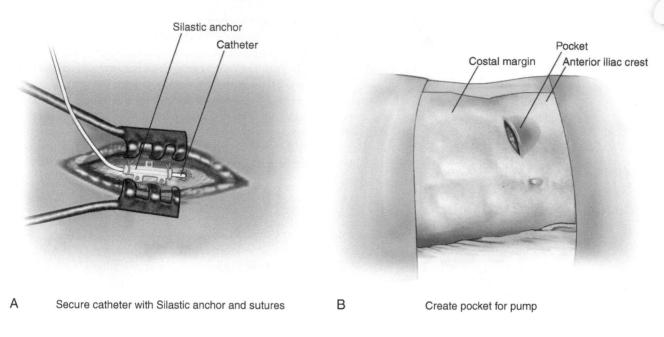

A — Secure catheter with Silastic anchor and sutures

B — Create pocket for pump

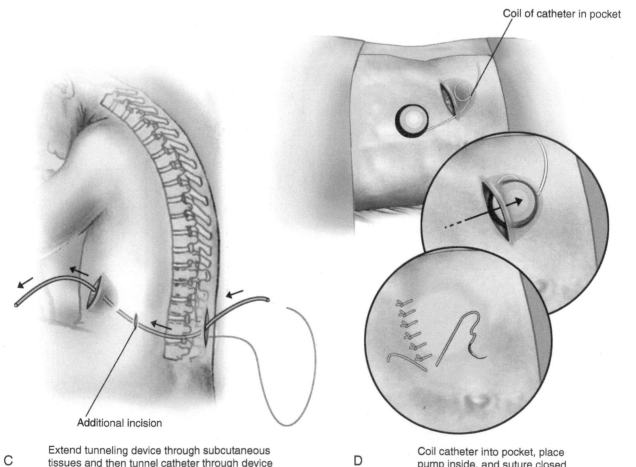

C — Extend tunneling device through subcutaneous tissues and then tunnel catheter through device

D — Coil catheter into pocket, place pump inside, and suture closed

Figure 5.16 Intrathecal pump implant. (From Brown, D. L. [2010]. *Atlas of regional anesthesia,* 4th ed. Philadelphia: Saunders.)

CHAPTER 6

Methods of Calculation

Objectives
- Determine the amount of drug needed for a specified time.
- Select a dosage formula, such as basic formula, ratio and proportion, fraction equation, or dimensional analysis, for solving drug dosage problems.
- Convert units of measurement to the same system and unit of measurement before calculating drug dosage.
- Calculate the dosage amount of tablets, capsules, and liquid volume (oral or parenteral) needed to administer the prescribed drug.

Outline **DRUG CALCULATION**

Before drug dosage can be calculated, units of measurement must be converted to one system. If the drug is ordered in grams and comes in milligrams, then grams are converted to milligrams or milligrams are converted to grams.

Four methods for calculating drug dosages include basic formula, ratio and proportion, fractional equation, and dimensional analysis. The ratio and proportion and fractional equation methods are similar. For drugs that require individualized dosing, body weight and body surface area are used. When body weight and body surface area calculations are used, one of the first four methods for calculation is necessary to determine the amount of drug needed from the container.

At some institutions, the nurse orders enough medication doses for a designated period. If the order requires 2 tablets, qid (4 times a day) for 5 days, then the number of tablets needed would be 2 tablets × 4 times a day × 5 days = 40 tablets.

DRUG CALCULATION

The four methods as mentioned for drug calculations are (1) basic formula, (2) ratio and proportion, (3) fractional equation, and (4) dimensional analysis (factor labeling).

Basic Formula

The following formula is often used to calculate drug dosages. The basic formula (BF) is the most commonly used method, and it is easy to remember.

$$\frac{D}{H} \times V = \text{Amount to give}$$

D or desired dose: drug dose ordered by physician or health care providers (HCPs)
H or on-hand dose: drug dose on label of container (bottle, vial, ampule)
V or vehicle: form and amount in which the drug comes (tablet, capsule, liquid)

EXAMPLES **PROBLEM 1:** Order: erythromycin (ERY-TAB) 0.5 g, po, q8h.
Drug available:

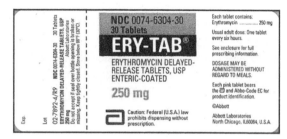

a. Both the dosage of the drug ordered and the dosage on the bottle are in the metric system; however, the units of measurement are different. Conversion is needed. To convert grams to milligrams, move the decimal point three spaces to the right (see Chapter 1: Systems Used for Drug Administration and Temperature Conversion):

$$0.5 \text{ g} = 0.500 \text{ mg} = 500 \text{ mg}$$

b. BF: $\dfrac{D}{H} \times V = \dfrac{\overset{2}{\cancel{500}} \text{ mg}}{\underset{1}{\cancel{250}} \text{ mg}} \times 1 \text{ tab} = 2 \text{ tablets}$

Answer: erythromycin 0.5 g = 2 tablets

PROBLEM 2: Order: loracarbef (Lorabid) 0.5 g, po, q12h for 7 days.
Drug available:

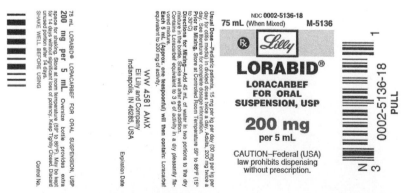

a. The unit of measurement ordered and the unit given on the bottle are in the same system but in different units; therefore conversion of units within the same system must be done first. To convert grams to milligrams, move the decimal point three spaces to the right (see Chapter 1).

$$0.5 \text{ g} = 0.500 \text{ mg} = 500 \text{ mg}$$

b. $\dfrac{D}{H} \times V = \dfrac{\overset{5}{\cancel{500}}}{\underset{2}{\cancel{200}}} \times 5 \text{ mL} = \dfrac{5}{2} \times 5 = \dfrac{25}{2} = 12.5 \text{ mL}$

Answer: Lorabid 0.5 g per dose = 12.5 mL

PROBLEM 3: Order: phenobarbital 120 mg, STAT.
Drug available: phenobarbital 30 mg per tablet.
a. Conversion of unit of measurement is NOT needed because both are of the same unit, milligrams.

b. BF: $\dfrac{D}{H} \times V = \dfrac{120}{30} \times 1 = \dfrac{120}{30} = 4 \text{ tablets}$

Answer: phenobarbital 120 mg = 4 tablets

PROBLEM 4: Order: meperidine (demerol) 35 mg, IM, STAT.
Drug Available:

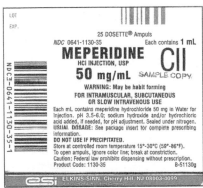

a. Conversion is not needed, because both are of the same unit of measurement.

b. BF: $\dfrac{D}{H} \times V = \dfrac{35}{50} \times 1 \text{ mL} = \dfrac{35}{50} = 0.7 \text{ mL}$

Answer: meperidine (Demerol) 35 mg = 0.7 mL

Ratio and Proportion

Ratio and proportion (RP) is the oldest method used for calculating dosage problems:

	Known			*Desired*	
H	:	V	::	D	:	X

on hand vehicle desired dose amount to give

means
extremes

H and **V**: On the left side of the equation are the known quantities, which are dose on hand and vehicle.
D and **X**: On the right side of the equation are the desired dose and the unknown amount to give.
Multiply the means and the extremes. Solve for **X**.

EXAMPLES   **PROBLEM 1:** Order: erythromycin (ERY-TAB) 0.5 g, po, q8h
Drug available:

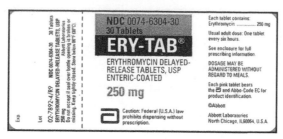

a. To convert grams to milligrams, move the decimal point three spaces to the right (see Chapter 1):

$$0.5 \text{ g} = 0.500 \text{ mg} = 500 \text{ mg}$$

b. RP: H : V :: D : X

250 mg : 1 tab :: 500 mg : X tab

$$250 \text{ X} = 500$$
$$\text{X} = 2 \text{ tablets}$$

Answer: erythromycin 0.5 g = 2 tablets

Note: With RP, the ratio on the left (milligrams to tablets) has the same relation as the ratio on the right (milligrams to tablets); the only difference is values.

PROBLEM 2: Order: aspirin (ASA) 650 mg, PRN.
Drug available: aspirin 325 mg per tablet.

RP :   H : V :: D : X

325 mg : 1 tablet :: 650 mg : X tablet

$$325 \text{ X} = 650$$
$$\text{X} = 2 \text{ tablets}$$

Answer: aspirin 650 mg = 2 tablets

PROBLEM 3: Order: amoxicillin 75 mg, po, qid.
Drug available:

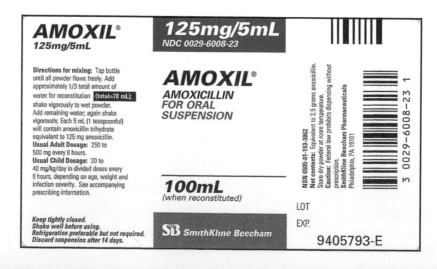

a. Conversion is not needed because both use the same unit of measurement.

b. RP :   H   :   V   ::   D   :   X

125 mg : 5 mL :: 75 mg : X mL

125 X = 375

X = 3 mL

Answer: amoxicillin 75 mg = 3 mL

PROBLEM 4: Order: meperidine (Demerol) 60 mg, IM, STAT.

Drug available:

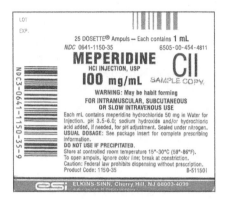

a. Conversion is not needed; the same unit of measurement is used.

b. RP :   H   :   V   ::   D   :   X

100 mg : 1 mL :: 60 mg : X mL

100 X = 60

X = 0.6 mL

Answer: meperidine (Demerol) 60 mg = 0.6 mL

Fractional Equation

The fractional equation (FE) method *is similar* to RP, except it is written as a fraction.

$$\frac{H}{V} = \frac{D}{X}$$

H: the dosage on hand or in the container
V: the vehicle or the form in which the drug comes (tablet, capsule, liquid)
D: the desired dosage
X: the unknown amount to give
Cross multiply and solve for X.

EXAMPLES   **PROBLEM 1:** Order: erythromycin (ERY-TAB) 750 mg, po, q8h.

Drug available:

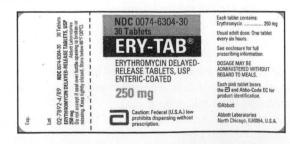

a. How many tablet(s) should the patient receive per dose? _____

FE: $\dfrac{H}{V} = \dfrac{D}{X}$ $\dfrac{250\ \text{mg}}{1\ \text{tab}} = \dfrac{750\ \text{mg}}{X} =$

(Cross multiply) $250\ X = 750$

$X = 3$ tablets per dose

b. How many tablet(s) should the patient receive per day? _____

3 tablets per dose $\times$ 3 times per day $= 9$ tablets per day

Answer: erythromycin: 9 tablets per day

PROBLEM 2: Order: valproic acid (Depakene) 100 mg, po, tid.
Drug available: valproic acid (Depakene) 250 mg/5 mL suspension.
a. No unit conversion is needed.

b. FE: $\dfrac{H}{V} = \dfrac{D}{X}$ $\dfrac{250}{5} = \dfrac{100}{X}$

(Cross multiply) $250\ X = 500$

$X = 2\ \text{mL}$

Answer: valproic acid (Depakene) 100 mg $= 2$ mL

PROBLEM 3: Order: atropine 0.6 mg, IM, STAT.
Drug available:

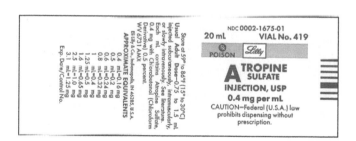

FE: $\dfrac{H}{V} = \dfrac{D}{X}$ $\dfrac{0.4\ \text{mg}}{1\ \text{mL}} = \dfrac{0.6\ \text{mg}}{X}$

(Cross multiply) $0.4\ X = 0.6$

$X = 1.5\ \text{mL}$

Answer: atropine 0.6 mg $= 1.5$ mL

Dimensional Analysis

Dimensional analysis (DA) is a calculation method known as units and conversions. The advantage of DA is that it decreases the number of steps required to calculate a drug dosage. It is set up as one long equation to answer a desired unit (e.g., mL, tab, or cap).

1. Identify the unit/form (tablet, capsule, mL) of the drug to be calculated. If the drug comes in tablet (unit), then tablet = (equal sign).

2. The known dose and unit/form from the drug label follow the equal sign.
Example order: Amoxicillin 500 mg. On the drug label: 250 mg per 1 capsule.

$$\text{capsule} = \frac{1\ \text{cap}}{250\ \text{mg}}\ (\text{unit})$$
$$(\text{drug label})$$

3. The milligram value (250 mg) is the **denominator** and it must match the NEXT **numerator,** which is 500 mg (desired dose or order). The NEXT denominator would be 1 (one) or blank.

$$\text{capsule} = \frac{1\ \text{cap} \times \overset{2}{\cancel{500\ \text{mg}}}}{\underset{1}{\cancel{250\ \text{mg}}} \times 1} =$$

4. Cancel out the mg, and reduce the 250 and 500. What remains is the capsule and 2. Answer: 2 capsules. When conversion is needed between milligrams (drug label) and grams (order), then a conversion factor is needed, which appears between the drug dose on hand (drug label) and the desired dose (order). You should REMEMBER the following:

Metric Equivalent
1 g = 1000 mg
1 mg = 1000 mcg

Also use Table 6.1 for metric and household conversions.

EXAMPLE Order: Amoxicillin 0.5 g.
Available: 250 mg = 1 capsule (drug label). A conversion is needed between grams and milligrams. Remember, 250 mg is the denominator; therefore 1000 mg (conversion factor, which is 1000 mg = 1 g) is the NEXT numerator and 1 g becomes the NEXT denominator. The third numerator is 0.5 g (desired dose), and the denominator is 1 (one) or blank.

$$\text{capsule} = \frac{1\ \text{cap} \quad \times \quad \overset{4}{\cancel{1000\ \text{mg}}} \times 0.5\ \cancel{g}}{\underset{1}{\cancel{250\ \text{mg}}} \times \quad 1\ \cancel{g} \quad \times \quad 1\ (\text{or blank})} = 2\ \text{capsules}$$
$$(\text{drug label}) \quad (\text{conversion}) \quad (\text{drug order})$$

If conversion from grams to milligrams is not needed, then the middle step can be omitted. The following are formulas for DA:

$$V\ (\text{form of drug}) = \frac{V\ (\text{drug form}) \times D\ (\text{desired dose})}{H\ (\text{on hand})(\text{drug label}) \times 1\ \text{or blank}\ (\text{drug order})}$$

For conversion: V (form of drug) =

$$\frac{V\ (\text{drug form}) \quad \times \quad C(H) \quad \times \quad D\ (\text{desired dose})}{H\ (\text{on hand}) \quad \times \quad C(D) \quad \times \quad 1\ (\text{or blank})}$$
$$\begin{array}{ccc} (\text{drug label}) & (\text{conversion} & (\text{drug order}) \\ & \text{factor}) & \end{array}$$

As with other methods for calculation, the three components are **D, H,** and **V.** With DA, the conversion factor is built into the equation and is included when the units of measurement of the drug order and the drug container differ. If the two are of the same units of measurement, the conversion factor is eliminated from the equation.

TABLE 6.1 Metric and Household Conversions

METRIC	
Grams (g)	Milligrams (mg)
1	1000
0.5	500
0.3	300 (325)
0.1	100
0.06	60 (64 or 65)
0.03	30 (32)
0.015	15 (16)
0.010	10
0.0006	0.6
0.0004	0.4
0.0003	0.3

Liquid (Approximate)
2230 mL = 1 oz = 2 tbsp (T) = 6 tsp (t)
15 mL = ½ oz = 1 T = 3 t
1000 mL = 1 quart (qt) = 1 liter (L)
500 mL = 1 pint (pt)
5 mL = 1 tsp (t)

EXAMPLES **PROBLEM 1:** Order: erythromycin (ERY-TAB) 1 g, po, q12h.
Drug available:

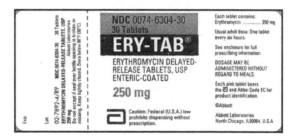

Drug label: 250 mg = 1 tablet
Drug order: 1 g
Conversion factor: 1 g = 1000 mg
a. How many tablets should the patient receive per dose?_____

$$\mathbf{DA:}\ tab = \frac{1\ tablet}{250\ mg} \times \frac{\overset{4}{1000\ mg}}{1\ g} \times \frac{1\ g}{1} = 4\ tablets$$

(drug label)   (conversion factor)   (drug order)

(cancel units and numbers from numerator and denominator)

Answer: erythromycin 1 g = 4 tablets
Give 4 tablets every 12 hours.

PROBLEM 2: Order: acetaminophen (Tylenol) 1 g, po, PRN.
Drug available:

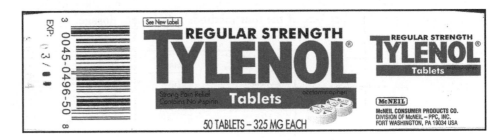

Drug label: 325 mg = 1 tablet
Conversion factor: 1000 mg = 1 g
How many tablet(s) would you give?

$$\textbf{DA: } \text{tab} = \frac{1 \text{ tab} \times 1000 \text{ mg} \times 1 \text{ g}}{325 \text{ mg} \times 1 \text{ g} \times 1} = \frac{1000}{325} = 3.07 \text{ tab or 3 tab (cannot round}$$
off in tenths for tablets)

Answer: acetaminophen 1 g = 3 tablets
Tylenol is also available in 500-mg (extra-strength) tablets.

PROBLEM 3: Order: ciprofloxacin (Cipro) 500 mg, po, q12h.
Drug available:

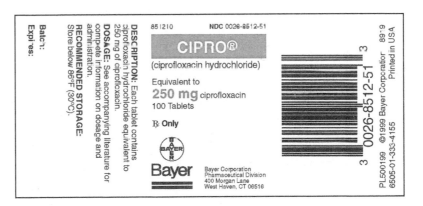

No conversion factor is needed because both are stated in milligrams (mg).

$$\textbf{DA: } \text{tab} = \frac{1 \text{ tab} \times \overset{2}{500} \text{ mg}}{\underset{1}{250} \text{ mg} \times 1} = 2 \text{ tablets}$$

Answer: Cipro 500 mg = 2 tablets

SUMMARY PRACTICE PROBLEMS

Answers can be found on pages 97 to 99.

Solve the following calculation problems. To convert units within the metric system (grams to milligrams), refer to Chapter 1. To convert apothecary to metric units and vice versa, refer to Chapter 2, Table 2.1. For reading drug labels, refer to Chapter 3. Several of the calculation problems have drug labels. Drug dosage and drug form are printed on the drug label.

Extra practice problems are available in the chapters on oral drugs, injectable drugs, and pediatric drug administration.

1. Order: doxycycline hyclate (Vibra-Tabs), po, initially 200 mg; then 50 mg, po, bid.
   Drug available: **Use one of the four methods to calculate dosage.**

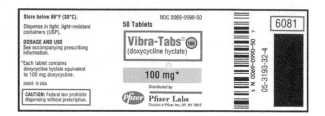

   a. How many tablet(s) would you give as the initial dose?_____

   b. How many tablets would you give for *each* dose after the initial dose? _____

2. Order: sulfisoxazole (Gantrisin) 1 g.
   Drug available: sulfisoxazole (Gantrisin) 250 mg per tablet.

   How many tablet(s) would you give? _____

3. Order: erythromycin 500 mg, po, q8h, for 7 days.
   Drug available:

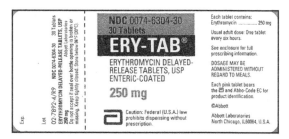

   a. How many tablets would you give every 8 hours? _____

   b. How many tablets would you order for 7 days? _____

4. Order: clarithromycin (Biaxin) 100 mg, po, q6h.
   Drug available:

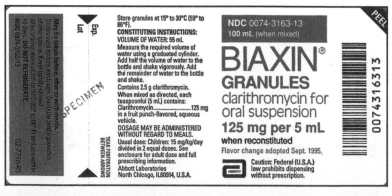

How many milliliters should the patient receive per dose? _____

5. Order: phenytoin (Dilantin) 50 mg, po, bid.
   Drug available:

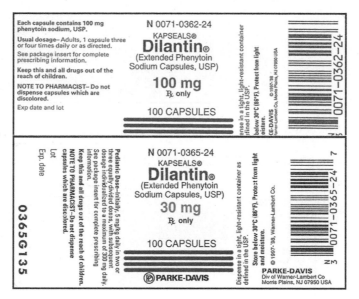

   a. Which Dilantin container would you select? _____

   b. How many Dilantin capsules would you give per dose? _____

6. Order: indomethacin (Indocin) 30 mg, po, tid.
   Drug available:

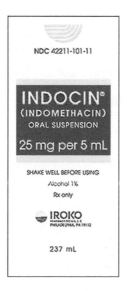

   a. How many milliliters would you give per dose? _____

   b. How many milligrams would the patient receive per day? _____

7. Order: dexamethasone (Decadron) 0.5 mg, po, qid.
   Drug available:

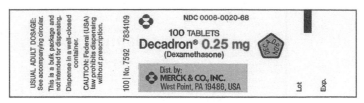

How many tablets would you give per dose? _____

8. Order: diltiazem (Cardizem) SR 120 mg, po, bid for hypertension.
   Drug available:

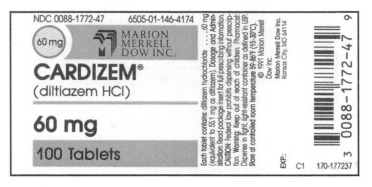

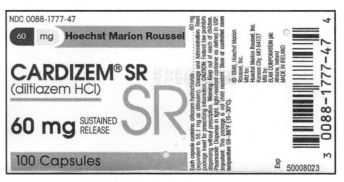

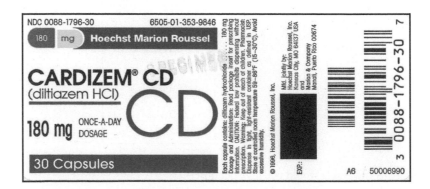

   a. Which drug bottle should be selected? _____
   b. How many tablet(s) should the patient receive per dose? _____

9. Order: cimetidine (Tagamet) 0.2 g, po, qid.
   Drug available:

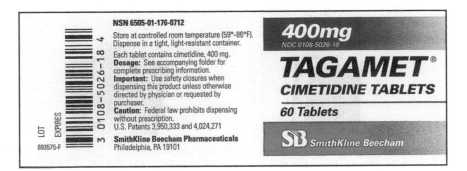

   How many tablet(s) would you give per dose? _____

10. Order: bisoprolol (Zebeta) 5 mg, po, daily for the first week. Increase Zebeta to 15 mg, po, daily starting with the second week.
    Drug available:

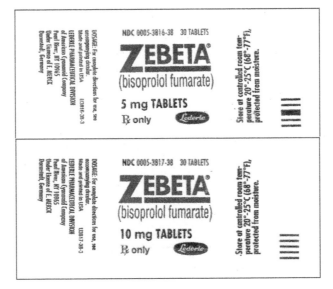

   a. Which drug bottle(s) would you select the first week and how many tablet(s) would you give?

   _____

   b. The dose is increased to 15 mg the second week. Explain which drug bottle(s) you would select
      and how many tablets you would give? _____

11. Order: fluoxetine (Prozac) 25 mg, po, in the AM.
    Drug available:

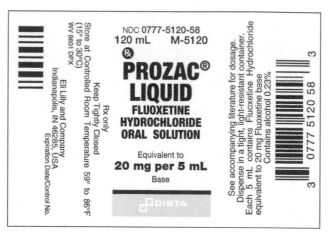

How many milliliters (mL) should the patient receive in the AM? _____

12. Order: methylprednisolone (Medrol) 75 mg, IM.
    Drug available: Medrol 125 mg per 2 mL per ampule.

How many milliliters would you give? _____

13. Order: atropine sulfate 0.3 mg, IM, STAT.
    Drug available:

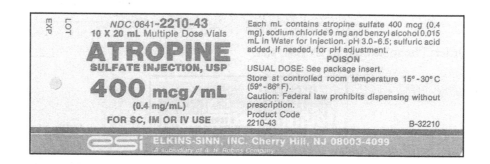

How many milliliters should the patient receive? _____

14. Order: Cefobid (cefoperazone NA) 1 g, IM, q12h.
    Drug available:

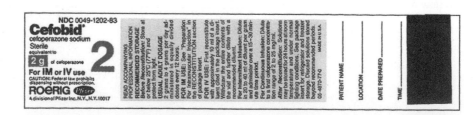

According to the drug administration instructions, 3.4 mL of sterile water should be added to drug to yield 4 mL of drug solution. How many milliliters (mL) would you administer per dose? _____

Additional Dimensional Analysis (Factor Labeling)

15. Order: aminocaproic acid 1.5 g, po, STAT.
Drug available: aminocaproic acid 500-mg tablet.
Drug label: 500 mg = tablet
Conversion factor: 1 g = 1000 mg

How many tablet(s) would you give? _____

16. Order: ampicillin (Principen) 50 mg/kg/day, po, in 4 divided doses (q6h).
Patient weighs 88 pounds, or 40 kg (88 ÷ 2.2 = 40 kg).
Drug available:

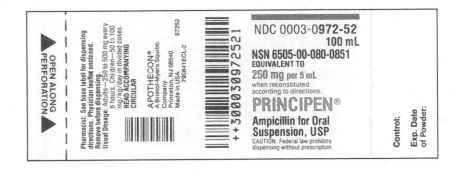

Drug label: 250 mg = 5 mL
Conversion factor: none (both are in milligrams)

a. How many milligrams per day should the patient receive? _____

b. How many milligrams per dose should the patient receive? _____

c. How many milliliters should the patient receive per dose (q6h)? _____

17. Order: cimetidine (Tagamet) 0.8 g, po, bedtime.
Drug available:

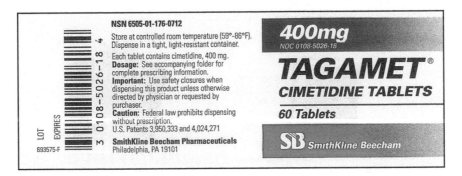

Drug label: 400 mg = 1 tablet
        0.8 g (drug order)
Conversion factor: 1 g = 1000 mg (units of measurements are not the same; conversion factor is needed)

How many tablet(s) would you give? _____

18. Order: Xanax (alprazolam) 0.125 mg, po, tid.
    Drug available:

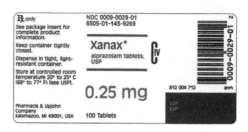

Xanax tablet is scored.

a. How many tablet(s) should the patient receive per dose? _____

b. How many tablet(s) should the patient receive per day? _____

19. Order: codeine 60 mg, po, STAT.
    Drug available:

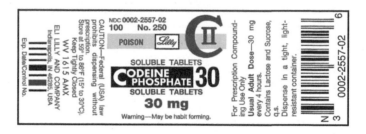

Drug label: 30 mg = 1 tablet
See Table 2.1 if needed.

How many tablet(s) would you give? _____

20. Order: Lasix (furosemide) 15 mg, IM, STAT.
    Drug available:

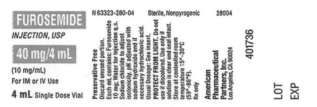

How many milliliters (mL) would you give? _____

ANSWERS   SUMMARY PRACTICE PROBLEMS

1. a. *Initially:*

$$\text{BF: } \frac{D}{H} \times V = \frac{200}{100} \times 1 =$$

$$2 \text{ tablets}$$

or

$$\text{FE} = \frac{100}{1} = \frac{200}{X}$$

$$100 \, X = 200$$
$$X = 2 \text{ tablets}$$

b. *Daily:*

$$\text{BF: } \frac{D}{H} \times V = \frac{50}{100} \times 1 = \frac{1}{2} \text{ tablet}$$

or

$$\text{FE} = \frac{100}{1} = \frac{50}{X} =$$

(Cross multiply) $100 \, X = 50$
$$X = \frac{1}{2} \text{ tablet}$$

or

RP: H :V∷ D :X
100 mg : 1 ∷ 200 mg : X

$$100 \, X = 200$$
$$X = 2 \text{ tablets}$$

or

DA: No conversion factor

$$\text{Tablet(s)} = \frac{1 \text{ tab} \times \overset{2}{\cancel{200}} \text{ mg}}{\underset{1}{\cancel{100}} \text{ mg} \times 1} = 2 \text{ tablets}$$

or

RP: H :V∷ D :X
100 mg : 1 ∷ 50 mg : X

$$100 \, X = 50$$
$$X = \frac{1}{2} \text{ tablet}$$

or

DA: No conversion factor

$$\text{Tablet(s)} = \frac{1 \text{ tab} \times \overset{1}{\cancel{50}} \text{ mg}}{\underset{2}{\cancel{100}} \text{ mg} \times 1} = \frac{1}{2} \text{ tablet}$$

2. 4 tablets

3. a. 2 tablets every 8 hours

b. 2 tablets × 3 doses per day × 7 days = 42 tablets per week

4. $\text{BF: } \dfrac{D}{H} \times V = \dfrac{100}{\underset{25}{\cancel{125}}} \times \overset{1}{\cancel{5}} = \dfrac{100}{25} = 4 \text{ mL}$

or

$$\text{DA: } \text{mL} = \frac{5 \text{ mL} \times \overset{4}{\cancel{100}} \text{ mg}}{\underset{5}{\cancel{125}} \text{ mg} \times 1} = \frac{20}{5} = 4 \text{ mL}$$

or

RP: H :V∷ D :X
125 : 5 ∷ 100 : X
125 X = 500
$$X = \frac{500}{125} = 4 \text{ mL}$$

or

$$\text{FE: } \frac{125}{5} = \frac{100}{X} =$$
(Cross multiply) 125 X = 500
$$X = 4 \text{ mL}$$

5. a. The nurse could *not* use either of the Dilantins.

b. A capsule *cannot* be cut in half. The physician should be notified. Dilantin dose should be changed.

6. a. $\text{BF: } \dfrac{D}{H} \times V = \dfrac{30 \text{ mg}}{25 \text{ mg}} \times 5 \text{ mL} = 6 \text{ mL}$

RP: H : V ∷ D :X
25 mg : 5 mL = 30 mg : X
25 X = 150
$$X = 6 \text{ mL}$$

$$\text{FE: } \frac{H}{V} = \frac{D}{X} = \frac{25 \text{ mg}}{5 \text{ mL}} = \frac{30 \text{ mg}}{X}$$

$$\text{DA: } \text{mL} = \frac{\overset{1}{\cancel{5}} \text{ mL} \times 30 \text{ mg}}{\underset{5}{\cancel{25}} \text{ mg} \times 1} = \frac{30}{5} = 6 \text{ mL}$$

$$25 \, X = 150$$
$$X = 6 \text{ mL}$$

b. 30 mg × 3 = 90 mg per day

7. **BF:** $\dfrac{D}{H} \times V = \dfrac{0.5}{0.25} \times 1$

or

RP: H : V :: D : X

0.25 : 1 tablet :: 0.5 : X tablets

$0.25 \overline{)0.50}^{\;2.} = 2$ tablets per dose

0.25 X = 0.5

X = 2 tablets per dose

8. **a.** Select Cardizem SR 60 mg
   b. 2 tablets per dose of Cardizem SR
9. Change grams to milligrams by moving the decimal three spaces to the right (see Chapter 1).

   0.2 g = 0.200 mg = 200 mg

   BF: $\dfrac{D}{H} \times V = \dfrac{200}{400} \times 1$ tablet

   $= \dfrac{200}{400} = $ ½ tablet

   or

   RP: H : V :: D : X

   400 mg : 1 tablet :: 200 mg : X tablet

   400 X = 200

   $X = \dfrac{200}{400} = 0.5$ or ½ tablet

   or

   DA: With conversion factor

   $$\text{Tablets} = \frac{1 \text{ tab} \times \overset{10}{\cancel{1000}} \text{ mg} \times 0.2 \cancel{g}}{\underset{4}{\cancel{400}} \text{ mg} \times 1 \cancel{g} \times 1} = \frac{2.0}{4} = \text{½ tablet}$$

10. **a.** Select Zebeta 5-mg bottle.

   BF: $\dfrac{D}{H} \times V = \dfrac{5 \text{ mg}}{5 \text{ mg}} \times 1 = 1$ tablet of Zebeta 5-mg bottle

   RP: H : V :: D : X

   5 : 1 :: 5 : X

   5 X = 5

   X = 1 tablet of Zebeta

   b. Select either Zebeta 5-mg bottle OR Zebeta 5-mg and Zebeta 10-mg bottles
   FE using Zebeta 5-mg bottle:

   $$\frac{H}{V} = \frac{D}{X} = \frac{5 \text{ mg}}{1} = \frac{15 \text{ mg}}{X}$$

   (Cross multiply) 5 X = 15

   X = 3 tablets of Zebeta

   If only the Zebeta 10-mg bottle was available, then give 1½ tablets.

11. **BF:** $\dfrac{D}{H} \times V = \dfrac{\overset{5}{\cancel{25}} \text{ mg}}{\underset{4}{\cancel{20}} \text{ mg}} \times 5 \text{ mL} = \dfrac{25}{4} = 6.25$ or 6.3 mL of Prozac

   FE: $\dfrac{H}{V} = \dfrac{D}{X} = \dfrac{20 \text{ mg}}{5 \text{ mL}} = \dfrac{25 \text{ mg}}{X}$

   (Cross multiply) 20 X = 125

   X = 6.25 OR 6.3 mL of Prozac

12. BF: $\dfrac{D}{H} \times V = \dfrac{75}{125} \times 2$

$\dfrac{150}{125} = 1.2 \text{ mL}$

or

FE: $\dfrac{125}{2} = \dfrac{75}{X}$

$125\,X = 150$

$X = 1.2 \text{ mL}$

13. BF: $\dfrac{D}{H} \times V = \dfrac{0.3 \text{ mg}}{0.4 \text{ mg}} \times 1 \text{ mL} =$

0.75 mL

or

FE: $\dfrac{0.4 \text{ mg}}{1} = \dfrac{0.3 \text{ mg}}{X} =$

$0.4 \text{ mg } X = 0.3 \text{ mg}$

$X = 0.75 \text{ mL}$

14. RP: H : V :: D : X

$2 \text{ g} : 4 \text{ mL} :: 1 \text{ g} : X$

$2\,X = 4$

$X = 2 \text{ mL of Cefobid per dose}$

or

RP: H : V :: D : X

$125 : 2 :: 75 : X$

$125\,X = 150$

$X = 1.2 \text{ mL}$

or

DA: No conversion factor needed

$mL = \dfrac{2 \text{ mL} \times \overset{3}{\cancel{75}} \text{ mg}}{\underset{5}{\cancel{125}} \text{ mg} \times 1} = \dfrac{6}{5} = 1.2 \text{ mL}$

or

RP: H : V :: D : X

$0.4 \text{ mg} : 1 \text{ mL} :: 0.3 \text{ mg} : X$

$0.4 \text{ mg } X = 0.3 \text{ mg}$

$X = 0.75 \text{ mL}$

or

DA: $mL = \dfrac{1 \text{ mL} \times 0.3 \cancel{\text{ mg}}}{0.4 \cancel{\text{ mg}} \times 1} = \dfrac{0.3}{0.4} = 0.75 \text{ mL}$

Additional Dimensional Analysis (Factor Labeling)

15. DA: $\text{Tablets} = \dfrac{1 \text{ tablet} \times \overset{2}{\cancel{1000}} \text{ mg} \times 1.5 \cancel{\text{ g}}}{\underset{1}{\cancel{500}} \text{ mg} \times 1 \cancel{\text{ g}} \times 1} = \dfrac{3.0}{1} = 3 \text{ tablets}$

16. **a.** 50 mg/kg/day

$50 \times 40 = 2000 \text{ mg}$

b. $2000 \text{ mg} \div 4 = 500 \text{ mg per dose}$

c. DA: $mL = \dfrac{5 \text{ mL} \times \overset{2}{\cancel{500}} \text{ mg}}{\underset{1}{\cancel{250}} \text{ mg} \times 1} = \dfrac{10}{1} = 10 \text{ mL}$

17. DA: $\text{Tablets} = \dfrac{1 \text{ tablet} \times \overset{10}{\cancel{1000}} \text{ mg} \times 0.8 \cancel{\text{ g}}}{\underset{4}{\cancel{400}} \text{ mg} \times 1 \cancel{\text{ g}} \times 1} = \dfrac{10 \times 0.8}{4} = \dfrac{8}{4} = 2 \text{ tablets}$

18. **a.** DA: $tab = \dfrac{1 \text{ tab} \times 0.125 \text{ mg}}{0.25 \text{ mg} \times 1} = \dfrac{0.125}{0.25} = \text{½ tablet of Xanax}$

b. ½ tablet $\times$ 3 (tid) = 1½ tablets per day

19. DA: $\text{Tablets} = \dfrac{1 \text{ tablet} \times \overset{2}{\cancel{60}} \text{ mg}}{\underset{1}{\cancel{30}} \text{ mg} \times 1 \cancel{\text{ gr}}} = 2 \text{ tablets}$

20. DA: $mL = \dfrac{1 \text{ mL} \times \overset{3}{\cancel{15}} \text{ mg}}{\underset{2}{\cancel{10}} \text{ mg} \times 1} = \dfrac{3}{2} = 1.5 \text{ mL of furosemide (Lasix)}$

CHAPTER 7

Methods of Calculation for Individualized Drug Dosing

Objectives
- State the differences between the weight formulas used for drug calculations.
- Calculate drug dosages according to body surface area.
- Calculate drug dosages according to body weight.
- List indications for use of ideal body weight, adjusted body weight, and lean body weight formulas.

Outline CALCULATION FOR INDIVIDUALIZED DRUG DOSING

CALCULATION FOR INDIVIDUALIZED DRUG DOSING

The two methods for individualizing drug dosing are body weight (BW) and body surface area (BSA). Other formulas that are associated with drug dosing, especially in bariatrics, are ideal body weight (IBW) and lean body weight (LBW).

Body Weight (BW)

Drug dosing by actual BW is the primary way medication is individualized for adults and children. Manufacturers supply dosing information in the package insert. The insert data provide the dosage based on the patient's weight in kilograms (kg). The first step is to convert pounds to kilograms (if necessary). The second step is to determine the drug dose per BW by multiplying drug dose × body weight (BW) × frequency (day or per day in divided doses). The third step is to choose one of the four methods of drug calculation for the amount of drug to be given.

EXAMPLES **PROBLEM 1:** Order: fluorouracil (5-FU), 12 mg/kg/day IV, not to exceed 800 mg/day. The adult weighs 140 pounds.

    a. Convert pounds to kilograms. Divide number of pounds by 2.2.
        Remember: 1 kg = 2.2 lbs

        140 lbs ÷ 2.2 lbs/kg = 64 kg

b. Dosage/BW: mg × kg × 1 day =

$$12 × 64 × 1 \quad = 768 \text{ mg IV per day}$$

Answer: fluorouracil (5-FU), 12 mg/kg/day = 768 mg or 770 mg

PROBLEM 2: Order: cefaclor (Ceclor), 20 mg/kg/day in three divided doses. The child weighs 20 pounds. Drug available:

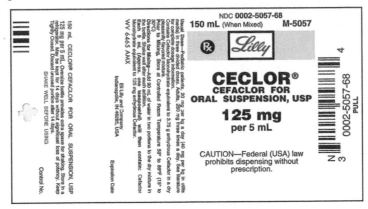

a. Convert pounds to kilograms.

$$20 \text{ lbs} ÷ 2.2 \text{ lbs/kg} = 9 \text{ kg}$$

b. Dosage/BW: 20 mg × 9 kg × 1 day = 180 mg per day

$$180 \text{ mg} ÷ 3 \text{ divided doses} = 60 \text{ mg}$$

BF: $\dfrac{D}{H} × V = \dfrac{60 \text{ mg}}{125 \text{ mg}} × 5 \text{ mL} =$

$$\dfrac{300}{125} = 2.4 \text{ mL}$$

or

RP: H : V :: D : X

125 mg : 5 mL :: 60 mg : X mL

125 X = 300

X = 2.4 mL

or

FE: $\dfrac{125 \text{ mg}}{5 \text{ mL}} = \dfrac{60 \text{ mg}}{X}$

125 X = 300

X = 2.4 mL

or

DA: mL $= \dfrac{\overset{1}{\cancel{5}} \text{ mL} × \overset{12}{\cancel{60}} \text{ mg}}{\underset{\underset{5}{25}}{\cancel{125}} \text{ mg} × 1} = \dfrac{12}{5} - 2.4 \text{ mL}$

Answer: cefaclor (Ceclor) 20 mg/kg/day = 2.4 mL per dose three times per day

Body Surface Area (BSA or m²)

Body surface area is an estimated mathematical function of height and weight measured in meters squared. BSA is considered to be the most accurate way to calculate drug dosages in that the correct dosage is more proportional to the surface area of the body. BSA is commonly used in chemotherapy and some drug dosages used for infants and children. There are two methods for calculating BSA. The first is the square root formula and the second is a nomogram derived from the square root formula.

 YOU MUST REMEMBER

Rounding Off Rule: Since calculators are used for working problems, round off at the final answer and not the steps in between. For BSA problems, round off answers to the nearest hundredth.

BSA With the Square Root

BSA can be calculated by using the square root and a fractional formula of height and weight divided by a constant, one for the metric system and another for inches and pounds. Now that calculators are readily available, the square root formula is easier to calculate than the longhand version. But errors can be made with calculators too; therefore a BSA nomogram can prove useful to verify answers. Follow institutional policy regarding BSA methods of calculation. When solving BSA problems, it is necessary to convert weight and height to the same system of measure.

BSA: Inch and Pound (lb) Formula

$$BSA = \sqrt{\frac{ht(in) \times wt(lb)}{3131}}$$

BSA: Metric Formula by Centimeters (cm) and Kilograms (kg)

$$BSA = \sqrt{\frac{ht(cm) \times wt(kg)}{3600}}$$

EXAMPLES **PROBLEM 1:** Order: melphalon (Alkeran) 16 mg/m^2 q 2 weeks. Patient is 68 inches tall and weighs 172 pounds. Use the BSA inches and pounds formula.

a. $BSA = \sqrt{\dfrac{68\ in \times 172\ lbs}{3131}}$

$BSA = \sqrt{\dfrac{11,696}{3131}}$

$BSA = \sqrt{3.73}$

$BSA = 1.9\ m^2$

b. 16 mg $\times$ 1.9 m^2 = 30.4 mg/m^2 or 30 mg/m^2

PROBLEM 2: Order: cisplatin (Platinol) 50 mg/m^2/cycle IV. Patient weighs 84.5 kg and is 168 cm tall. Use the BSA metric formula.

a. $BSA = \sqrt{\dfrac{168\ cm \times 84.5\ kg}{3600}}$

$BSA = \sqrt{\dfrac{14,196}{3600}}$

$BSA = \sqrt{3.94}$

$BSA = 1.99\ m^2$

b. 50 mg $\times$ 1.99 m^2 = 99.5 mg/m^2, or 100 mg/m^2

BSA With a Nomogram

The BSA in square meters (m^2) is determined by the person's height and weight and where these points intersect on the nomogram scale (Figures 7.1 and 7.2). The nomogram charts were developed from the square root formula and were correlated with heights and weights to provide a quick and simple method for drug dosing before calculators were readily available. There are separate nomograms for infants, children, and adults. When a nomogram is used, points on the scale must be carefully plotted and a straight line drawn connecting the two points. An error in plotting points or drawing intersecting lines can lead to reading of the incorrect BSA, resulting in dosing errors. Although there are slight discrepancies between the nomogram and square root method, the trend in medication safety is to use the nomogram to verify the calculator-generated square root.

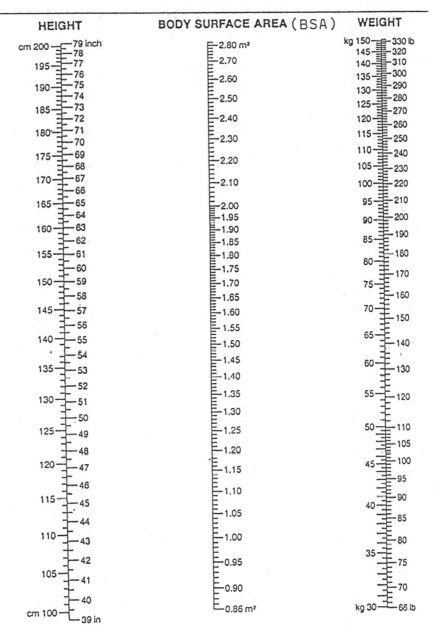

Figure 7.1 Body surface area (BSA) nomogram for adults. Directions: (1) find height, (2) find weight, (3) draw a straight line connecting the height and weight. Where the line intersects on the BSA column is the body surface area (m²). (From Deglin, H., Vallerand, A. H., & Russin, M. M. [1991]. *Davis' drug guide for nurses,* 2nd ed. Philadelphia: F. A. Davis, p. 1218. Used with permission from Lentner, C. [1991]. *Geigy scientific tables,* 8th ed., vol. 1, Basel, Switzerland: Ciba-Geigy, pp. 226-227.)

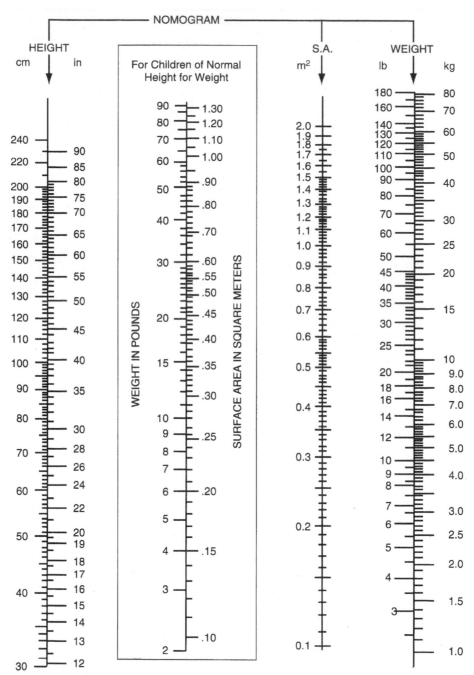

Figure 7.2 West nomogram for infants and children. Directions: (1) find height, (2) find weight, (3) draw a straight line connecting the height and weight. Where the line intersects on the SA column is the body surface area (m²). (From Kliegman RM, St. Geme JW, Blum NJ, et al: *Nelson textbook of pediatrics,* ed. 21, Philadelphia, 2020, Saunders.)

To calculate the dosage by BSA obtained with nomogram, multiply the drug dose $\times$ m^2, e.g., 100 mg $\times$ 1.6 m^2 = 160 mg/m^2. The advantage of using the nomogram is that no conversions from pounds to kilograms or inches to centimeters are needed.

EXAMPLES **PROBLEM 1:** Order: cyclophosphamide (Cytoxan) 100 mg/m^2/day, po. Patient weighs 150 pounds and is 5'8" (68 inches) tall.
a. 68 inches and 150 pounds intersect the nomogram scale at 1.88 m^2 (BSA) (see the red line in Figure 7.3).
b. BSA: 100 mg $\times$ 1.9 m^2 = 190 mg/m^2/day of Cytoxan

$$1.88 \text{ m}^2 = 188 \text{ mg/m}^2/\text{day or } 190 \text{ mg/m}^2/\text{day}$$

PROBLEM 2: Order: cytarabine (cytosine arabinoside) 200 mg/m^2/day IV $\times$ 5 days for a patient with myelocytic leukemia. The patient is 64 inches tall and weighs 130 pounds.
a. 64 inches and 130 pounds intersect the nomogram scale at 1.69 m^2 (BSA) (see the blue line in Figure 7.3).
b. BSA: 200 mg $\times$ 1.69 m^2 = 340 mg/m^2 IV daily for 5 days

$$1.69 \text{ m}^2 = 338 \text{ mg/m}^2 \text{ or } 340 \text{ mg/m}^2$$

Ideal Body Weight (IBW)

Drug dosing by ideal body weight (IBW) or lean body weight/mass (LBW)/(LBM) formulas is used for medications that are poorly absorbed and distributed throughout the body fat. The ideal body weight formula is based on height and can be adjusted for weight and is used for nutritional assessment. The lean body weight/mass formula is based upon height and weight but is less frequently used because it may predict insufficient doses in obese patients.

IBW Formula

Male: 50 kg + 2.3 kg for **EACH** inch over 5 feet
Female: 45.5 kg + 2.3 kg for **EACH** inch over 5 feet

EXAMPLE Female is 5 feet 2 inches (2 inches $\times$ 2.3 kg)
IBW: 45.5 kg + 2 (2.3 kg) = 45.5 kg + 4.6 kg = 50.1 kg

Adjusted Body Weight (ABW)

Adjusted body weight (ABW) is used for dosing some medication for obese individuals or pregnant women. ABW is better for nutritional assessment of obese individuals because it prevents overfeeding. The ABW formula uses both the IBW and the actual body weight with adjustments for male and female.

ABW Formula

Male: IBW + 0.4 (Actual Body Weight [kg] − IBW [kg]) = ABW
Female: IBW + 0.4 (Actual Body Weight [kg] − IBW [kg]) = ABW

EXAMPLE Female is 5 feet 2 inches and weighs 100.5 kg
50.1 kg + 0.4 (100.5 − 50.1 kg) =
50.1 kg + 0.4 (50.4 kg) =
50.1 kg + 20.16 kg = 70.26 kg or 70.3 kg

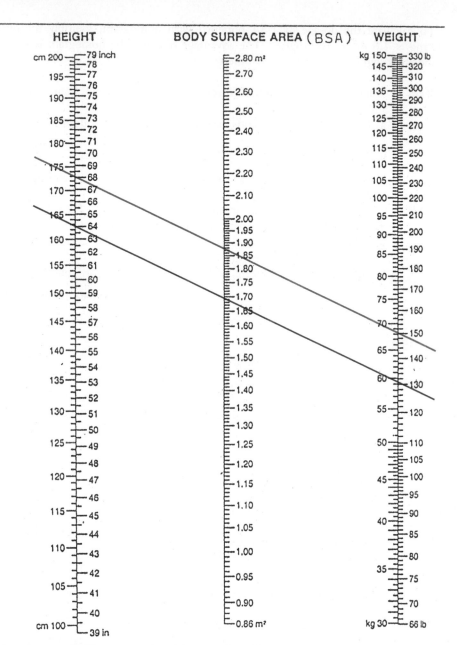

HEIGHT   **BODY SURFACE AREA (BSA)**   **WEIGHT**

Figure 7.3 Body surface area (BSA) nomogram for adults. Example Problem 1: a. 68 inches and 150 pounds intersect the nomogram BSA scale at 1.88 m² (red line). Example Problem 2: a. 64 inches and 130 pounds intersect nomogram BSA scale at 1.69 m² (blue line).

Lean Body Weight (LBW)

Lean body weight (LBW) is the weight of bone, muscle, and organs without any fat. LBW is used for the dosing of some medications and can be used as an indicator of overall health for patients with chronic diseases.

LBW Formula

Lean body weight in kilograms (males over 16 years of age) = (0.32810 × [body weight in kg] + 0.33929 × [height in centimeters]) − 29.5336

Lean body weight in kilograms (women over 30) = (0.29569 × [body weight in kg] + 0.41813 × [height in centimeters]) − 43.2933

EXAMPLE Female is 5 feet 2 inches, weighs 100.5 kg, and is 55 years old.

(0.29569 × [100.5 kg] + ([0.41813 × (62″ × 2.54 cm)])) − 43.2933 =

29.71 + (0.41813 × 157.48) − 43.2933 =

29.71 + 65.84 − 43.2933 =

95.55 − 43.2933 = 52.26 kg

SUMMARY PRACTICE PROBLEMS

Answers can be found on pages 112 to 116.

Body Weight

1. Order: trimethoprim-sulfamethoxazole 6 mg/kg/day, po, q12h.
   Patient weighs 44 pounds.

   How many milligrams should the patient receive per dose? _____

2. Order: azithromycin (Zithromax), po. First day: 10 mg/kg/day; next 4 days: 5 mg/kg/day. Patient weighs 44 pounds.
   Drug available:

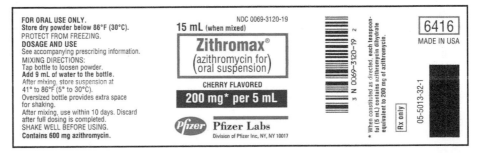

   a. How much does the child weigh in kilograms? _____
   b. How many milliliters should the child receive for the first day? _____
   c. How many milliliters should the child receive each day for the next 4 days (second to fifth days)? _____

3. Order: ticarcillin disodium (Ticar), 200 mg/kg/day in 4 divided doses, IV. Patient weighs 176 pounds.
   Max dose: 24 g every day
   Drug available:

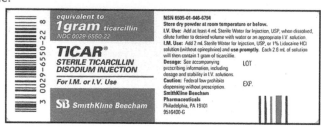

a. How many kilograms does the patient weigh?_____

b. How many milligrams per day should the patient receive? How many milligrams per dose? _____ mg, q6h. Or how many grams per dose? _____ g, q6h

4. Order: tobramycin 5.1 mg/kg/day in 3 divided doses (q8h), IV. The patient weighs 180 pounds.
   Drug available:

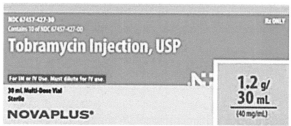

a. How many kilograms does the patient weigh? _____

b. How many milligrams should the patient receive per day? _____

c. How many milliliters should the patient receive per dose? _____

5. Order: sulfisoxazole (Gantrisin) 2 g/m² daily in 4 divided doses (q6h). The patient weighs 110 pounds and is 60 inches tall. Use nomogram.
   How many milligrams should the patient receive per dose? _____

6. Order: doxorubicin (Adriamycin) 60 mg/m² IV per month. Patient weighs 120 pounds and is 5'2" (62 inches) tall. Use nomogram.
   How many milligrams should the patient receive? _____

7. Order: etoposide (VePesid) 100 mg/m^2/day × 5 days. Patient weighs 180 pounds and is 70 inches tall. Use nomogram.
   Drug available:

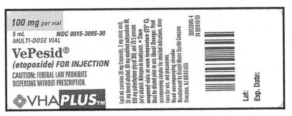

   a. What is the BSA? _____

   b. How many milligrams should the patient receive? _____

   c. How many milliliters are needed? _____

BSA by Square Root

8. Order: vinblastine sulfate (Velban) 7.4 mg/m^2 IV × 1. Patient's height is 115 cm and weight is 52 kg. Use the BSA metric formula to determine dosage.
   Drug available:

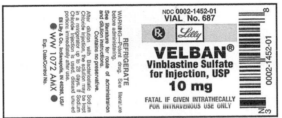

   How many milligrams should the patient receive?_____

9. Order: etoposide (VePesid) 50 mg/m^2 day IV. Patient's height is 72 inches and weight is 180 pounds.

   How many milligrams should the patient receive? _____

10. Patient with advanced colorectal cancer
    Order: Fluorouracil 250 mg/m^2/day × 7 days
    Patient's height and weight: 6′2″, 218 lbs.

    a. What is patient's BSA in square meters? _____ (use square root)

    b. What is the daily dose? _____

    c. What is the total dosage for 7 days? _____

11. Order: docetaxel (Taxotene) 60 mg/m^2/dose in 200 mL of normal saline solution over 60 minutes.
    Patient's height and weight: 5′8″, 136 lbs.

    a. What is patient's BSA in square meters? _____

    b. What is the total dosage of docetaxel? _____

    c. What is the concentration per milliliter? _____

12. Order: gemcitabine (Gemzar) 800 mg/m^2/dose in 100 mL of normal saline solution over 30 minutes. Patient's height and weight: 6'6", 150 lbs.
    Drug available: gemcitabine 1 g/25 mL

    a. What is patient's BSA in square meters? _____

    b. What is the total dose of gemcitabine? _____

    c. How many milliliters should you prepare? _____

13. Order: Liposomal doxorubicin 20 mg/m^2 in 250 mL D$_5$W IV over 30 minutes. Patient's height and weight: 6', 129 lbs.
    Drug available: Doxorubicin 20 mg/10 mL

    a. What is patient's BSA in square meters? _____

    b. What is the total dose of doxorubicin? _____

    c. How many milliliters should you prepare? _____

14. Order: irinotecan (Camptosar) 60 mg/m^2 in 500 mL D5 ½NS IV over 90 minutes. Patient's height and weight: 6', 202 lbs.
    Drug available: irinotecan 20 mg/mL

    a. What is patient's BSA in square meters? _____

    b. What is the total dose of irinotecan? _____

    c. How many milliliters should you prepare? _____

15. Order: Cisplatin 80 mg/m^2 in 500 mL normal saline solution over 90 minutes. Patient's height and weight: 6', 200 lbs.
    Drug available: Cisplatin 1 mg/mL

    a. What is patient's BSA in square meters?_____

    b. What is the total dose of cisplatin?_____

16. Order: Adriamycin 50 mg/m^2 in 3 individual doses mixed with 1000 mL normal saline solution per dose continuous infusion over 24 hr. Patient's height and weight: 5'8", 139 lbs.
    Drug available: Adriamycin 10 mg/5 mL

    a. What is patient's BSA in square meters? _____

    b. What is the total dosage? _____

    c. What is the divided dose? _____

17. Order: Paclitaxel 100 mg/m^2 in 250 mL D$_5$W over 3 hrs. Pt's height and weight: 68.5", 218 lbs.
    Drug available: Paclitaxel 300 mg/50 mL

    a. What is the patient's BSA in square meters? _____

    b. What is the total dose of paclitaxel? _____

18. Order: bortezomib 1.3 mg/m^2 subcutaneously. Pt height and weight: 70″, 191.6 lbs.
Drug available: Bortezomib 3.5 mg dilute with 1.4 mL sterile saline to produce a
concentration of 2.5 mg/mL.

   a. What is the patient's BSA in square meters? _____
   b. What is the total dose of bortezomib? _____
   c. How many milliliters should the patient receive per dose? _____

19. Order: petetrexed 500 mg/m^2 in 100 mL NS over 10 minutes. Pt's height and weight: 6′2″, 230.4 lbs.
Drug available: petetrexed 500 mg vial, dilute with 20 mL sodium chloride.

   a. What is the patient's BSA in square meters? _____
   b. What is the total dose of petetrexed? _____
   c. How many milliliters should the patient receive per dose? _____

20. Order: Erbitux 400 mg/m^2 initial dose in 250 NS over 120 minutes. Pt's height and weight: 74″,
198 lbs. Convert to metric.
Drug available: Erbitux 200 mg/100 mL.

   a. What is the patient's BSA in square meters? _____
   b. What is the total dose of Erbitux? _____
   c. How many milliliters should the patient receive per dose? _____

Ideal Body Weight (IBW) and Adjusted Body Weight (ABW)

21. What is the IBW and ABW for a male weighing 385 lbs and 5′8″ tall? _____

22. What is the IBW and ABW for a female weighing 370 lbs and 5′2″ tall? _____

23. What is the IBW and ABW for a female weighing 290 lbs and 5′3″ tall? _____

24. What is the IBW and ABW for a male weighing 310 lbs and 5′10″ tall? _____

Lean Body Weight (LBW)

25. What is the LBW for a 50-year-old male weighing 385 lbs and 5′8″ tall? _____

26. What is the LBW for a 60-year-old female weighing 385 lbs and 5′2″ tall? _____

27. What is the LBW for a 30-year-old male weighing 134 lbs and 6′ tall? _____

28. What is the LBW for a 65-year-old female weighing 99 lbs and 5′2″ tall? _____

ANSWERS   SUMMARY PRACTICE PROBLEMS

Body Weight

1. $44 \text{ lbs} \div 2.2 \text{ lbs/kg} = 20 \text{ kg}$

   $20 \text{ kg} \times 6 \text{ mg/kg/day} = 120 \text{ mg} \div 2 \text{ doses} = 60 \text{ mg/dose trimethoprim-sulfamethoxazole}$

2. **a.** 20 kg

   b. First day: $10 \text{ mg} \times 20 \text{ kg} = 200 \text{ mg}$

   $$\text{BF:} \frac{D}{H} \times V = \frac{\overset{1}{\cancel{200 \text{ mg}}}}{\underset{1}{\cancel{200 \text{ mg}}}} \times 5 \text{ mL} = 5 \text{ mL}$$

   or

   $$\text{RP:} \quad H \ : \ V \ :: \ D \ :X$$
   $$200 \text{ mg} : 5 \text{ mL} :: 200 \text{ mg} : X$$
   $$200 X = 1000$$
   $$X = 5 \text{ mL}$$

   $$\text{DA: mL} = \frac{5 \text{ mL} \times \overset{1}{\cancel{200 \text{ mg}}}}{\underset{1}{\cancel{200 \text{ mg}}} \times 1} = 5 \text{ mL}$$

   or

   $$\text{FE} = \frac{200 \text{ mg}}{5 \text{ mL}} = \frac{200 \text{ mg}}{X} = 200 X = 1000$$
   $$X = 5 \text{ mL}$$

   First day give 5 mL.

   c. Second to fifth days (next 4 days): $5 \text{ mg} \times 20 \text{ kg} = 100 \text{ mg}$
   Give 2.5 mL/day.

3. **a.** Client weighs 80 kg.

   b. $200 \text{ mg} \times 80 = 16,000 \text{ mg per day}$; 4000 mg per dose or 4 g per dose (q6h)

4. Tobramycin: $1.2 \text{ g} = 1200 \text{ mg}$

   a. $180 \text{ lbs} \div 2.2 \text{ kg} = 81.8 \text{ kg}$

   $5.1 \text{ mg} \times 81.8 \text{ kg} = 417.2 \text{ mg/day}$

   b. $417.2 \text{ mg} \div 3 \text{ doses/day} = 139 \text{ mg/dose or } 140 \text{ mg/dose}$

   c. $\text{BF:} \dfrac{D}{H} \times V = \dfrac{140 \text{ mg}}{1200 \text{ mg}} \times 30 \text{ mL} = \dfrac{4200}{1200} = 3.5 \text{ mL}$

   or

   $$\text{RP:} \quad H \ : \ V \ :: \ D \ :X$$
   $$1200 \text{ mg} : 30 \text{ mL} :: 140 \text{ mg} : X$$
   $$1200 X = 4200$$
   $$X = 3.5 \text{ mL of tobramycin}$$

   $$\text{DA: mL} = \frac{30 \text{ mL} \times 140 \text{ mg}}{1200 \text{ mg} \times 1} = \frac{4200}{1200} = 3.5 \text{ mL of tobramycin}$$

5. 60 inches and 110 pounds intersect the nomogram scale at 1.5 m^2.
   BSA: $2 \text{ g} \times 1.5 \text{ m}^2 = 3 \text{ g or } 3000 \text{ mg per day}$
   $3000 \text{ mg} \div 4 \text{ times per day} = 750 \text{ mg}$

6. 62 inches and 120 pounds intersect the nomogram scale at 1.6 m^2.
   BSA: $60 \text{ mg} \times 1.6 \text{ m}^2 = 96 \text{ mg of Adriamycin}$

7. **a.** With the use of the nomogram, the BSA is 2.06.

   b. $100 \text{ mg} \times 2.06 = 206 \text{ mg or } 200 \text{ mg}$.

   c. The amount of VePesid administered should be 10 mL.

   $$\text{BF:} \frac{D}{H} \times V = \frac{200 \text{ mg}}{100 \text{ mg}} \times 5 \text{ mL} = 10 \text{ mL}$$

   or

   $$\text{RP:} \ 100 \text{ mg} : 5 \text{ mL} :: 200 \text{ mg} : X$$
   $$100 X = 1000$$
   $$X = 10 \text{ mL}$$

   or

   $$\text{DA: mL} = \frac{5 \text{ mL} \times \overset{2}{\cancel{200 \text{ mg}}}}{\underset{1}{\cancel{100 \text{ mg}}} \times 1} = 10 \text{ mL}$$

BSA by Square Root

8. $\text{BSA} = \sqrt{\dfrac{115 \text{ cm} \times 52 \text{ kg}}{3600}}$

$\text{BSA} = \sqrt{\dfrac{5980}{3600}}$

$\text{BSA} = \sqrt{1.66}$

$\text{BSA} = 1.29 \text{ m}^2$

$7.4 \text{ mg} \times 1.29 \text{m}^2 = 9.5 \text{ mg/m}^2$

9. $\text{BSA} = \sqrt{\dfrac{72 \text{ in} \times 180 \text{ lbs}}{3131}}$

$\text{BSA} = \sqrt{\dfrac{12,960}{3131}}$

$\text{BSA} = \sqrt{4.13}$

$\text{BSA} = 2.0 \text{ m}^2$

$50 \text{ mg/m}^2 \times 2\text{m}^2 = 100 \text{ mg}$

10.
a. $\sqrt{\dfrac{74 \times 218}{3131}} = 2.27 \text{ m}^2$
b. $250 \text{ mg} \times 2.27 \text{ m}^2 = 567.5$ or 568 mg
c. $568 \text{ mg} \times 7 = 3976 \text{ mg}$

11.
a. $\sqrt{\dfrac{68 \times 136}{3131}} - 1.7 \text{ m}^2$
b. $60 \text{ mg/m}^2 \times 1.7 \text{ m}^2 = 102 \text{ mg}$
c. $\dfrac{102 \text{ mg}}{200 \text{ mL}} = 0.51 \text{ mg/mL}$

12.
a. $\sqrt{\dfrac{78 \times 150}{3131}} - 1.9 \text{ m}^2$
b. $800 \text{ mg/m}^2 \times 1.9 \text{ m}^2 = 1520 \text{ mg}$
c. $1 \text{ g} = 1000 \text{ mg}$

$\text{BF:} \dfrac{D}{H} \times V = \dfrac{1520 \text{ mg}}{1000 \text{ mg}} \times \dfrac{25 \text{ mL}}{1} =$

$\dfrac{38,000}{1000} = 38 \text{ mL}$

or

$\text{DA: mL} = \dfrac{25 \text{ mL} \times 1520 \text{ mg}}{1000 \text{ mg} \times 1} = 38 \text{ mL}$

or

$\text{RP: } 1000 \text{ mg}:25 \text{ mL}::1520 \text{ mg}:X$
$1000 X = 38,000$
$X = 38 \text{ mL}$

or

$\text{FE: } \dfrac{1000 \text{ mg}}{25 \text{ mL}} = \dfrac{1520 \text{ mg}}{X}$
$1000 X = 38,000$
$X = 38 \text{ mL}$

13. **a.** $\sqrt{\dfrac{72 \times 129}{3131}} = 1.72 \text{ m}^2$

b. $20 \text{ mg/m}^2 \times 1.72 \text{ m}^2 = 34 \text{ mg}$

c. BF: $\dfrac{D}{H} \times V = \dfrac{34 \text{ mg}}{20 \text{ mg}} \times 10 \text{ mL}$

$\dfrac{340}{20} = 17 \text{ mL}$

or

DA: $\text{mL} = \dfrac{10 \text{ mL} \times 34 \text{ mg}}{20 \text{ mg} \times 1} = 17 \text{ mL}$

or

RP: $20 \text{ mg} : 10 \text{ mL} :: 34 \text{ mg} : X$

$20 X = 340$

$X = 17 \text{ mL}$

or

FE: $\dfrac{20 \text{ mg}}{10 \text{ mL}} = \dfrac{34 \text{ mg}}{X} = 20X = 340$

$X = 17 \text{ mL}$

14. **a.** $\sqrt{\dfrac{72 \times 202}{3131}} = 21.5 \text{ m}^2$

b. $60 \text{ mg} \times 2.15 \text{ m}^2 = 129 \text{ mg or } 130 \text{ mg/m}^2$

c. BF: $\dfrac{D}{H} \times V = \dfrac{130 \text{ mg}}{20 \text{ mg}} \times 1 \text{ mL} =$

$\dfrac{130}{20} = 6.5 \text{ mL}$

or

DA: $\text{mL} = \dfrac{1 \text{ mL} \times 130 \text{ mg}}{20 \text{ mg} \times 1} = 6.5 \text{ mL}$

or

RP: $20 \text{ mg} : 1 \text{ mL} :: 130 \text{ mg} : X$

$20 X = 130$

$X = 6.5 \text{ mL}$

or

FE: $\dfrac{20 \text{ mg}}{1 \text{ mL}} = \dfrac{130 \text{ mg}}{X}$

$20 X = 130$

$X = 6.5 \text{ mL}$

15. **a.** $\sqrt{\dfrac{72 \times 200}{3131}} = 2.14 \text{ m}^2$

b. $80 \text{ mg/m}^2 \times 2.14 \text{ m}^2 = 171 \text{ mg or } 170 \text{ mg}$

16. **a.** $\sqrt{\dfrac{68 \times 139}{3131}} = 1.73 \text{ m}^2$

b. $50 \text{ mg/m}^2 \times 1.73 \text{ m}^2 = 86.5 \text{ mg}$

c. $86.5 \text{ mg/3 doses} = 28.8 \text{ mg}$

17. $\sqrt{\dfrac{68.5 \times 218}{3131}} = \sqrt{\dfrac{14,933}{3131}} = 2.18 \text{ m}^2 \quad 100 \text{ mg/m}^2 \times 2.18 \text{ m}^2 = 218 \text{ mg}$

18. **a.** $\sqrt{\dfrac{17.78 \, m \times 7.09 \, kg}{3600}} = \sqrt{\dfrac{15,484.6}{3600}} = 2.07 \text{ m}^2$ **b.** $1.3 \text{ mg/m}^2 \times 2.07 \text{ m}^2 = 2.7 \text{ mg}$

c. BF: $\dfrac{D}{F} \times V = \dfrac{2.7 \, mg}{2.5 \, mg} \times \dfrac{1 \, mL}{1} = 1.08 \, mL \text{ or } \mathbf{1.1} \, \mathbf{mL}$

DA: $\text{mL} = \dfrac{1 \, mL \times 2.7 \, mg}{25 \, mg \times 1} = \dfrac{2.7}{2.5} = 1.08 \, mL \text{ or } 1.1 \, mL$

RP: $2.5 \text{ mg} : 1 \text{ mL} :: 2.7 \text{ mg} : X$

$2.5 X = 2.7$

$X = 1.08 \, mL \text{ or } 1.1 \, mL$

FE: $\dfrac{2.5 \, mg}{1} = \dfrac{2.7 \, mg}{X}$

$2.5 X = 2.7$

$X = 1.08 \text{ or } 1.1 mL$

19. $6'2'' = 74''$

a. $\dfrac{\sqrt{74'' \times 230.4\ lbs}}{3131} = \dfrac{\sqrt{17,049.6}}{3131} = 2.33\ m^2$ b. $500\ mg/m^2 \times 2.33\ m^2 = 1165\ mg$

c. **BF:** $\dfrac{D}{H} \times V = \dfrac{1165\ mg}{500\ mg} \times \dfrac{20\ mL}{1} = \dfrac{1165}{25} = 46.6\ mL$ or

DA: $mL = \dfrac{20\ mL \times 1165\ mg}{500\ mg \times 1} = \dfrac{1165}{25} = 46.6\ mL$ or

RP: $500\ mg : 20\ mL :: 1165\ mg : X$ or   **FE:** $\dfrac{500\ mg}{20\ mL} = \dfrac{1165}{X}$

$500\ X = 23,300$ $25\ X = 1165$

$X = 46.6\ mL$ $X = 46.6 mL$

20. $74'' \times 0.0254 = 160\ cm$ $198\ lbs \div 2.2 = 90\ kg$

a. $\sqrt{\dfrac{160\ cm \times 90\ kg}{3600}} = \sqrt{\dfrac{14,400}{3600}} = \sqrt{4} = 2\ m^2$ b. $400\ mg/m^2 \times 2\ m^2 = 800\ mg$

c. **BF:** $\dfrac{D}{H} \times V = \dfrac{800\ mg}{200\ mg} \times 100\ mL = 400\ mL$ or

DA: $mL = \dfrac{100\ mL}{200\ mg} \times \dfrac{800\ mg}{1} \times 400\ mL$ or

RP: $200\ mg : 100\ mL :: 800\ mg : X$ or   **FE:** $\dfrac{200\ mg}{100\ mL} = \dfrac{800\ mg}{X}$

$200\ X = 80,000$ $200\ X = 80,000$

$X = 400\ mL$ $X = 400\ mL$

Ideal Body Weight (IBW) and Adjusted Body Weight (ABW)

21. $385\ lbs \div 2.2 = 175\ kg$

IBW $= 50\ kg + 2.3\ kg(8\ inches) =$

$50\ kg + 18.4\ kg = 68.4\ kg$

Adjusted Body Weight $68.4\ kg + 0.4(175\ kg - 68.4) =$

$68.4\ kg + 0.4(106.6\ kg) =$

$68.4\ kg + 42.64\ kg = 111.04\ kg$

22. $370\ lbs \div 2.2 = 168.2\ kg$

IBW $= 45.5\ kg + 2.3(2\ inches) =$

$45.5\ kg + 4.6\ kg = 50.1\ kg$

$Adjusted\ Body\ Weight$ $50.1\ kg + 0.4(168.2\ kg - 50.1) =$

$$50.1\ kg + 0.4(118.1\ kg) =$$

$$50.1\ kg + 47.24\ kg = 97.34\ kg$$

23. $290\ lbs \div 2.2 = 131.8\ kg$

$IBW = 45.5\ kg + 2.3(3\ inches) =$

$$45.5\ kg + 6.9\ kg = 52.4\ kg$$

$Adjusted\ Body\ Weight$ $52.4\ kg + 0.4(131.8\ kg - 52.4) =$

$$52.4\ kg + 0.4(79.4\ kg) =$$

$$52.4\ kg + 31.76\ kg = 84.16\ or\ 84.2\ kg$$

24. $310\ lbs \div 2.2 = 141\ kg$

$IBW = 50\ kg + 2.3\ kg(10\ inches) =$

$$50\ kg + 23\ kg = 73\ kg$$

$Adjusted\ Body\ Weight$ $73\ kg + 0.4(141\ kg - 73) =$

$$73\ kg + 0.4(68) =$$

$$73\ kg + 27.2 = 100.2\ kg$$

Lean Body Weight (LBW)

25. $0.32810 \times (385\ lbs \div 2.2) + 0.33929 \times (68'' \times 2.54) - 29.5336 =$

$0.32810 \times (175\ kg) + 0.3329 \times (172.72\ cm) - 29.5336 =$

$$57.4 + 58.6 - 29.5336 =$$

$$116 - 29.5336 = 86.46\ kg$$

26. $0.29569 \times (385\ lbs \div 2.2) + 0.41813 \times (62'' \times 2.54) - 29.5336 =$

$0.29569 \times (175\ kg) + 0.41813 \times (157.48\ cm) - 43.2933 =$

$$51.7 + 65.84 - 43.2933 =$$

$$117.54 - 43.2933 = 74.246\ or\ 74.25\ kg$$

27. $(0.32810 \times (135\ lbs \div 2.2) + 0.33929 \times [72'' \times 2.54]) - 29.5336 =$

$0.32810 \times (61.3\ kg) + 0.3329 \times (182.79\ cm) - 29.5336 =$

$$20.11253 + 62.05614 - 29.5336 =$$

$$82.16867 - 29.5336 = 52.63507\ kg\ or\ 52.64\ kg$$

28. $(0.29569 \times [99\ lbs \div 2.2] + 0.41813 \times [60'' \times 2.54]) - 43.2933 =$

$0.29569 \times (45\ kg) + 0.41813 \times (152.4\ cm) - 43.2933 =$

$$13.306 + 63.7230 - 43.2933 =$$

$$77.0290 - 43.2933 = 33.7357\ kg\ or\ 33.74\ kg$$

NGN® PREP

1. A 56-year-old man has been receiving chemotherapy for liver cancer. At the beginning of his treatment his weight was 278lbs and his height is 6 feet 2 inches and his body surface area was A . After his third round of chemotherapy, his weight has dropped 43lbs, and he has not gained any weight. His current BSA is needed for the fourth round of chemotherapy and is B .

Option A	Option B
$2.7m^2$	$2.35m^2$
$2.56m^2$	$2.85m^2$
$3.56m^2$	$3.8m^2$
$2.9m^2$	$2.25m^2$

2. A 5-year-old with congestive heart failure from cardiac myopathy and is starting digoxin therapy. She weighs 34 lbs and has been prescribed digoxin 1mg per day in divided doses. Her weight in kg is A . The safe therapeutic range for digoxin for her age is 0.02 to 0.035mg/kg. Safe dose range for Mary is B .

Option A	Option B
16.9kg	0.5mg to 0.7mg
15.5kg	0.3mg to 0.54mg
18kg	0.4mg to 0.7mg
14.5kg	4mg to 6mg

3. A 4-year-old female with central adrenal insufficiency is in the preoperative area being checked in for major surgery. The patient weighs 15.4kg and is 100.3cm tall. The patient's outpatient hydrocortisone dose is currently $7mg/m^2$/day by mouth in 3 divided doses with food. Because of her glucocorticoid deficiency, the dose of hydrocortisone will need to be increased due to the high level of stress from major surgery. Prior to major surgery, she will receive a $50mg/m^2$ hydrocortisone bolus pre-anesthesia intravenously (IV) 30 to 60 minutes prior to surgery. She will then receive $50mg/m^2$ IV divided every 6 hours for at least 24 hours to help account for the increased stress-state from surgery. Each dosage of hydrocortisone she takes at home is A mg. Preoperatively the patient will receive B mg intravenously. Post-operative the patient will receive C per dose.
Chose the correct option from those presented below.

Option A	Option B	Option C
15mg	3mg	38mg
1.5mg	2.3mg	8mg
20.2mg	32.7mg	23mg
2.2mg	23mg	2mg

ANSWERS – NGN® PREP

1. **Option A:** $\sqrt{\dfrac{(74'' X 278lbs)}{3131}} = \sqrt{\dfrac{20,572}{3131}} = \sqrt{6.57} = 2.56m^2$

   Option B: 278lbs-43lbs = 235lbs

   $\sqrt{\dfrac{(74'' X 235lbs)}{3131}} = \sqrt{\dfrac{17,390}{3131}} = \sqrt{5.55} = 2.35m^2$

2. **Option A:** 34kg ÷ 2.2lbs/kg = 15.5kg

   Option B: 15.5kg X 0.02mg/kg = 0.310mg
   15.5kg X 0.035mg/kg = 0.5425mg

3. **Option A:** $\sqrt{\dfrac{15.4 \text{ kg X } 100.3cm}{3600}} = \sqrt{\dfrac{1544.92}{3600}} = \sqrt{.429} = 0.6549m^2$ 0.6549m²

   X 7mg/m²/day

   4.5843mg or 4.6mg/day

   4.6mg/day ÷3 = 1.533 *or* 1.5*mg per dose*

   Option B: 0.6549m² X 50mg/m² = 32.7mg

   Option C: 32.7mg ÷4 times in 24hrs = 8.17 or 8mg/per dose

PART III

CALCULATIONS FOR ORAL, INJECTABLE, AND INTRAVENOUS DRUGS

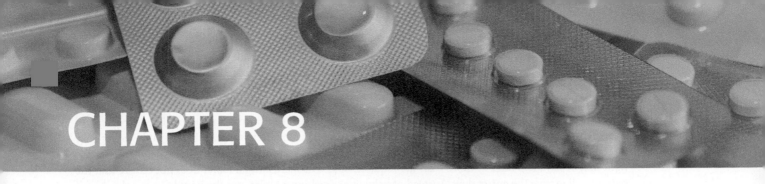

CHAPTER 8

Oral and Enteral Preparations With Clinical Applications

Objectives
- State the advantages and disadvantages of administering oral medications.
- Calculate oral dosages from tablets, capsules, and liquids using given formulas.
- Give the rationale for diluting and not diluting oral liquid medications.
- Explain the method for administering sublingual medication.
- Calculate the amount of oral drug to be given per day in divided doses.

Outline
SOLID ORAL MEDICATIONS
LIQUIDS
BUCCAL TABLETS
SUBLINGUAL TABLETS
FILM STRIPS
ENTERAL NUTRITION AND DRUG ADMINISTRATION

Enteral medications are administered via the gastrointestinal tract. They can be administered orally, rectally, or by a tube inserted into the stomach via the nasal passage (nasogastric tube or dobhoff tube) as well as directly into the intestines (percutaneous gastrostomy tube or jejunal feeding tube). Orally administered medications are the most common form of enteral medication given.

Oral administration of drugs is considered a convenient, less invasive, and economical method of giving medications. Oral drugs are available as tablets, capsules, powders, and liquids. Oral medications are referred to as po (per os, or by mouth) drugs and are absorbed by the gastrointestinal tract, mainly from the small intestine.

There are some disadvantages in administering oral medications, such as (1) variation in absorption rate caused by gastric and intestinal pH and food consumption within the gastrointestinal tract; (2) irritation of the gastric mucosa causing nausea, vomiting, or ulceration (e.g., with oral potassium chloride); (3) retention or inactivation of the drug in the body because of reduced liver function; (4) destruction of drugs by digestive enzymes; (5) aspiration of drugs into the lungs by seriously ill or confused patients; and (6) discoloration of tooth enamel (e.g., with a saturated solution of potassium iodide [SSKI]). Oral administration is an effective way to give medications in many instances, and at times it is the route of choice.

Body weight and body surface area are discussed in Chapter 7. When solving drug problems that require body weight or body surface area, refer to Chapter 7.

Enteral nutrition and non-oral forms of enteral medication are discussed toward the end of the chapter.

SOLID ORAL MEDICATIONS

TABLETS: Tablets are powdered medications that are compressed into a variety of shapes, types, and sizes. Most tablets are scored and can be broken in half or in quarters (Figure 8.1). Half a tablet may be indicated when the drug does not come in a lesser strength. If the tablet is not broken equally, the patient may receive less than or more than the required dose. Also, crushing a tablet does not ensure that the patient will receive the entire dose. Instead of halving or crushing a tablet, use the liquid form of the drug if available. If a tablet is not scored, then it should NOT be broken or altered.

CHEWABLE TABLETS: Tablets that are meant to be chewed rather than swallowed to be effective.

ENTERIC-COATED TABLETS: Tablets that are coated to prevent gastric secretions from dissolving the medication in the stomach rather than the small intestines.

CAPSULES/CAPLETS: Capsules are gelatin shells containing powder or time pellets. Many drugs that come in capsule form also come in liquid form. When a smaller dose is indicated and is not available in tablet or capsule form, the liquid form of the drug is used (Figure 8.2). Caplets (solid-looking capsules are hard-shelled capsules. Sprinkle capsules have small granules inside that may be opened and sprinkled on food. They may also be swallowed whole.

EXTENDED-RELEASE/TIME-RELEASE: Extended and time-release tablets and capsules release medication over a period of time and should never be halved or crushed.

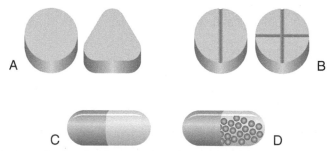

Figure 8.1 A and **B,** Some shapes of tablets. **C** and **D,** Shapes of capsules. (From Kee, J. L., Hayes, E. R., & McCuistion, L. E. [2015]. *Pharmacology: a patient-centered nursing process approach,* 8th ed. Philadelphia: Elsevier.)

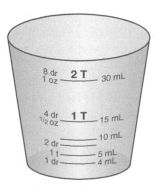

Figure 8.2 Medicine cup for liquid measurement. (From Kee, J. L., Hayes, E. R., & McCuistion, L. E. [2015]. *Pharmacology: a patient-centered nursing process approach,* 8th ed. Philadelphia: Elsevier.)

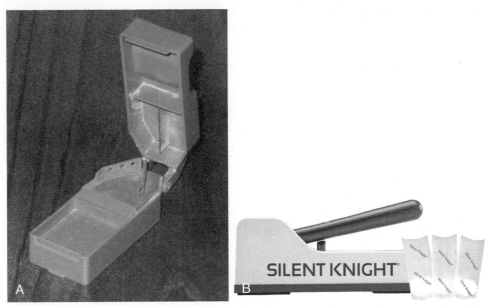

Figure 8.3 A, Pill/tablet cutter. **B,** Silent Knight tablet crushing system. (**B,** Used with permission from Links Medical Products, Inc., Irvine, California.)

Pill/Tablet Cutter and Crusher

A pill or tablet cutter can be used to evenly split or divide a scored or unscored tablet. The pill cutter *cannot* be used to cut/divide enteric-coated tablets or capsules, time-released, sustained-released, or controlled-released capsules. Pill/tablet cutters can be purchased at a drug-store (Figure 8.3). If the patient cannot swallow pills or tablets, best practice is to consult with the prescriber or pharmacist to find if a liquid form of the drug is available. If the medication is not manufactured in liquid form, then a pill crusher (see Figure 8-3, *B*) can be used to reduce tablets to a powdered form that can be mixed with water, juice, fruit sauce, or ice cream. Not all pills can be crushed; see Caution below.

> **! CAUTION**
> - Enteric-coated tablets have a special coating that allows them to move through the stomach and be dissolved in the small intestine so that the medication doesn't irritate the gastric mucosa.
> - Time-released, sustained-release, or controlled-release tablets slowly release drug over a period of time.
> - Layered tablets have medications that may be released at different times. The outer coating dissolves quickly, and the tablet core will dissolve slowly.

Calculation of Tablets and Capsules

The following steps should be taken to determine the drug dose:
1. Check the drug order.
2. Determine the drug available (generic name, brand name, and dosage per drug form).
3. Set up the method for drug calculation (basic formula, ratio and proportion, fraction equation, or dimensional analysis).
4. Convert to like units of measurement within the same system before solving the problem. Use the unit of measure on the drug container to calculate the drug dose.
5. Solve for the unknown (X).

Decide which of the methods of calculation you wish to use, and then use that same method for calculating all dosages. In the following examples, the basic formula, the ratio and proportion, fraction equation, and dimensional analysis methods are used (see Chapter 6).

Basic Formula (BF)

$$\frac{D \text{ (desired dose)}}{H \text{ (on-hand dose)}} \times V \text{ (vehicle)} = X$$

Fraction Equation (FE)

$$\frac{H \text{ (on hand)}}{V \text{ (Vehicle)}} = \frac{D \text{ (desired dose)}}{X \text{ (unknown)}}$$

(Cross multiply)

Ratio and Proportion (RP)

$$\underbrace{H}_{\text{on hand}} : \underbrace{V}_{\text{vehicle}} :: \underbrace{D}_{\text{desired dose}} : \underbrace{X}_{X}$$

Dimensional Analysis (DA)

$$V = \frac{V \times C(H) \times D}{H \times C(D) \times 1}$$

Note: C = conversion factor if needed.

EXAMPLES **PROBLEM 1:** Order: pravastatin sodium (pravachol) 20 mg, daily.
Drug available:

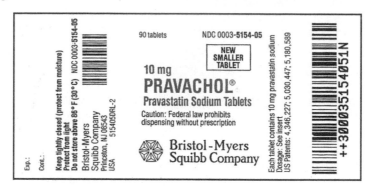

Method: **BF:** $\dfrac{D}{H} \times V$

$$\frac{20 \text{ mg}}{10 \text{ mg}} \times 1 \text{ tab} = 2 \text{ tablets}$$

or

RP: H : V :: D : X
10 mg : 1 tab :: 20 mg : X tab
$$10\,X = 20$$
$$X = 2 \text{ tablets}$$

or

FE: $\dfrac{H}{V} = \dfrac{D}{X} =$

$$\frac{10 \text{ mg}}{1 \text{ tab}} = \frac{20 \text{ mg}}{X} =$$

$$10\,X = 20$$
$$X = 2 \text{ tablets}$$

or

DA: no conversion factor

$$\text{tab} = \frac{1 \text{ tab} \times \overset{2}{20 \text{ mg}}}{\underset{1}{10 \text{ mg}} \times 1} = 2 \text{ tablets}$$

Answer: Pravachol 20 mg = 2 tablets, daily

PROBLEM 2: Order: erythromycin (ERY-TAB) 0.5 g, qid (four times a day).
Drug available:

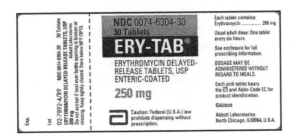

Note: Grams (g) and milligrams (mg) are units in the metric system. *Remember:* When changing grams (larger unit) to milligrams (smaller unit), move the decimal point three spaces to the right. Refer to Chapter 1, Table 1-2. Because the drug dose on the drug label is in milligrams, conversion should be from grams to milligrams.

Methods: 0.5 g = 0.500 mg or 500 mg

BF: $\dfrac{D}{H} \times V = \dfrac{500 \text{ mg}}{250 \text{ mg}} \times 1$ tab

$= \dfrac{500}{250} = 2$ tablets

or

FE: $\dfrac{250 \text{ mg}}{1 \text{ tab}} = \dfrac{500 \text{ mg}}{X}$

$250 \, X = 500$

$X = 2$ tablets

or

RP: H   :   V   ::   D   :   X
250 mg : 1 tab :: 500 mg : X tab
$250 \, X = 500$
$X = 2$ tablets

or

DA: tablet $= \dfrac{1 \text{ tab} \quad \times \quad \overset{4}{\cancel{1000}} \text{ mg} \times 0.5 \cancel{g}}{\underset{1}{\cancel{250}} \cancel{mg} \times \quad 1 \cancel{g} \quad \times \quad 1}$

$4 \times 0.5 = 2$ tablets

Answer: ERY-TAB 0.5 g = 2 tablets

PROBLEM 3: Order: aspirin 650 mg, po, STAT.
Drug available: aspirin 325 mg per tablet.

Methods:

BF: $\dfrac{D}{H} \times V = \dfrac{\overset{2}{\cancel{650}} \text{ mg}}{\underset{1}{\cancel{325}} \text{ mg}} \times 1 = \dfrac{2}{1} = 2$ tablets

or

RP: H   :   V   ::   D   :   X
325 mg : 1 tab :: 650 mg : X tab
$325 \, X = 650$
$X = 2$ tablets

or

FE: $\dfrac{H}{V} = \dfrac{D}{X} =$

$\dfrac{325 \text{ mg}}{1} = \dfrac{650 \text{ mg}}{X} =$

$325 \, X = 650$

$X = 2$ tablets

or

DA: tablet $= \dfrac{1 \text{ tab} \quad \times \quad \overset{2}{\cancel{650}} \text{ mg}}{\underset{1}{\cancel{325}} \text{ mg} \times \quad 1} = 2$ tablets

Answer: Aspirin 650 mg = 2 tablets

LIQUIDS

Liquid medications come as tinctures, extracts, elixirs, suspensions, and syrups. Some liquid medications are irritating to the gastric mucosa and must be well diluted before being given (e.g., potassium chloride [KCl]). Medications in tincture form are always diluted or should be diluted. Liquid medication can be poured into a calibrated measuring cup or drawn up into a syringe (Figure 8.4) when greater accuracy is required (i.e., liquid narcotics).

Liquids are designed to be taken orally or through an enteral tube and are made palatable by the addition of sweeteners such as suctrose, aspartame, saccharin, fructose, and sorbitol. Unpalatable liquid drugs can be mixed with 30 to 60 mL of fruit juice. Grapefruit juice interacts with many medications. Check with the pharmacist before choosing which juice to mix with the drug.

> **! CAUTION**
>
> - Concentrated liquid medication that can irritate the gastric mucosa should be diluted in *at least* 6 ounces of fluid, preferably 8 ounces of fluid.
> - Liquid medication that can discolor the teeth *should be well diluted* and taken through a drinking straw.

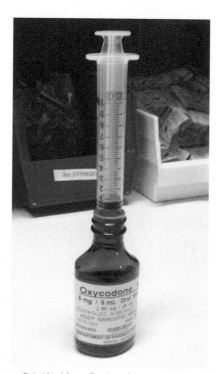

Figure 8.4 Liquid medication drawn up into a syringe.

Calculation of Liquid Medications

EXAMPLES **PROBLEM 1:** Order: potassium chloride (KCl) 20 mEq, po, bid.
Drug available: liquid potassium chloride 10 mEq per 5 mL.

Methods: **BF:** $\dfrac{D}{H} \times V = \dfrac{20\ mEq}{10\ mEq} \times 5\ mL = \dfrac{100}{10} = 10\ mL$

or
RP: H : V :: D : X
    10 mEq : 5 mL :: 20 mEq : X mL
           10 X = 100
              X = 10 mL

or
FE: $\dfrac{H}{V} = \dfrac{D}{X} =$

$\dfrac{10\ mEq}{5\ mL} = \dfrac{20\ mEq}{X}$

    10 X = 100
       X = 10 mL

or
DA: no conversion factor

$mL = \dfrac{5\ mL \times \overset{2}{\cancel{20}}\ mEq}{\underset{1}{\cancel{10}}\ mEq \times 1} = 10\ mL$

Answer: potassium chloride 20 mEq = 10 mL

PROBLEM 2: Order: amoxicillin (Amoxil) 0.25 g, po, tid.
Drug available:

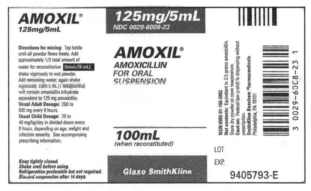

Change grams to milligrams: 0.25 g = 0.250 mg or 250 mg

Methods: **BF:** $\dfrac{D}{H} \times V = \dfrac{250\ mg}{125\ mg} \times 5 = \dfrac{1250}{125} = 10\ mL$

or
RP: H : V :: D : X
    125 mg : 5 mL :: 250 mg : X mL
       125 X = 1250
          X = 10 mL

or
FE: $\dfrac{H}{V} = \dfrac{D}{X} =$

$\dfrac{125\ mg}{5} = \dfrac{250\ mg}{X} =$

    125 X = 1250
       X = 10 mL

or
DA: $mL = \dfrac{5\ mL \times \overset{8}{\cancel{1000}}\ mg \times \overset{1}{\cancel{0.25}}\ g}{\underset{1}{\cancel{125}}\ mg \times \underset{4}{\cancel{1}}\ g \times 1} = \dfrac{40}{4} = 10\ mL$

Answer: Amoxil 0.25 g = 10 mL

PROBLEM 3: Order: SSKI 300 mg, q6h, diluted in water.
Drug available: saturated solution of potassium iodide, 50 mg per drop (gt).

Methods: **BF:** $\dfrac{D}{H} \times V = \dfrac{300 \text{ mg}}{50 \text{ mg}} \times 1 \text{ drop} = \dfrac{300}{50} = 6 \text{ drops}$

or

RP: $\begin{array}{cccc} H & : V & :: & D & :X \\ \end{array}$
50 mg : 1 drop :: 300 mg : X drop
50 X = 300
X = 6 drops

or

FE: $\dfrac{H}{V} = \dfrac{D}{X} =$

$\dfrac{50 \text{ mg}}{1 \text{ drop}} = \dfrac{300 \text{ mg}}{X} =$

50 X = 300
X = 6 drops

or

DA: $gtt = \dfrac{1 \text{ gt} \times \overset{6}{\cancel{300} \text{ mg}}}{\underset{1}{\cancel{50} \text{ mg}} \times 1} = 6 \text{ drops}$

Answer: SSKI 300 mg = 6 drops (gtt)

BUCCAL TABLETS

Buccal tablets are dissolved when held between the cheek and gum, permitting direct absorption of the active ingredient through the oral mucosa. The buccal tablet should be placed in the buccal cavity, above the rear molar between the upper cheek and gum.

> **! CAUTION**
>
> The patient should not split, crush, or chew the tablet.

EXAMPLE PROBLEM 1: Order: fentanyl buccal tablet, 100 mcg, STAT.
Drug available: fentanyl tablet (Fentora) 100 mcg tablet in a blister package. Dissolve 1 tablet in the buccal cavity over 30 minutes.

SUBLINGUAL TABLETS

Drugs that are administered under the tongue are called sublingual tablets. They are small and soluble and are quickly absorbed by the numerous capillaries on the underside of the tongue. Sublingual tablets are also referred to as "orally disintegrating tablets". Medications given by the sublingual route include steroids, enzymes, anti-nausea medications, antipsychotics, and cardiovascular drugs.

> **! CAUTION**
>
>
> • A sublingual tablet (e.g., nitroglycerin [NTG]) should not be swallowed. If the drug is swallowed, the desired immediate action of the drug is decreased or lost.
> • Fluids *should not* be taken until the drug has dissolved.

Calculation of Sublingual Medications

EXAMPLES **PROBLEM 1:** Order: nitroglycerin (Nitrostat) 0.6 mg, sublingually (SL).
Drug available:

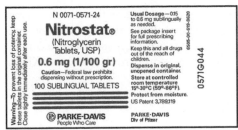

Methods: $\mathbf{BF:}\ \dfrac{D}{H} \times V = \dfrac{0.6\ mg}{0.6\ mg} \times 1\ tab = \dfrac{0.6}{0.6} = 1$ SL tablet

or
DA: no conversion factor

$$SL\ tab = \dfrac{1\ tab \times \overset{1}{\cancel{0.6\ mg}}}{\underset{1}{\cancel{0.6\ mg}} \times 1} = 1\ SL\ tablet$$

or
RP: H : V :: D : X
0.6 mg : 1 tab :: 0.6 mg : X
0.6 X = 0.6
X = 1 tab

or
$\mathbf{FE:}\ \dfrac{H}{V} = \dfrac{D}{X}$

$\dfrac{0.6\ mg}{1\ tab} = \dfrac{0.6\ mg}{X}$

0.6 X = 0.6
X = 1 tab

Answer: nitroglycerin (Nitrostat) 0.6 mg = 1 SL tablet

PROBLEM 2: Order. Order: isosorbide dinitrate (Isordil) 5 mg, SL.
Drug available: isordil 2.5 mg per tablet.

Methods: $\mathbf{BF:}\ \dfrac{D}{H} \times V = \dfrac{5\ mg}{2.5\ mg} \times 1 = 2$ SL tablets

or
RP: H : V :: D : X
2.5 mg : 1 tab :: 5 mg : X tab
2.5 X = 5
X = 2 SL tablets

or
$\mathbf{FE:}\ \dfrac{H}{V} = \dfrac{D}{X} = \dfrac{2.5\ mg}{1} = \dfrac{5\ mg}{X}$

2.5 X = 5
X = 2 SL tablets

or
DA: no conversion factor

$$SL\ tablets = \dfrac{1\ SL\ tab \times \overset{2}{\cancel{5\ mg}}}{\underset{1}{\cancel{2.5\ mg}} \times 1} = 2\ SL\ tablets$$

Answer: isordil 5 mg = 2 SL tablets

PROBLEM 3: Order: olanzapine (Zyprexa, Zydis) 5 mg, SL daily.
Drug available: olanzapine 2.5-, 5-, 7.5-, 10-, 20-mg orally disintegrating blister packet.
a. Which tablet in the blister pack of olanzapine would you select?
b. Explain how the orally disintegrating (SL) olanzapine tablet is administered.

Answer
a. Select 5-mg tablet from the olanzapine blister pack.
b. Have the patient place the sublingual tablet under the tongue, where it will be dissolved and absorbed by the oral mucosa.

FILM STRIPS

Drug films are strips of medication that dissolve in seconds when in contact with wet mucosa. They were originally designed for children, the elderly, or for anyone who has difficulty swallowing. Films are convenient, have high dosage accuracy, and improve compliance. Strips are not to be torn or cut. Examples of drugs that come in film form are Benadryl and Klonopin.

EXAMPLE PROBLEM 1: Order: Suboxone 24 mg/6 mg sublingual film daily

Drug available:

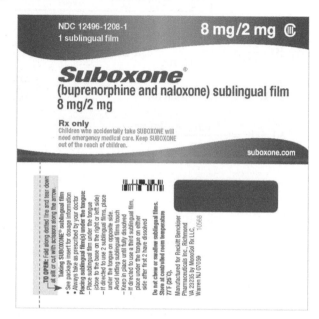

Methods: $BF: \dfrac{D}{H} \times V = \dfrac{24\ mg/6\ mg}{6\ mg/2\ mg} \times 1 = \dfrac{3}{3} = 3$

Answer: 3 sublingual film strips

PRACTICE PROBLEMS ▶ ORAL MEDICATIONS

Answers can be found on pages 152 to 158.

Note: Tablets: Round off tenths to whole numbers; Liquid: Round off to hundredths and then to tenths. For each question, calculate the correct dosage that should be administered.

1. Order: doxycycline hyclate (Vibra-Tabs) 50 mg, po, q12h.
   Drug available:

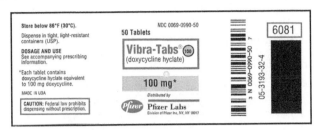

   How many tablets(s) would you give for each dose?_____

2. Order: trimethoprim/sulfamethexazole (Septra) 40 mg/200 mg, po, bid.
   Drug available:

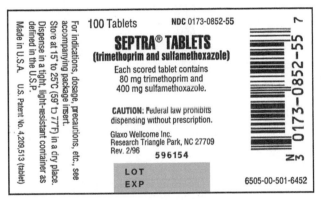

   a. The drug label states that each tablet is _____.

   b. How many tablet(s) would you give? _____

3. Order: digoxin (Lanoxin) 0.5 mg.
   Drug available:

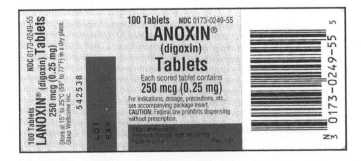

   How many tablets should the patient receive? _____

4. Order: furosemide (Lasix) 20 mg, po, daily.
   Drug available: Drug is scored.

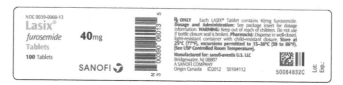

How many tablet(s) would you give? _____

5. Order: Diovan HCT (valsartan and hydrochlorothiazide) 160 mg/25 mg, po, daily.
   Drug available:

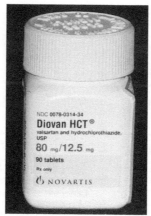

How many tablets would you give? _____

6. Order: potassium chloride 20 mEq, po.
   Drug available:

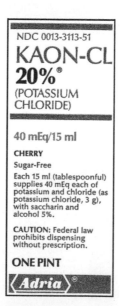

How many milliliters should the patient receive? _____

7. Order: cefaclor (Ceclor) 250 mg, q8h.

Drug available:

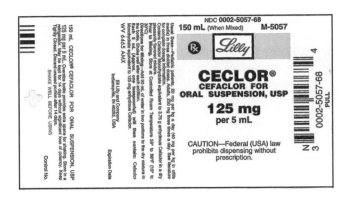

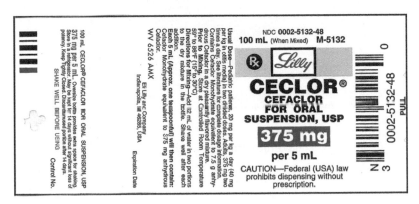

    a. Which Ceclor bottle would you select? Why? _____

    b. How many milliliters per dose should the patient receive? _____

8. Order: ProSom (estazolam) 2 mg, po, at bedtime.

Drug available: 1 mg tablet.

How many tablet(s) should be given? _____

9. Order: cefuroxime axetil (Ceftin) 400 mg, po, q12h.

   Drug available:

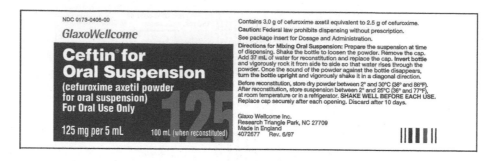

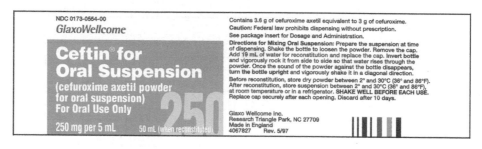

a. How many milliliters should the patient receive? _____

b. Which drug bottle would you use? _____

   Why? _____

10. Order: zidovudine (Retrovir) 300 mg, po, q12h.

    Drug available:

240 mL   NDC 0173-0113-18

RETROVIR®
(zidovudine)
Syrup

For indications, dosage, pre-cautions, etc., see accompanying package insert.
Store at 15° to 25°C (59° to 77°F).

Each 5 mL (1 teaspoonful) contains zidovudine 50 mg and sodium ben-zoate 0.2% added as a preservative.

Made in U.S.A.   Rev. 5/96   587023

CAUTION: Federal law prohibits dispensing without prescription.

U.S. Patent Nos. 4818538 (Product Patent);
4724232, 4833130, and 4837208 (Use Patents)

GlaxoWellcome
Glaxo Wellcome Inc.
Research Triangle Park, NC 27709

LOT
EXP

a. How many milligrams would you give per day? _____

b. How many milliliters would you give per dose? _____

11. Order: Depakene 750 mg, po, daily.
Drug available:

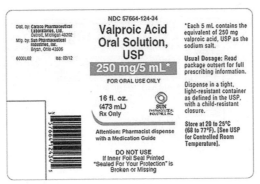

How many milliliters would the patient receive? _____

12. Order: HydroDiuril 50 mg, po, daily.
Drug available:

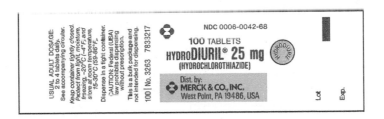

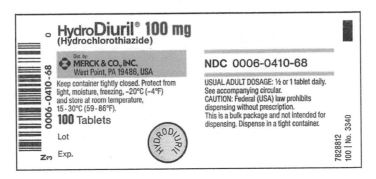

a. Which drug bottle would you use? _____

b. How many tablet(s) would you give, if the tablet(s) are not scored?

_____

Explain. _____

13. Order: simvastatin (Zocor) 30 mg, po, daily.
Drug available:

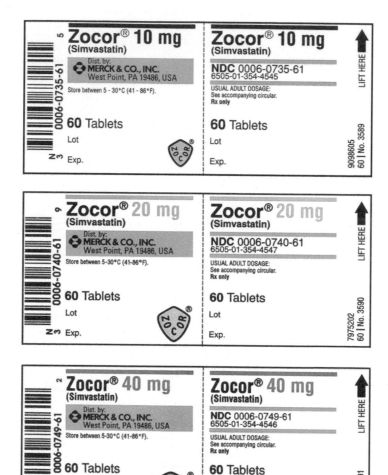

a. Which bottle(s) of Zocor would you select? Why? _____

b. How many tablet(s) should the patient receive? _____

14. Order: oxycodone hydrochloride, 15 mg, po, q6h, PRN for pain.
    Drug available:

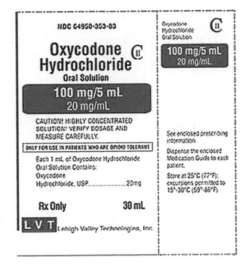

How many milliliters (mL) should the patient receive? _____

15. Order: phenobarbital gr ½ (apothecary system). See Table 2.1.
    Drug available: phenobarbital 15 mg per tablet.

    How many tablet(s) should the patient receive? _____

16. Order: cefprozil (Cefzil) 100 mg, po, q12h.
    Drug available:

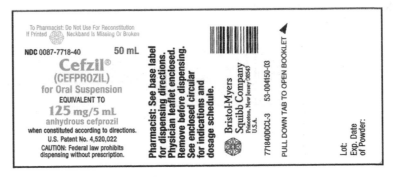

How many milliliters should the patient receive per dose? _____

17. Order: Crestor 20 mg, po, daily.
Drug available:

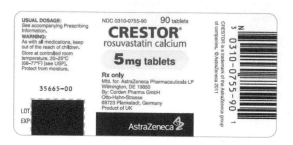
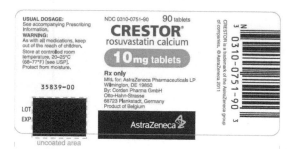

a. Which Crestor bottle(s) would you select? _____

b. How many tablet(s) would you give? _____

18. Order: nitroglycerin 0.4 mg SL, STAT.
Drug available:

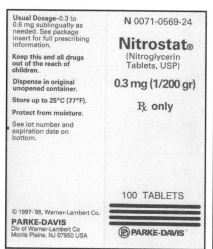
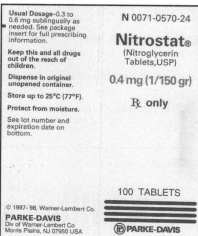
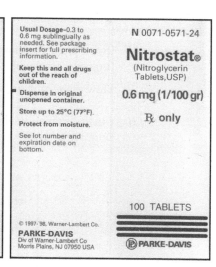

Which Nitrostat SL tablet would you give? _____

19. Order: cefixime 0.4 g, po, daily.
Drug available:

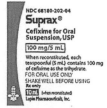

How many milliliters would the patient receive? _____

20. Order: digoxin (Lanoxin) 0.25 mg, po, daily.

Drug available:

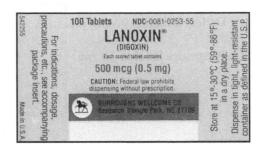

a. Which Lanoxin bottle would you select? _____

b. How many tablet(s) would you give? _____

21. Order: diazepam (Valium) 2½ mg.

Drug available: Valium 5 mg scored tablet.

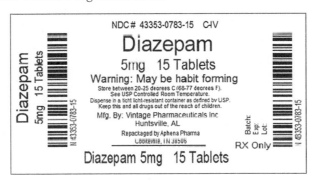

How many tablet(s) would you give? _____

22. Order: ondansetron HCl (Zofran) 6 mg, po, 30 min before chemotherapy, then q8h × 2 more doses

Drug available:

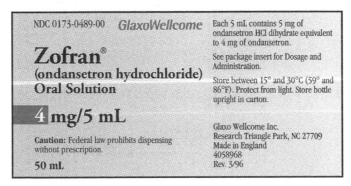

How many milliliters would you give per dose? _____

23. Order: allopurinol 450 mg, po, daily.

Drug available: allopurinol 300 mg scored tablet.

How many tablet(s) would you give? _____

24. Order: captopril (Capoten) 25 mg, po, bid, for an elderly patient with heart failure.
Drug available:

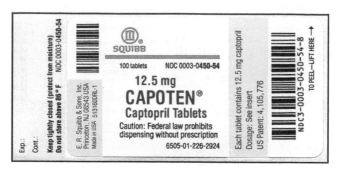

a. How many milligrams should the patient receive per day? _____

b. How many tablet(s) would you give? _____

25. Order: Cogentin 1.5 mg, initially (first day); then 1 mg, po, daily starting second day.
Drug available:

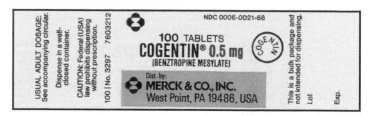

a. How many tablet(s) should the patient receive initially (first day)? _____

b. How many tablet(s) should the patient receive the second day? _____

26. Order: fluconazole (Diflucan) 120 mg, po, daily for 4 weeks.
Drug available:

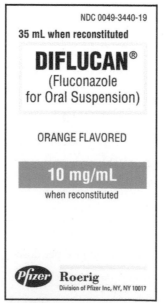

How many milliliters should the patient receive per dose? _____

27. Order: lithium carbonate 600 mg, po, tid.

Drug available:

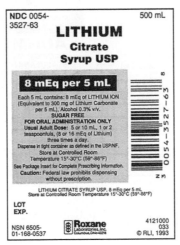

a. Drug label states that 8 mEq per 5 mL of lithium citrate is equivalent to _____ of lithium carbonate.

b. How many milliliters per dose should the patient receive? _____

c. How many milligrams should the patient receive per day? _____

28. Order: furosemide 100 mg, po, as a loading dose, then furosemide 20 mg, po, q12h.

Drug available:

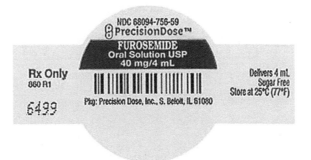

a. How many milliliters would be given as the loading dose? _____

b. How many milliliters would be given for the next scheduled dose? _____

29. Order: amoxicillin/clavulanate potassium (Augmentin) 0.5 g, po, q8h.

Drug available:

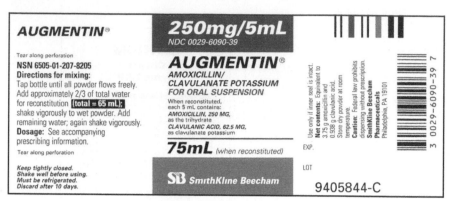

How many milliliters should the patient receive per dose? _____

30. Order: Prozac 30 mg, po, daily.

Drug available:

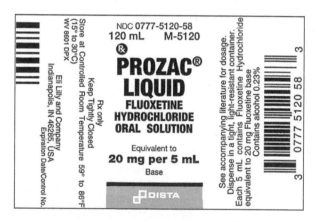

How many milliliters should the client receive? _____

Solve **questions 31 to 39** with Additional Dimensional Analysis (factor labeling). Refer to Chapter 6 as necessary.

31. Order: Ativan 1.5 mg, po, bid.

Drug available:

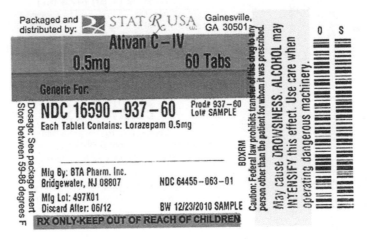

How many milligrams should the patient receive per dose? _____

32. Order: Vasotec 5 mg, po, bid.

Drug available:

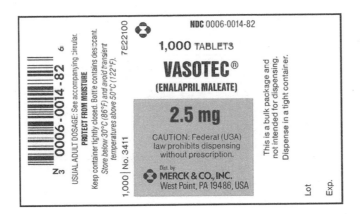

Factors: 2.5 mg = 1 tablet (drug label); 5 mg/1 (drug order)

Conversion factor: none.

How many tablet(s) should the patient receive? _____

33. Order: Phenobarbital 60 mg, po, daily.

Drug available:

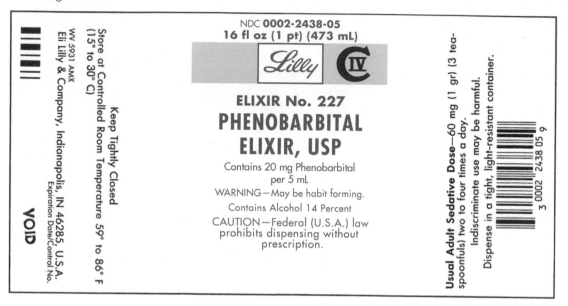

How many milliliters would you give? _____

34. Order: cephalexin (Keflex) 1 g, po, 1 hour before dental cleaning.

Drug available:

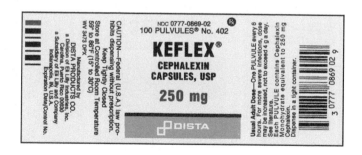

a. Conversion factor: 1 g = 1000 mg

b. How many capsules would you give 1 hour before dental cleaning? _____

35. Order: metoprolol (Lopressor) 0.1 g, po, daily.

Drug available:

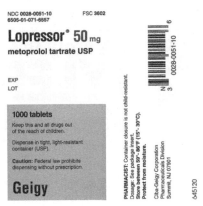

Conversion factor: 1 g = 1000 mg

How many tablet(s) would you give? _____

36. Order: amoxicillin (Amoxil) 0.4 g, po, q6h.

Drug available:

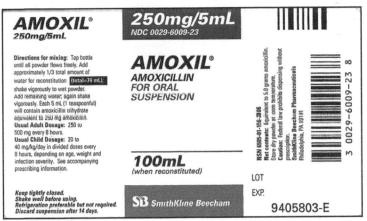

Factors: 250 mg/5 mL (drug label); 0.4 g/1 (drug order)

Conversion factor: 1 g = 1000 mg

How many milliliters would you give? _____

37. Order: acetaminophen (Tylenol) 650 mg, po.
Drug available:

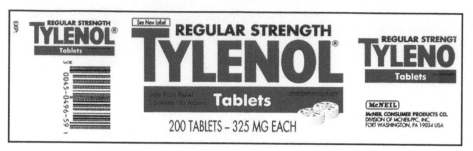

How many acetaminophen tablets would you give? _____

38. Order: atenolol (Tenormin) 50 mg, po, daily for the first 2 weeks and then increase to 100 mg, po, daily starting the third week.
Drug available:

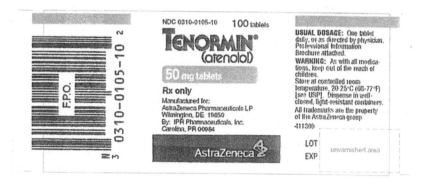

Conversion factor: none

a. How many tablet(s) should the patient receive for the first 2 weeks? _____

b. How many tablet(s) should the patient receive after the second week? _____

39. Order: lactulose 25 g, po × 1 dose.
Drug available:

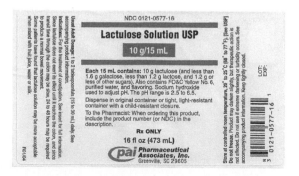

How many milliliters would the patient receive? _____

Questions 40 to 44 relate to body weight and body surface area. Refer to Chapter 7 as necessary.

40. Order: valproic acid (Depakene) 10 mg/kg/day in three divided doses (tid), po. Patient weighs 165 pounds. How much Depakene should be administered tid? _____

41. Order: cyclophosphamide (Cytoxan) 4 mg/kg/day, po. Patient weighs 154 pounds. How much Cytoxan would you give per day? _____

42. Order: mercaptopurine 2.5 mg/kg/day po or 100 mg/m^2 body surface area po. The patient weighs 132 pounds and is 64 inches tall. The estimated body surface area according to the nomogram is 1.7 m^2. The amount of drug the patient should receive according to body weight is_____ and according to body surface area is_____

43. Order: ethosuximide (Zarontin) 20 mg/kg/day in 2 divided doses (q12h). Patient weighs 110 pounds (110 ÷ 2.2 = 50 kg).

Drug available:

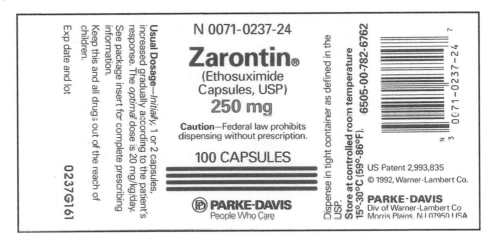

a. How many milligrams should the patient receive per day? _____

b. How many tablet(s) should the patient receive per dose? _____

44. Order: minocycline HCl (Minocin) 4 mg/kg/day in 2 divided doses (q12h). Patient weighs 132 pounds (132 ÷ 2.2 = 60 kg).

Drug available: Minocin 50 mg/5 mL.

a. How many milligrams should the patient receive per day? _____

b. How many milliliters should the patient receive per dose? _____

45. Order: Pradaxa 150 mg, po, q12h.

Drug available: Pradaxa 75 mg tablet.

How many tablets should the patient receive? _____

46. Order: Xarelto 10 mg, po, daily.

Drug available: Xarelto 20 mg tablet.

How many tablets should the patient receive? _____

ENTERAL NUTRITION AND DRUG ADMINISTRATION

When the patient is unable to take nourishment by mouth, enteral feeding (tube feeding) is usually preferred over parenteral (intravenous) nutrition. Candidates for enteral feedings include patients who suffer from neurological deficits and have swallowing problems; patients who are debilitated; have burns; suffer from malnutrition disorders; and those who have undergone radical head and neck surgery. The cost of enteral nutrition is much less than the use of intravenous therapy. Enteral nutrition also carries considerably less risk of infection.

Drugs that can be administered orally (with the exception of sustained-release and extended-release drugs) can also be given through the enteral feeding tube. The drug must be in liquid form or dissolved into a liquid.

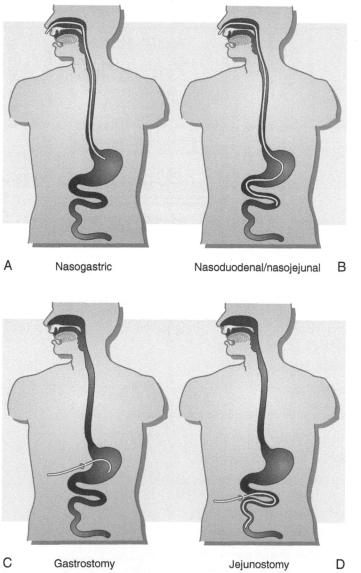

A   Nasogastric   Nasoduodenal/nasojejunal   B

C   Gastrostomy   Jejunostomy   D

Figure 8.5 Types of gastrointestinal tubes for enteral feedings. (From Kee, J. L., Hayes, E. R., & McCuistion, L. E. [2015]. *Pharmacology: a nursing process approach,* 8th ed. Philadelphia: Saunders.)

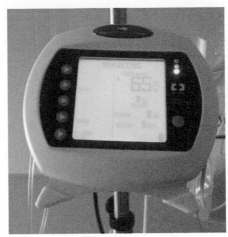

Figure 8.6 Kangaroo pump.

Enteral Feedings

Enteral nutrition may be provided by a gastric, jejunal, or nasogastric tube. Enteral feeding tubes can be identified by their anatomical insertion site and the location of the tip (Figure 8.5). Gastrostomy and jejunostomy routes are used for long-term feeding and require a surgical procedure for insertion. There are two types of nasogastric tubes: the flexible small-bore tube that has a small diameter (4-8 Fr), and the rigid large bore tube with a larger diameter (10-18 Fr). All tubes inserted orally or nasally are primarily for short-term use and may cause nasal or pharyngeal irritation if the use is prolonged. Large-bore tubes are less likely to clog than smallbore tubes. It is essential to flush any feeding tube before and after feedings and between medications.

Enteral feedings may be given as a bolus (intermittent) or as a continuous drip feeding over a specific time period. Continuous feedings can be given by gravity flow from a bag or by infusion pump (Figure 8.6). With bolus feedings, the amount of solution administered is approximately 200 mL or less and feeding times per day are more frequent.

Although enteral feeding solutions (Table 8.1) are formulated to be given at full strength, this may not be tolerated. Solutions that are highly concentrated (hyperosmolar or hypertonic) when given in full strength can cause vomiting, cramping, or excessive diarrhea. In many situations, clients have better gastrointestinal tolerance when the strength of the solution is gradually increased. Continuous feedings are usually started slowly and advanced as tolerated by approximately 10 mL/hr to the goal feeding rate.

If diarrhea continues, changing to a fiber-containing formula may decrease or eliminate it. With some patients, hypoalbuminemia could be a cause of diarrhea, which can lead to malabsorption in the intestines. The prealbumin level is a better indicator of hypoalbuminemia than is the serum albumin test. Other causes of diarrhea may include fecal impaction, *Clostridium difficile,* pseudomembranous colitis, and gut atrophy.

Blood sugar levels should be monitored during enteral therapy. This is important for patients who are acutely ill, have septic conditions, are recovering from acute trauma, or who are receiving steroids. If hyperglycemia occurs, decreasing the tube feeding rate or concentration may help.

Enteral feedings may be ordered in a percentage (%), which is less than the full strength. The nurse must calculate the amount of feeding solution and the amount of water that should be given. After enteral feeding, the tube is always flushed with water (usually 30 mL) to prevent clogging of the tube.

TABLE 8.1 Common Enteral Formulations

Ensure	Isocal	Nephro
Ensure Plus	Sustacal	Ultracal
Ensure HN	Sustacal HC	Jevity
Osmolite	Vital	Criticare
Osmolite HN	Pulmocare	Promote

Calculation of Percent for Enteral Feeding Solutions

Percent (%) of a solution indicates its strength. Percent is a portion of 100, e.g., 20% is 20 of 100%. The basic formula, ratio and proportion, or a percentage problem can be used to determine percent.

D: desired percent
H: on hand volume (100)
V: desired total volume
X: unknown amount of solution

EXAMPLES **PROBLEM 1:** Order: The patient is to receive 250 mL of 70% Osmolite solution q6h.
How much Osmolite solution and water should be mixed to equal 250 mL?
Methods: 0% solution is 70 of 100%.

$$\text{BF:} \frac{D}{H} \times V = \frac{70}{100} \times 250 = \frac{17,500}{100} = 175 \text{ mL of Osmolite}$$

or

$$\text{RP:} H: \quad V \quad :: D : X$$

$$100 : 250 \text{ mL} :: 70 : X \text{ mL}$$

$$100\,X = 17,500$$

$$X = 175 \text{ mL of Osmolite}$$

How much water should he added?;.

$$\text{Total amount} - \text{Amount of TF} = \text{Amount of water}$$
$$250 \text{ mL} - 175 \text{ mL} \qquad = 75 \text{ mL}$$

Answer: 175 mL of Osmolite + 75 mL of water

PROBLEM 2: Order: The patient is to receive 250 mL of 40% Ensure Plus.
How much Ensure Plus and water should be mixed to equal 250 mL?
Methods: 40% solution is 40 or 100%.

$$\text{BF:} \frac{D}{H} \times V = \frac{40}{100} \times 250 = \frac{10,000}{100} = 100 \text{ mL of Ensure Plus}$$

or

$$\text{RP:} H: \quad V \quad :: D : X$$

$$100 : 250 \text{ mL} :: 40 : X \text{ mL}$$

$$100\,X = 10,000$$

$$X = 100 \text{ mL of Ensure Plus}$$

How much water should be added?

$$\text{Total amount} - \text{Amount of TF} = \text{Amount of water}$$
$$250 \text{ mL} - 100 \text{ mL.} \qquad = 150 \text{ mL}$$

Answer: 100 mL of Ensure Plus + 150 mL of water

Enteral Medications

Oral medications in liquid, tablet, or capsule form may be administered through a feeding tube when diluted with 30 to 60 mL of water. Tablets or capsules that can be crushed should be pulverized into a fine powder and then mixed in enough water to form a slurry. The slurry can be given through a large-bore feeding tube with a catheter-tip syringe; 30 to 60 mL of water is flushed through the feeding tube between medications. Some new feeding pumps are designed to include a flush bag that periodically clears the feeding tube and prevents clogging.

 CAUTION

- Use caution with crushing devices, such as a mortar and pestle, to avoid cross-contamination and possible allergic reactions, which may occur if the device is not cleaned or if the medication being crushed is not shielded.

 CAUTION

- Medications in time-released, enteric-coated, or sublingual form and bulk-forming laxatives cannot be crushed or administered enterally.

PRACTICE PROBLEMS > CASE

1. A 77-year-old male patient with a past medical history of chronic hypertension, dementia, and chronic kidney disease was admitted to the Rehabilitation Facility post left hip replacement. Vital signs reported to the RN during the first assessment of the are the following: B/P 172/90, HR 56, Temp 98.4, RR 15 and SaO2 98%. The RN retakes the B/P in R arm, 176/96 and L arm 174/90. The HCP is contacted and a medication order for Hydralazine 50mg PO now, is given. Hydralazine 20mg tablets are available from the pharmacy. How many tablets should be given?
   a. Give 3 tablets now
   b. Give 2 tablets and wait for a 10mg tablet to arrive later
   c. Give 2 tablets now
   d. Give 2 ½ tablets now

ANSWERS

Oral Medications

1. **BF:** $\dfrac{D}{H} \times V = \dfrac{50 \text{ mg}}{100 \text{ mg}} \times 1 \text{ tab} = 0.5 = \frac{1}{2} \text{ tablet}$

   FE: $\dfrac{H}{V} = \dfrac{D}{X} = \dfrac{100 \text{ mg}}{1} = \dfrac{50 \text{ mg}}{X}$

   $$100 \, X = 50$$
   $$X = 0.5 \text{ or } \frac{1}{2} \text{ tablet}$$

   or

   RP: H : V :: D : X
   100 mg : 1 tab :: 50 mg : X tab
   $$100 \, X = 50$$
   $$X = 0.5 \text{ or } \frac{1}{2} \text{ tablet}$$

   or

   DA: no conversion factor

   $$\text{tab} = \dfrac{1 \text{ tab} \times \overset{1}{\cancel{50 \text{ mg}}}}{\underset{2}{\cancel{100 \text{ mg}}} \times 1} = \frac{1}{2} \text{ tablet}$$

2. **a.** scored
   b. ½ tablet

3. 2 tablets

4. **BF:** $\dfrac{D}{H} \times V = \dfrac{\overset{1}{\cancel{20 \text{ mg}}}}{\underset{2}{\cancel{40 \text{ mg}}}} \times 1 = \frac{1}{2} \text{ tablet of Lasix}$

   RP: H : V :: D : X
   40 mg : 1 tab :: 20 mg : X
   $$40 \, X = 20$$
   $$X = \frac{1}{2} \text{ tablet of Lasix}$$

   FE: $\dfrac{H}{V} = \dfrac{D}{X} = \dfrac{40 \text{ mg}}{1} = \dfrac{20 \text{ mg}}{X}$

   $$40 \, X = 20$$
   $$X = \frac{1}{2} \text{ tablet of Lasix}$$

5. 2 tablets daily

6. 7.5 mL

7. **a.** Select the 125-mg/5-mL bottle. It is a fractional dosage with the 375-mg/5-mL bottle (3.3 mL).

   b. **BF:** $\dfrac{D}{H} \times V = \dfrac{250 \text{ mg}}{125 \text{ mg}} \times 5 \text{ mL} = \dfrac{1250}{125} = 10 \text{ mL of Ceclor}$

   or

   RP: H : V :: D : X
   125 mg : 5 mL :: 250 mg : X
   $$125 \, X = 1250$$
   $$X = 10 \text{ mL of Ceclor}$$

   or

   DA: $\text{mL} = \dfrac{5 \text{ mL} \times \overset{2}{\cancel{250 \text{ mg}}}}{\underset{1}{\cancel{125 \text{ mg}}} \times 1} = 10 \text{ mL of Ceclor}$

8. 2 tablets of ProSom

9. a. BF: $\dfrac{D}{H} \times V = \dfrac{400 \text{ mg}}{125 \text{ mg}} \times 5 \text{ mL} = \dfrac{2000}{125} = 16$ mL of Ceftin

or

BF: $\dfrac{D}{H} \times V = \dfrac{400 \text{ mg}}{250 \text{ mg}} \times 5 \text{ mL} = \dfrac{2000}{250} = 8$ mL of Ceftin

b. Either Ceftin bottle could be used. For fewer milliliters, select the 250-mg/5-mL bottle.

10. a. 600 mg per day

b. BF: $\dfrac{D}{H} \times V = \dfrac{300 \text{ mg}}{50 \text{ mg}} \times 5 \text{ mL}$

$= 30$ mL per dose

or

RP: H : V :: D : X
   50 mg : 5 mL :: 300 mg : X mL
       50 X = 1500
           X = 30 mL

or

FE: $\dfrac{H}{V} = \dfrac{D}{X} = \dfrac{50 \text{ mg}}{5 \text{ mL}} = \dfrac{300 \text{ mg}}{X} =$

50 X = 1500
    X = 30 mL per dose

or

DA: mL $= \dfrac{5 \text{ mL} \times \overset{6}{\cancel{300} \text{ mg}}}{\underset{1}{\cancel{50} \text{ mg}} \times 1} = 30$ mL per dose

11. BF: $\dfrac{D}{H} \times V = \dfrac{750 \text{ mg}}{250 \text{ mg}} \times 5 \text{ mL} = 15$ mL

or

RP: H : V :: D : X
   250 : 5 :: 750 : X
   250 X = 3750
       X = 15 mL

or

FE: $\dfrac{H}{V} = \dfrac{D}{H} = \dfrac{250 \text{ mg}}{5 \text{ mL}} = \dfrac{750 \text{ mg}}{X}$

250 X = 3750
    X = 15 mL

or

DA: mL $= \dfrac{5 \text{ mL} \times 750 \text{ mg}}{250 \text{ mg} \times 1} = 15$ mg

12. a. The HydroDiuril 25-mg tablet bottle is preferred. A half-tablet from the HydroDiuril 100-mg tablet bottle can be used; however, breaking or cutting the 100-mg tablet can result in an inaccurate dose.

b. From the HydroDiuril 25-mg bottle, give 2 tablets. From the HydroDiuril 100-mg bottle, give ½ tablet (if the tablet is scored).

13. a. Select a 10-mg and 20-mg Zocor bottle. The 40-mg tablet would not be selected because breaking or cutting the tablet can result in an inaccurate dose.

b. Give 1 tablet from each bottle.

14. BF: $\dfrac{D}{H} \times V = \dfrac{15 \text{ mg}}{20 \text{ mg}} \times 1 \text{ mL} = 0.75 \text{ mL}$

or

RP: H   :V ::   D   :X
   20 mg: 1 :: 15 mg:X
      20 X = 15
         X = 0.75 mL

or

FE: $\dfrac{H}{V} = \dfrac{D}{X} = \dfrac{20 \text{ mg}}{1} = \dfrac{15 \text{ mg}}{X}$

20 X = 15
   X = 0.75 mL

or

DA: $\text{mL} = \dfrac{1 \text{ mL} \times 15 \text{ mg}}{20 \text{ mg} \times 1} = 0.75 \text{ mL}$

15. Use the metric system. Give 2 tablets (gr ½ = 30 mg).

16. BF: $\dfrac{D}{H} \times V = \dfrac{100}{125} \times 5 \text{ mL} = \dfrac{500}{125} = 4 \text{ mL}$

or

RP: H   :   V   ::   D   :X
   125 mg:5 mL::100 mg:X
      125 X = 500
         X = 4 mL

or

FE: $\dfrac{125 \text{ mg}}{5 \text{ mL}} = \dfrac{100 \text{ mg}}{X} = 125 \text{ X} = 500$

X = 4 mL

or

DA: no conversion factor

$\text{mL} = \dfrac{5 \text{ mL} \times \overset{4}{\cancel{100 \text{ mg}}}}{\underset{5}{\cancel{125 \text{ mg}}} \times 1} = \dfrac{20}{5} = 4 \text{ mL}$

17. a. Preferred the selection of Crestor 10-mg bottle. Could select Crestor 5-mg bottle; however, the number of tablets given would have to be increased.

b. 2 tablets from Crestor 10-mg bottle. If Crestor 5-mg bottle was selected, then 4 tablets.

18. Nitrostat 0.4 mg

19. Change grams to milligrams: 0.400 g = 400 mg

BF: $\dfrac{D}{H} \times V = \dfrac{400 \text{ mg}}{100 \text{ mg}} \times 5 \text{ mL} = 20 \text{ mL}$

or

RP: H :V ::   D   : X
   100 : 5 :: 400 : X
   100 X = 2000
      X = 20 mL

or

FE: $\dfrac{H}{V} = \dfrac{D}{X} = \dfrac{100 \text{ mg}}{5 \text{ mL}} = \dfrac{400 \text{ mg}}{X}$

100 X = 2000
   X = 20 mL

or

DA: $\text{mL} = \dfrac{5 \text{ mL} \times 400 \text{ mg}}{100 \text{ mg} \times 1} = 20 \text{ mL}$

20. a. Preferred: the selection of Lanoxin 0.125-mg (125-mcg) bottle. Could select Lanoxin 0.5-mg (500-mcg) bottle because the tablets are scored.

b. 2 tablets from the Lanoxin 0.125-mg bottle or ½ tablet from the Lanoxin 0.5-mg bottle.

21. ½ tablet

22. BF: $\dfrac{D}{H} \times V = \dfrac{6 \text{ mg}}{4 \text{ mg}} \times 5 \text{ mL} = \dfrac{30}{4} = 7.5 \text{ mL of Zofran}$

23. 1½ tablets

24. a. 50 mg per day

b. BF: $\dfrac{D}{H} \times V = \dfrac{25 \text{ mg}}{12.5 \text{ mg}} \times 1 \text{ tab} = 2 \text{ tablets}$

or

RP: H   :   V   ::   D   :   X
12.5 mg : 1 tab :: 25 mg : X tab
12.5 mg X = 25 mg
X = 2 tablets

or

FE: $\dfrac{H}{V} = \dfrac{D}{X} = \dfrac{12.5 \text{ mg}}{1 \text{ tablet}} = \dfrac{25 \text{ mg}}{X} =$

12.5 X = 25
X = 2 tablets

or

DA: tablets $= \dfrac{1 \text{ tab} \times \overset{2}{\cancel{25 \text{ mg}}}}{\underset{1}{\cancel{12.5 \text{ mg}}} \times 1} = 2 \text{ tablets}$

25. a. Initially, first day

BF: $\dfrac{D}{H} \times V = \dfrac{\overset{3}{\cancel{1.5 \text{ mg}}}}{\underset{1}{\cancel{0.5 \text{ mg}}}} \times 1 = 3 \text{ tablets}$

or

RP: H   :   V   ::   D   :X
0.5 mg : 1 tab :: 1.5 mg : X
0.5 X = 1.5
X = 3 tablets of Cogentin

b. Second day and ON

FE: $\dfrac{H}{V} = \dfrac{D}{X} = \dfrac{0.5 \text{ mg}}{1} = \dfrac{1 \text{ mg}}{X}$

0.5 X = 1
X = 2 tablets

or

DA: tablet $= \dfrac{1 \text{ tab} \times \overset{2}{\cancel{1 \text{ mg}}}}{\underset{1}{\cancel{0.5 \text{ mg}}} \times 1} = 2 \text{ tablets of Cogentin}$

26. 12 mL of Diflucan

27. a. 300 mg per 5 mL

b. BF: $\dfrac{D}{H} \times V = \dfrac{\overset{2}{\cancel{600 \text{ mg}}}}{\underset{1}{\cancel{300 \text{ mg}}}} \times 5 \text{ mL} = 10 \text{ mL of lithium}$

or

RP: H   :   V   ::   D   :X
300 mg : 5 mL :: 600 mg : X
300 X = 3000
X = 10 mL

or

FE: $\dfrac{H}{V} = \dfrac{D}{X} = \dfrac{300 \text{ mg}}{5 \text{ mL}} = \dfrac{600 \text{ mg}}{X}$

300 X = 3000
X = 10 mL of lithium

or

DA: mL $= \dfrac{5 \text{ mL} \times \overset{2}{\cancel{600 \text{ mg}}}}{\underset{1}{\cancel{300 \text{ mg}}} \times 1} = 10 \text{ mL}$

c. 600 mg × 3 (tid) = 1800 mg per day

28. a. Loading dose

BF: $\dfrac{D}{H} \times V = \dfrac{100 \text{ mg}}{40 \text{ mg}} \times 4 \text{ mL} =$

$\dfrac{400}{40} = 10 \text{ mL of furosemide}$

or

RP: H   :   V   ::   D   :X
40 mg : 4 mL :: 100 mg : X
40 X = 400
X = 10 mL

b. Per dose

FE: $\dfrac{H}{V} = \dfrac{D}{X} = \dfrac{40 \text{ mg}}{4 \text{ mL}} = \dfrac{20 \text{ mg}}{X}$

40 X = 80
X = 2 mL

or

DA: mL $= \dfrac{4 \text{ mL} \times \overset{1}{\cancel{20 \text{ mg}}}}{\underset{2}{\cancel{40 \text{ mg}}} \times 1} = \dfrac{4}{2} = 2 \text{ mL of furosemide}$

29. 10 mL

30. **BF:** $\dfrac{D}{H} \times V = \dfrac{30 \text{ mg}}{20 \text{ mg}} \times 5 \text{ mL} =$

$\dfrac{150}{20} = 7.5$ mL of Prozac

or

DA: $\text{mL} = \dfrac{5 \text{ mL} \times \overset{3}{\cancel{30 \text{ mg}}}}{\underset{2}{\cancel{20 \text{ mg}}} \times 1} = \dfrac{15}{2} = 7.5$ mL of Prozac

Additional Dimensional Analysis

31. **DA:** $\text{tab} = \dfrac{1 \text{ tab} \times 1.5 \text{ mg}}{0.5 \text{ mg} \times 1} = \dfrac{1.5}{0.5} = 3$ tablets of Ativan

32. $\text{tablets} = \dfrac{1 \times \overset{2}{\cancel{5.0 \text{ mg}}}}{\underset{1}{\cancel{2.5 \text{ mg}}} \times 1} = 2$ tablets of Vasotec

33. **BF:** $\dfrac{D}{H} \times V = \dfrac{60 \text{ mg}}{20 \text{ mg}} \times 5 \text{ mL} = 15 \text{ mL}$

FE: $\dfrac{H}{V} = \dfrac{D}{X} = \dfrac{20 \text{ mg}}{5 \text{ mL}} = \dfrac{60 \text{ mg}}{X}$

$20 X = 300$

$X = 15 \text{ mL}$

or

RP: $H : V :: D : X$

$20 \text{ mg} : 5 \text{ mL} :: 60 \text{ mg} : X$

$20 X \boxtimes 300$

$X \boxtimes 15 \text{ mL}$

or

DA: no conversion factor

$\text{mL} = \dfrac{5 \text{ mL} \times 60 \text{ mg}}{20 \text{ mg} \times 1} = 15 \text{ mL}$

34. **DA:** $\text{cap} = \dfrac{1 \text{ cap} \times \overset{4}{\cancel{1000 \text{ mg}}} \times 1 \text{ g}}{\underset{1}{\cancel{250 \text{ mg}}} \times 1 \text{ g} \times 1} = 4$ capsules of Keflex

35. **DA:** $\text{tab} = \dfrac{1 \text{ tab} \times \overset{20}{\cancel{1000 \text{ mg}}} \times 0.1 \cancel{\text{ g}}}{\underset{1}{\cancel{50 \text{ mg}}} \times 1 \cancel{\text{ g}} \times 1} = \dfrac{20 \times 0.1}{1} = 2$ tablets of Lopressor

36. **DA:** $\text{mL} = \dfrac{5 \text{ mL} \times \overset{4}{\cancel{1000 \text{ mg}}} \times 0.4 \cancel{\text{ g}}}{\underset{1}{\cancel{250 \text{ mg}}} \times 1 \cancel{\text{ g}} \times 1} = 8 \text{ mL}$

Give 8 mL per dose of amoxicillin.

37. Drug label: 325 mg = 1 tablet

DA: $\text{tablet} = \dfrac{1 \text{ tab} \times \overset{2}{\cancel{650 \text{ mg}}}}{\underset{1}{\cancel{325 \text{ mg}}} \times 1} = 2$ tablets

38. **a.** 1 tablet of Tenormin

b. DA: $\text{tablet} = \dfrac{1 \text{ tablet} \times \overset{2}{\cancel{100 \text{ mg}}}}{\underset{1}{\cancel{50 \text{ mg}}} \times 1} = 2$ tablets of Tenormin

39. BF: $\dfrac{D}{H} \times V = \dfrac{25\,g}{10\,g} \times 15\,mL = 37.5\,mL$

or
RP: $H : V :: D :X$
$\qquad 10\,g:15\,mL::25\,g:X$
$\qquad\qquad 10\,X = 375$
$\qquad\qquad\quad X = 37.5\,mL$

or
FE: $\dfrac{H}{V} = \dfrac{D}{X} = \dfrac{10\,g}{15\,mL} = \dfrac{25\,g}{X}$

(Cross multiply) $10\,X = 375$
$\qquad\qquad\qquad X = 37.5\,mL$

or
DA: $mL = \dfrac{15\,mL \times 25\,mg}{10\,mg \times \quad 1} = 37.5\,mL$

40. 165 lbs = 75 kg (change pounds to kilograms by dividing by 2.2 into 165 pounds, or 165 ÷ 2.2)
    10 mg/kg/day $\times$ 75 = 750 mg/day
    750 ÷ 3 = 250 mg, tid
41. 154 lbs = 70 kg
    4 mg/kg/day $\times$ 70 kg = 280 mg/day
42. 132 lbs = 60 kg
    2.5 mg/kg/day $\times$ 60 kg = 150 mg **or** 100 mg/m^2 $\times$ 1.7 m^2 = 170 mg
43. **a.** 20 mg/50 kg/day = 20 $\times$ 50 = 1000 mg per day
    b. 2 tablets of Zarontin per dose (500 mg per dose)
44. **a.** 4 mg/60 kg/day = 4 $\times$ 60 = 240 mg per day **or** 120 mg, q12h

b. BF: $\dfrac{D}{H} \times V = \dfrac{120\,mg}{\underset{10}{\cancel{50}\,mg}} \times \cancel{5}^{\,1}\,mL = \dfrac{120}{10} = 12\,mL$

or
RP: $\quad H : V :: D :X$
$\qquad 50\,mg . 5\,mL::120\,mg:X$
$\qquad\qquad 50\,X = 600$
$\qquad\qquad\quad X = \dfrac{600}{50} = 12\,mL$

or
DA: $mL = \dfrac{5\,mL \times \overset{12}{\cancel{120}\,mg}}{\underset{5}{\cancel{50}\,mg} \times \quad 1} = \dfrac{60}{5} = 12\,mL$

Give 12 mL per dose of minocycline.

45. BF: $\dfrac{D}{H} \times V = \dfrac{150\,mg}{75\,mg} \times 1\,tab = 2\,tablets$

or
RP: $\quad H : V :: D :X$
$\qquad 75\,mg:1\,tab::150\,mg:X$
$\qquad\qquad 75\,X = 150$
$\qquad\qquad\quad X = 2\,tablets$

46. BF: $\dfrac{D}{H} \times V = \dfrac{10\,mg}{20\,mg} \times 1\,tab = 0.5\ or\ \tfrac{1}{2}\,tablet$

or
RP: $\quad H : V :: D :X$
$\qquad 20\,mg:1\,tab::10\,mg:X$
$\qquad\qquad 20\,X = 10$
$\qquad\qquad\quad X = 0.5\ or\ \tfrac{1}{2}\,tablet$

Case

1. d. Give 2 ½ tablets now

$$\frac{D}{H} = \frac{50\ mg}{20\ mg} \times 1\ \text{tab} = 2\frac{1}{2}\ Tablets$$

For additional practice problems, refer to the Oral Dosages section of the Elsevier's Interactive Drug Calculation Application, Version 1 on Evolve.

CHAPTER 9

Injectable Preparations
With Clinical Applications

Objectives
- Select the correct syringe and needle for a prescribed injectable drug.
- Calculate dosages of drugs for subcutaneous and intramuscular routes from solutions in vials and ampules.
- Explain the procedure for preparing and calculating medications in powder form for injectable use.
- State the various sites for intramuscular injection.
- Explain how to administer intradermal, subcutaneous, and intramuscular injections.

Outline
INJECTABLE PREPARATIONS
INTRADERMAL INJECTIONS
SUBCUTANEOUS INJECTIONS
INTRAMUSCULAR INJECTIONS
MIXING OF INJECTABLE DRUGS

Parenteral medications are those that are administered by any route other than the gastrointestinal tract and include all injectable medications. The parenteral route may be preferred if the patient cannot take oral medications. They are also absorbed more rapidly than the enteral route, and they are useful when patients are unconscious or uncooperative. The most common parenteral routes are:

Intradermal (ID): The needle is inserted just under the epidermis in the dermal layer of the skin.
Subcutaneous (subcut, subQ, SC, and SQ): The needle is placed farther into the fatty tissue of the skin.
Intramuscular (IM): The needle is inserted directly into the muscle.
Intravenous (IV): The needle or medication is injected directly into the vein. (Intravenous injectables are discussed in Chapter 10.)

Because these routes are commonly used in drug orders, they are often abbreviated. It is essential that injectable drugs be given by the correct route. Any use of abbreviations should follow institutional policies and protocols.

Injectable drugs are ordered in grams, milligrams, micrograms, or international units. The drug manufacturer prepares the medication as either a liquid or a powder according to the stability of the compound. The nurse's responsibility is to have working knowledge of all types of injectable preparations, the equipment for injections, and the routes of administration.

INJECTABLE PREPARATIONS

Vials and Ampules

Drugs are packaged in vials (sealed rubber-top containers) for single and multiple doses and in ampules (sealed glass containers) for a single dose. Multiple-dose vials can be used more than once because of their self-sealing rubber top; however, ampules are used only once after the glass-necked container is opened. A 15-gauge filtered needle should be used with a glass ampule to prevent aspiration of small glass particles. The drug is available in either liquid or powder form in vials and ampules. When drugs in solution deteriorate rapidly, they are packaged in dry form, and solvent (diluent) is added before administration. If the drug is in powdered form, mixing instructions and dose equivalents such as milligrams (mg) per milliliter (mL) are usually given; if not, check the drug information insert. After the dry form of the drug is reconstituted with sterile water, bacteriostatic water (sterile water with a small amount of benzyl alcohol to prevent bacterial growth), or saline solution, the drug must be used immediately or refrigerated. Usually, the reconstituted drug in the vial is used within 48 hours to 1 week; check the drug information insert. A Mix-O-Vial has two containers, one holding a diluent and the other holding a powdered drug. When pressure is applied to the top of the vial, the liquid is released, which dissolves the powdered drug. A vial, a Mix-O-Vial, and an ampule are shown in Figure 9.1.

The route by which the injectable drug can be given, such as subcut or SQ, IM, or IV, is printed on the drug label.

Syringes

There are three types of syringes for injection: hypodermic, tuberculin, and insulin (insulin syringes are discussed in Chapter 10). Syringes come in a variety of sizes from 0.3 mL to 60 mL or greater. The 3-mL and 5-mL syringes are used most commonly with injectable medications. Syringes that hold more than 5 mL are used mostly for drug preparation. A syringe is composed of a barrel (outer shell); a plunger (inner part); and the tip, where the needle joins the syringe (Figure 9.2).

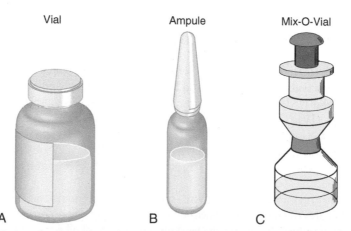

Vial   Ampule   Mix-O-Vial

A   B   C

Figure 9.1 A, Vial. **B,** Ampule. (From Kee, J. L., Hayes, E. R., & McCuistion, L. E. [2015]. *Pharmacology: a patient-centered nursing process approach,* 8th ed., Philadelphia: Elsevier.) **C,** Mix-O-vial. (From Clayton BD, Willihnganz M: *Basic pharmacology for nurses,* ed 17, St Louis, 2017, Mosby.)

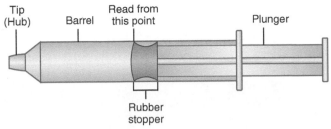

Figure 9.2 Parts of a syringe.

Three-Milliliter Syringe

The 3-mL syringe is calibrated in tenths (0.1 mL). The amount of fluid in the syringe is determined by the rubber end of the plunger that is closer to the tip of the syringe (Figure 9.3). An advance in safety needle technology is the SafetyGlide shielding hypodermic needle (Figure 9.4). The purpose of this type of needle is to reduce needlestick injuries. Needles should never be recapped by hand and should always be disposed of in a sharps container (Figure 9.5).

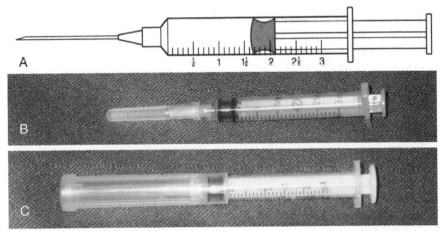

Figure 9.3 Three-milliliter syringes: **A,** 3-mL syringe with 0.1-mL markings. **B,** 3-mL syringe with a needle cover. **C,** 3-mL syringe with a protective cover over the needle after injection. (**B** and **C** from Kee, J. L., Hayes, E. R., & McCuistion, L. E. [2015]. *Pharmacology: a patient-centered nursing process approach.* 8th ed., Philadelphia: Elsevier.)

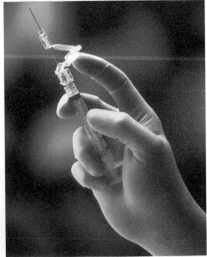

Figure 9.4 BD SafetyGlide™ needle. (Courtesy and © Becton, Dickinson and Company)

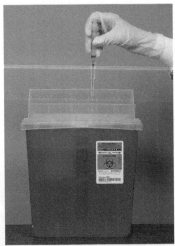

Figure 9.5 Sharps container. (From Clayton BD, Willihnganz M: *Basic pharmacology for nurses,* ed 17, St Louis, 2017, Mosby.)

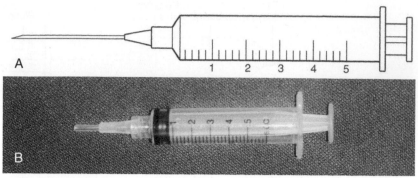

Figure 9.6 Five-milliliter syringes. **A,** 5-mL syringe with 0.2-mL markings. **B,** Needleless 5-mL syringe that can penetrate a rubber-top vial. (**B** from Kee, J. L., Hayes, E. R., & McCuistion, L. E. [2015]. *Pharmacology: a patient-centered nursing process approach.* 8th ed., Philadelphia: Elsevier.)

Five-Milliliter Syringe

The 5-mL syringe is calibrated in 0.2 mL increments. A 5-mL syringe usually is used when the fluid needed is more than 2½ mL. This syringe is frequently used to draw up appropriate solution to dilute the dry form of a drug in a vial because the volume needed for reconstitution is generally more than 2½ mL. Figure 9.6 shows the 5-mL syringe and its markings and the 5-mL needleless syringe.

Tuberculin Syringe

The tuberculin syringe has a capacity of either 0.5-mL or 1-mL. It is calibrated in tenths (0.1 mL) and in hundredths (0.01 mL) (Figure 9.7). This syringe is used when the amount of drug solution to be administered is less than 1 mL. Tuberculin syringes are commonly used for skin testing as well as pediatric and heparin dosages. Figure 9.8 shows the 0.5-mL and 1-mL tuberculin syringes.

Pre-filled Drug Cartridge and Syringe

Many injectable drugs are packaged in pre-filled disposable cartridges. The disposable cartridge is placed into a reusable metal or plastic holder. A pre-filled cartridge usually contains 0.1 to 0.2 mL of excess drug solution. On the basis of the amount of drug to be administered, the excess solution must be expelled before administration. Injectables are also supplied by pharmaceutical companies in ready-to-use pre-filled syringes that do not require a holder. Figure 9.9, *A,* shows a Carpuject syringe. Figure 9.9, *B,* shows a Tubex syringe. Figure 9.9, *C,* shows a pre-filled Lovenox syringe.

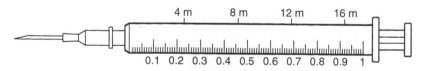

Figure 9.7 Tuberculin syringe.

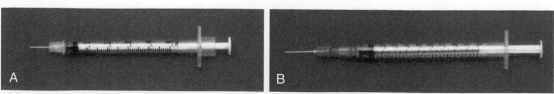

Figure 9.8 Two types of tuberculin syringes: **A,** ½-mL tuberculin syringe with a permanently attached needle. **B,** 1-mL tuberculin syringe with a detachable needle. (Courtesy and © Becton, Dickinson and Company)

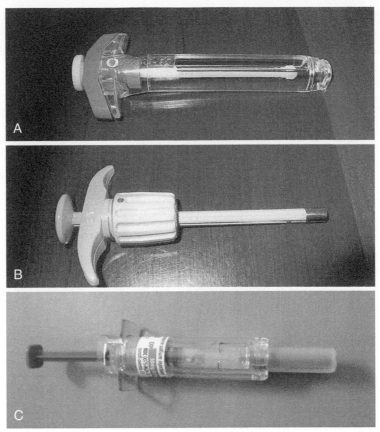

Figure 9.9 A, Carpuject syringe. **B,** Tubex syringe. (From Kee, J. L., Hayes, E. R., & McCuistion, L. E. [2015]. *Pharmacology: a patient-centered nursing process approach.* 8th ed., Elsevier: Saunders.) **C,** Lovenox syringe.

Needles

A needle consists of a hub (large metal or plastic part attached to the tip of the syringe), a shaft (thin needle length), and a bevel (end of the needle). Figure 9.10 shows the parts of a needle.

Needle size is determined by gauge (diameter of the shaft) and by length. Higher gauge numbers indicate a smaller needle diameter, and lower gauge numbers indicate a wider needle diameter. Needle selection depends on a variety of factors including size of the patient, location to be administered, viscosity of medication, and the condition of the skin. For example, when administering blood products, a lower gauge needle (higher shaft diameter) is preferred due to the high viscosity of blood. Table 9.1 lists the sizes and lengths of needles used in intradermal, subcutaneous, and intramuscular injections.

Pre-filled cartridges have permanently attached needles. With other syringes, needle sizes can be changed. Needle gauge and length are indicated on the syringe package or on the top cover of the syringe. These values appear as gauge/length, such as 21 g/1½ inch. Figure 9.11 shows two types of needle gauge and length.

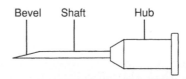

Figure 9.10 Parts of a needle. (From Kee, J. L., Hayes, E. R., & McCuistion, L. E. [2015]. *Pharmacology: a patient-centered nursing process approach.* 8th ed., Philadelphia: Elsevier.)

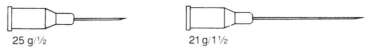

TABLE 9.1 Needle Size and Length		
Type of Injection	**Needle Gauge**	**Needle Lengths (inch)**
Intradermal	25, 26	$^3/_8$, $^1/_2$, $^5/_8$
Subcutaneous	23, 25, 26	$^3/_8$, $^1/_2$, $^5/_8$
Intramuscular	18, 19, 20, 21, 22	1, 1½, 2

25 g/½ 21 g/1½

Figure 9.11 Two combinations of needle gauge and length.

Research has shown that after an injection, medication remains in the hub of the syringe, where the needle joins the syringe. This volume can be as much as 0.2 mL. There is controversy as to whether air should be added to the syringe before administration to ensure that the total volume is given. The best practice is to follow the institution's policy.

Angles for Injection

For injections, the needle enters the skin at different angles. Intradermal injections are given at a 10- to 15-degree angle; subcutaneous injections, at a 45- to 90-degree angle; and intramuscular injections, at a 90-degree angle. Figure 9.12 shows the angles for intradermal, subcutaneous, and intramuscular injections.

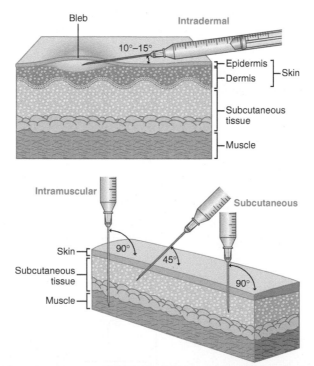

Figure 9.12 Angles of injection. (From Kee, J. L., Hayes, E. R., & McCuistion, L. E. [2015]. *Pharmacology: a patient-centered nursing process approach.*. 8th ed., Philadelphia: Elsevier.)

PRACTICE PROBLEMS ▶ | NEEDLES

Answers can be found on page 191.

1. Which would have the larger needle lumen: a 21-gauge needle or a 25-gauge needle?

_____

2. Which would have the smaller needle lumen: an 18-gauge needle or a 26-gauge needle?

_____

3. Which needle would have a length of 1½ inches: a 20-gauge needle or a 25-gauge needle?

_____

4. Which needle would have a length of ⅝ inch: a 21-gauge needle or a 25-gauge needle?

_____

5. Which needle would be used for an intramuscular injection: a 21-gauge needle with a 1½-inch length or a 25-gauge needle with a ⅝-inch length?

_____

INTRADERMAL INJECTIONS

Intradermal injections (ID) are designed to deliver medication into the dermis, just below the epidermis. This route has the longest absorption time of all the parenteral routes. It is typically used for skin testing (tuberculin and allergy tests). It is also used for local anesthesia to the skin. Tuberculin syringes are commonly used for ID injections. The dosage given is usually less than 0.5 mL.

The inner aspect of the forearm is often used for diagnostic testing because there is less hair in the area and the test results are easily seen. The upper back can also be used as a testing site. The needle is inserted with the bevel upward at a 5 to 15-degree angle. Do not aspirate. The injected fluid creates a wheal or blister that is slowly absorbed. For allergy testing, results are usually read in minutes to 24 hours after the injection. For tuberculin testing, results are read 48-72 hours after the injection. A reddened or raised hardened area, called the area of induration, indicates a positive reaction.

SUBCUTANEOUS INJECTIONS

Drugs injected into the subcutaneous (fatty) tissue are absorbed slowly because there are fewer blood vessels in the fatty tissue. The amount of drug solution administered subcutaneously is generally 0.5 to mL at a 45-, 60-, or 90-degree angle. Irritating drug solutions are given intramuscularly because they could cause sloughing of the subcutaneous tissue.

The two types of syringes used for subcutaneous injection are the tuberculin syringe (1 mL), which is calibrated in 0.1 and 0.01 mL, and the 3-mL syringe, which is calibrated in 0.1 mL (Figure 9.13). The needle gauge commonly used is 25 or 26 gauge, and the length is usually ⅜ to ⅝ inch. Insulin and heparin are both administered subcutaneously and will be discussed in Chapters 10 and 12, respectively.

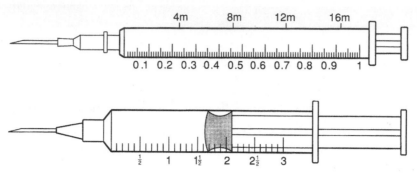

Figure 9.13 Syringes used for subcutaneous injections.

Calculations for Subcutaneous Injections

Types of formulas for calculating small dosages include the following: (1) basic formula, (2) ratio and proportion, (3) fractional equation, and (4) dimensional analysis (see Chapter 6).

EXAMPLES **PROBLEM 1:** Order: Hydromorphone 1 mg, subcut.
Drug available:

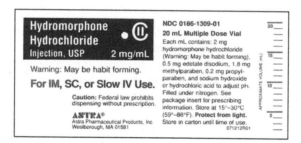

Methods: **BF:**

$$\frac{D}{H} \times V = \frac{1}{2} \times 1 = \frac{1}{2} = 0.5 \text{ mL}$$

RP:

$$H : V :: D : X$$
$$2 : 1 :: 1 : X$$
$$2\,X = 1$$
$$X = 0.5 \text{ mL}$$

FE:

$$\frac{H}{V} = \frac{D}{X} = \frac{2}{1} = \frac{1}{X} =$$

(Cross multiply) $2\,X = 1$

$$X = 0.5 \text{ mL}$$

DA:

$$V = \frac{V}{H} \times \frac{D}{1} = \frac{1}{2} \times \frac{1}{1} = \frac{1}{2} = 0.5 \text{ mL}$$

Answer: 0.5 mL

PROBLEM 2: Order: morphine 10 mg, subcut.
Drug available:

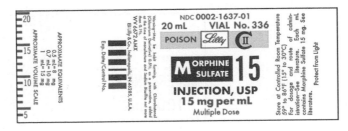

See label with approximate equivalents.

Methods: **BF**: $\dfrac{D}{H} \times V = \dfrac{10 \text{ mg}}{15 \text{ mg}} \times 1 \text{ mL} = \dfrac{2}{3} = 0.67 \text{ mL or } 0.7 \text{ mL} \left(\text{round off in tenths}\right)$

or

RP: $\text{H} \; : \; \text{V} \; :: \; \text{D} \; : \; \text{X}$

$15 \text{ mg} : 1 \text{ mL} :: 10 \text{ mg} : \text{X mL}$

$15 \text{ X} = 10$

$\text{X} = \dfrac{\overset{2}{\cancel{10}}}{\underset{3}{\cancel{15}}} = \dfrac{2}{3} = 0.67 \text{ mL or } 0.7 \text{ mL}$

or

FE: $\dfrac{\text{H}}{\text{V}} = \dfrac{\text{D}}{\text{X}} = \dfrac{15 \text{ mg}}{1 \text{ mL}} = \dfrac{10 \text{ mg}}{\text{X}} =$

(Cross multiply) $15 \text{ X} = 10$

$\text{X} = \dfrac{10}{15} = \dfrac{2}{3} =$

$0.67 \text{ or } 0.7 \text{ mL}$

or

DA: no conversion factor

$\text{mL} = \dfrac{1 \text{ mL} \times \overset{2}{\cancel{10 \text{ mg}}}}{\underset{3}{\cancel{15 \text{ mg}}} \times 1} = \dfrac{2}{3} \text{ or } 0.7 \text{ mL}$

Answer: morphine 10 mg = 0.67 or 0.7 mL (use a tuberculin syringe or a 3-mL syringe). (Round off in tenths.)

PRACTICE PROBLEMS ▶ II SUBCUTANEOUS INACTIONS

Answers can be found on pages 191 to 192.

Use the formula you chose for calculating oral drug dosages in Chapter 8.

Note: Answers should be rounded off in tenths or whole numbers.

1. Which needle gauge and length should be used for a subcutaneous injection?

   a. 25 g/⁵⁄₈ inch or 26 g/³⁄₈ inch?_____

2. Order: Meperidine 75 mg, subcut.
   Drug available:

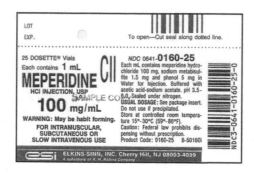

   a. How many milliliters of Meperidine would you give?_____

   b. At what angle would you administer the drug?_____

3. Order: Narcan 0.2 mg, subcut.
   Drug available:

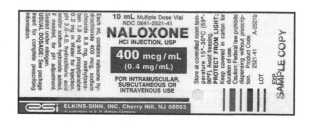

How many milliliters of narcan would you give?_____

4. Order: Epogen 13,000 units, subcut.
   Drug available:

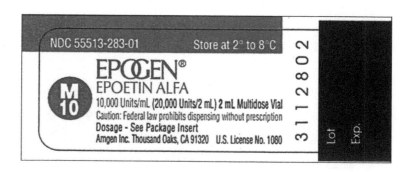

How many units of epogen would you give?_____

5. Order: atropine sulfate 0.6 mg, subcut.
Drug available:

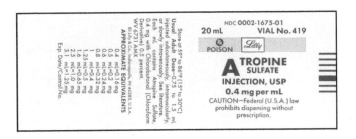

How many milliliters of atropine would you give?_____

6. Order: Relistor 8 mg, subcut.
Drug available: 12 mg/0.6 mL single dose vial

How many milliliters would you give?_____

7. Order: filgrastim (Neupogen) 6 mcg/kg, subcut, bid.
Drug available:

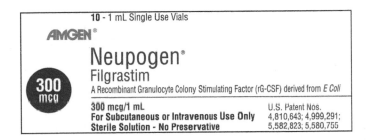

Patient weighs 198 pounds.

   a. How many kilograms does the patient weigh?_____

   b. How many micrograms (mcg) would you give? _____

   c. How many milliliters would you give? _____

   d. Explain how the drug should be drawn up. _____

8. Order: Epinephrine 0.3 mg, subcut.
Drug available: 30 mL multi-dose vial contains 1 mg epinephrine per 1 mL.

How many milliliters would you give? _____

9. Order: morphine 8 mg, subcut, × 1 dose.
Drug available:

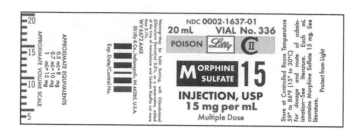

How many milliliters would the patient receive? _____

10. Order: Fragmin 120 units/kg, subcut, q12h.
Drug available:

> 10 x 0.4 mL single dose syringes,   NDC 62856-100-10
> preassembled with needle guards   Rx only
>
> **Fragmin®**
> dalteparin sodium injection
>
> For subcutaneous injection
>
> **10,000 IU (anti-Xa) per 0.4 mL***
>
> Eisai Inc.   Pfizer Inc

Patient weighs 65 kg.

a. How many international units (IU) would the patient receive per dose?_____

b. How many milliliters would the patient receive per dose?_____

INTRAMUSCULAR INJECTIONS

The IM injection is a common method of administering injectable drugs. The muscle has many blood vessels (more than fatty tissue), so medications given by IM injection are absorbed more rapidly than those given by subcutaneous injection. The volume of solution for an IM injection is 0.5 to 3.0 mL, with the average being 1 to 2 mL. A volume of drug solution greater than 3 mL causes increased muscle tissue displacement and possible tissue damage. Occasionally, 5 mL of certain drugs, such as magnesium sulfate, may be injected into a large muscle, such as the ventrogluteal. Dosages greater than 3 mL are usually divided and are given at two different sites.

Needle gauges for IM injections containing thick solutions are 19 gauge and 20 gauge, and for thin solutions, 20 gauge to 21 gauge. IM injections are administered at a 90-degree angle. The needle length depends on the amount of adipose (fat) and muscle tissue; the average needle length is 1½ inches.

The *Z*-track injection technique delivers medication intramuscularly in a method that prevents the drug from leaking back into the subcutaneous tissue (Figure 9.14). This method is ordered for medications that could cause irritation to the subcutaneous tissue or discoloration to the skin. When preparing the medication, a needle change is made after the drug has been drawn up into the syringe and before it is injected into the patient. The large gluteal muscle is frequently used for *Z*-track injections.

Common sites for IM injections are the deltoid, dorsogluteal, ventrogluteal, and vastus lateralis muscles. Figure 9.15 displays the sites for each muscle used with IM injection. Table 9.2 gives the volume for drug administration, common needle size, patient's position, and angle of injection for the four IM injection sites.

Note: Some institutions may prohibit using the dorsogluteal for intramuscular injections due to the close proximity of the sciatic nerve to the injection site. Always check institutional policy and procedures.

Drug Solutions for Injection

Commercially premixed drug solutions are stored in vials and ampules for immediate use. At times, enough drug solution may be left in a vial for another dose, and the vial may be saved. The balance of a drug solution in an ampule is *always* discarded after the ampule has been opened and used. For multi-dose vials, injecting air into the vial, equivalent to the volume of medication to be given, will aid in aspirating the medication from the vial.

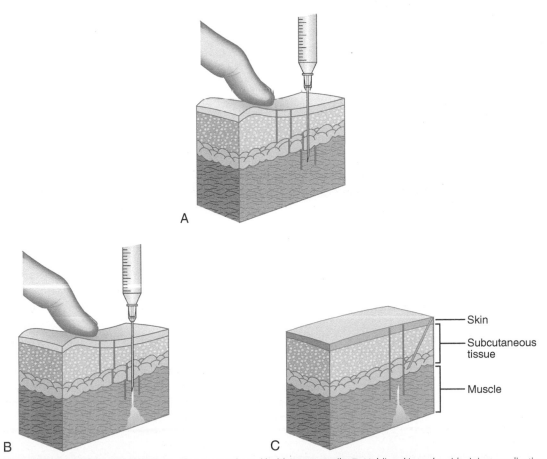

Figure 9.14 Z-track injection. **A,** Pull the skin to one side and hold; insert needle. **B,** Holding skin to the side, inject medication. **C,** Withdraw needle and release skin. This technique prevents medication from entering subcutaneous tissue. (From Kee, J. L., Hayes, E. R., & McCuistion, L. E. [2015]. *Pharmacology: a patient-centered nursing process approach,* 8th ed., Philadelphia: Elsevier.)

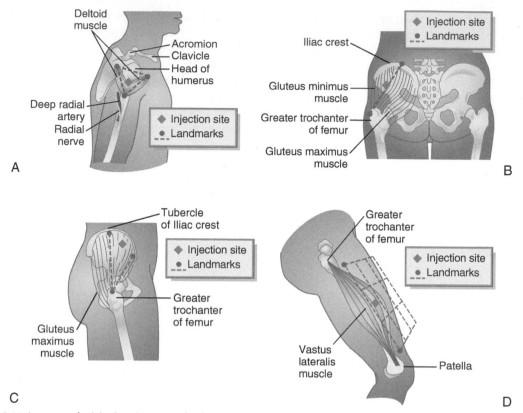

Figure 9.15 Intramuscular injection sites. **A,** Deltoid. **B,** Dorsogluteal. **C,** Ventrogluteal. **D,** Vastus lateralis. (From Kee, J. L., Hayes, E. R., & McCuistion, L. E. [2015]. *Pharmacology: a patient-centered nursing process approach., 8th ed.,* Philadelphia: Elsevier.)

TABLE 9.2 Intramuscular Injection Sites in the Adult

	Deltoid	Dorsogluteal	Ventrogluteal	Vastus Lateralis
Volume for drug Administration	*Usual:* 0.5 to1 mL *Maximum:* 2.0 mL	*Usual:* 1.0 to 3 mL *Maximum:* 3 mL; 5 mL gamma globulin	*Usual:* 1 to 3 mL *Maximum:* 3 to4 mL	*Usual:* 1 to 3 mL Maximum: 3 to 4 mL
Common needle size	23 to 25 gauge; $^5/_8$ to 1½ inches	18 to 23 gauge; 1¼ to 3 inches	20 to 23 gauge; 1¼ to 2½ inches	20 to 23 gauge; 1¼ to 1½ inches
Patient's position	Sitting; supine; prone	Prone	Supine; lateral	Sitting (dorsiflex foot); supine
Angle of injection	90-degree angle, angled slightly toward the acromion	90-degree angle to flat surface; upper outer quadrant of the buttock *or* outer aspect of line from the posterior iliac crest to the greater trochanter of the femur	80- to 90-degree angle; angle the needle slightly toward the iliac crest	80- to 90-degree angle For thin person: 60- to 75-degree angle

EXAMPLES Here are two problems for calculating IM dosage, using all four methods and rounded to the nearest tenths.

   PROBLEM 1: Order: gentamycin (Garamycin) 60 mg, IM, q12h.
               Drug available:

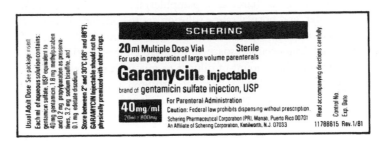

Methods: **BF:** $\dfrac{D}{H} \times V = \dfrac{60 \text{ mg}}{40 \text{ mg}} \times 1 \text{ mL} = \dfrac{3}{2}$ **or**   **RP:**   H : V :: D : X
$$= 1.5 \text{ mL of gentamycin}$$

   40 mg : 1 mL :: 60 mg : X mL
   40 X = 60
   X = 1.5 mL

or
FE: $\dfrac{H}{V} = \dfrac{D}{X} = \dfrac{40 \text{ mg}}{1 \text{ mL}} = \dfrac{60 \text{ mg}}{X} =$ **or**   **DA:** mL $= \dfrac{1 \text{ mL} \times \overset{3}{\cancel{60}} \text{ mg}}{\underset{2}{\cancel{40}} \text{ mg} \times 1} = \dfrac{3}{2}$

(Cross multiply) 40 X = 60
            X = 1.5 mL of gentamycin

$= 1.5 \text{ mL of gentamycin}$

Answer: gentamycin 60 mg = 1.5 mL

   PROBLEM 2: Order: Naloxone 0.5 mg, IM, STAT.
               Drug available:

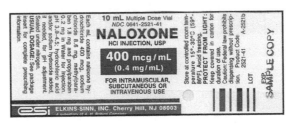

Methods: **BF:** $\dfrac{D}{H} \times V = \dfrac{0.5 \text{ mg}}{0.4 \text{ mg}} \times 1 \text{ mL} = 1.25 \text{ mL}$ **or**   **FE:** $\dfrac{H}{V} = \dfrac{D}{X}$

or

RP: H : V :: D : X

   0.4 mg : 1 mL :: 0.5 mg : X

$\dfrac{0.4 \text{ mg}}{1 \text{ mL}} = \dfrac{0.5 \text{ mg}}{X}$

0.4 X = 0.5
      X = 1.25 mL

   0.4 X = 0.5
      X = 1.25 mL

or
DA: mL $= \dfrac{1 \text{ mL} \times \overset{10}{\cancel{1000}} \text{ mcg} \times 0.5 \text{ mg}}{\underset{4}{\cancel{400}} \text{ mcg} \times 1 \text{ mg} \times 1} = \dfrac{10 \times 0.5}{4} = \dfrac{5}{4} = 1.25 \text{ mL}$

Answer: Naloxone 0.5 mg = 1.25 mL

Reconstitution of Powdered Drugs

Certain drugs lose their potency in liquid form. Therefore manufacturers package these drugs in powdered form, and they are reconstituted before administration. To reconstitute a drug, look on the drug label or in the drug information insert (circular or pamphlet) for the type and amount of diluent to use. Sterile water, bacteriostatic water, and normal saline solution are the primary diluents. If the type and amount of diluent are not specified on the drug label or in the drug information insert, call the pharmacy.

The powdered drug occupies space and therefore increases the volume of drug solution. Usually, manufacturers determine the amount of diluent to mix with the drug powder to yield 1 to 2 mL per desired dose. After the powdered drug has been reconstituted, the unused drug solution should be dated, initialed, and refrigerated. Most drugs retain their potency for 48 hours to 1 week when refrigerated. Check the drug information insert or drug label to see how long the reconstituted drug may be used.

EXAMPLES **PROBLEM 1:** Order: Tazicef 500 mg, IM, q8h.

Drug available:

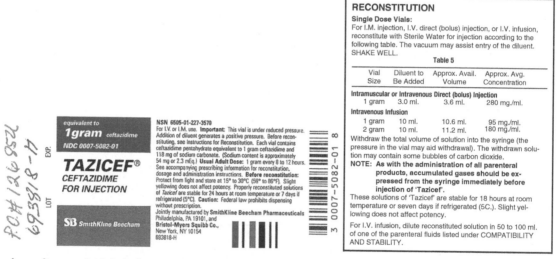

According to the label, the amount of powdered drug is 1 g. The drug label states for IM injection add 3 mL of sterile water (diluent) to the vial to yield a volume of 1 g/3.6 mL or 280 mg/mL.

Note: The diluent amount is different for IM versus IV formulation.

Milligrams

$$\text{BF: } \frac{D}{H} \times V = \frac{500 \text{ mg}}{280 \text{ mg}} \times 1 \text{ mL} = 1.78 \text{ mL} \qquad \textbf{or} \qquad \text{RP: } H \ : \ V \ :: \ D \ :X$$

or 1.8 mL

$$280 \text{ mg} : 1 \text{ mL} :: 500 \text{ mg} : X$$
$$280 \, X = 500$$
$$X = 1.78 \text{ mL or } 1.8 \text{ mL}$$

Grams

$$\text{DA: mL} = \frac{3.6 \text{ mL} \times \quad \cancel{1 \text{ g}} \quad \times \overset{1}{\cancel{500 \text{ mg}}}}{\cancel{1 \text{ g}} \times \underset{2}{\cancel{1000 \text{ mg}}} \times 1} = \frac{3.6}{2} \qquad \textbf{or} \qquad \text{FE: } \frac{H}{V} = \frac{D}{X} = \frac{280 \text{ mg}}{1 \text{ mL}} = \frac{500 \text{ mg}}{X}$$

$$= 1.8 \text{ mL}$$

(Cross multiply)
$$280 \, X = 500$$
$$X = 1.78 \text{ mL}$$
or 1.8 mL

Answer: Tazicef 500 mg = 1.8 mL

PROBLEM 2: Order: methylprednisolone 250 mg IM × 1 dose.
Drug available:

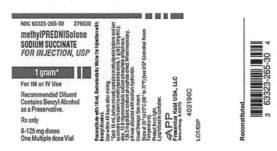

The drug label says to add 16 mL bacteriostatic water to reconstitute 1 g of methyl-prednisolone.

Change grams to milligrams (1 g = 1000 mg).

BF: $\dfrac{D}{H} \times V = \dfrac{250 \text{ mg}}{1000 \text{ mg}} \times 16 \text{ mL} = 4 \text{ mL}$ **or**   **RP:**   H : V :: D :X

$$1000 \text{ mg}:16 \text{ mg}::250 \text{ mg}:\text{X}$$
$$1000 \text{ X} = 4000$$
$$\text{X} = 4 \text{ mL}$$

FE: $\dfrac{H}{V} = \dfrac{D}{X}$ **or**   **DA:** $\text{mL} = \dfrac{16 \text{ mL} \times \quad \cancel{1\text{g}} \quad \times \overset{1}{\cancel{250 \text{ mg}}}}{\cancel{1\text{g}} \quad \times \underset{4}{\cancel{1000 \text{ mg}}} \times \quad 1} = \dfrac{16}{4} = 4 \text{ mL}$

$$\dfrac{1000 \text{ mg}}{16 \text{ mL}} = \dfrac{250 \text{ mg}}{\text{X}}$$
$$1000 \text{ X} = 4000$$
$$\text{X} = 4 \text{ mL}$$

Answer: methylprednisolone 250 mg = 4 mL. Since the volume of the ordered drug is greater than 3 mL, the dose should be divided into 2 mL per injection site.

MIXING OF INJECTABLE DRUGS

Drugs mixed together in the same syringe must be compatible to prevent precipitation. To determine drug compatibility, check drug references or check with a pharmacist. When in doubt about compatibility, do *not* mix drugs.

The three methods of drug mixing are (1) mixing two drugs in the same syringe from two vials, (2) mixing two drugs in the same syringe from one vial and one ampule, and (3) mixing two drugs in a pre-filled cartridge from a vial.

▶ Method 1
Mixing Two Drugs in the Same Syringe From Two Vials
1. Draw air into the syringe to equal the amount of solution to be withdrawn from the first vial, and inject the air into the first vial. Do *not* allow the needle to come into contact with the solution. Remove the needle.
2. Draw air into the syringe to equal the amount of solution to be withdrawn from the second vial. Invert the second vial and inject the air.
3. Withdraw the desired amount of solution from the second vial.
4. Change the needle unless you will use the entire volume in the first vial.
5. Invert the first vial and withdraw the desired amount of solution.

or

1. Draw air into the syringe to equal the amount of solution to be withdrawn, and inject the air into the first vial. Withdraw the desired drug dose.
2. Insert a 25-gauge needle into the rubber top (not in the center) of the second vial. This acts as an air vent. Injecting air into the second vial is *not* necessary.
3. Insert the needle in the center of the rubber-top vial (beside the 25-g needle—air vent), invert the second vial, and withdraw the desired drug dose.

▶ **Method 2**

Mixing Two Drugs in the Same Syringe From One Vial and One Ampule (same "prep" as Method 1).
1. Remove the amount of desired solution from the vial.
2. Aspirate the amount of desired solution from the ampule.

▶ **Method 3**

Mixing Two Drugs in a Pre-filled Cartridge From a Vial
1. Check the drug dose and the amount of solution in the pre-filled cartridge. If a smaller dose is needed, expel the excess solution.
2. Draw air into the cartridge to equal the amount of solution to be withdrawn from the vial. Invert the vial and inject the air.
3. Withdraw the desired amount of solution from the vial. Make sure the needle remains in the fluid and do *not* take more solution than needed.

EXAMPLES   Mixing drugs in the same syringe.

PROBLEM 1: Order: meperidine (Demerol) 60 mg and atropine sulfate 0.4 mg IM.
The two drugs are compatible.
Drug available:

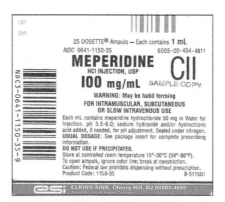

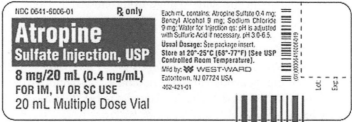

Note: Meperidine is in an ampule and atropine sulfate is in a vial.

How many milliliters of each drug would you give? Explain how to mix the two drugs.

Methods: meperidine

$$\text{BF:}\frac{D}{H} \times V = \frac{60 \text{ mg}}{100 \text{ mg}} \times 1 \text{ mL} = 0.6 \text{ mL}$$

or
RP: H : V :: D : X
       100 mg : 1 mL :: 60 mg : X mL
            100 X = 60
                X = 0.6 mL

or
FE: $\frac{H}{V} = \frac{D}{X} = \frac{100 \text{ mg}}{1 \text{ mL}} = \frac{60 \text{ mg}}{X}$
   (Cross multiply) 100 X = 60
                X = 0.6 mL

or
DA: no conversion factor

$$\text{mL} = \frac{1 \text{ mL} \times 60 \text{ mg}}{100 \text{ mg} \times 1} = \frac{60}{100} = 0.6 \text{ mL}$$

atropine SO_4 = 0.4 mg

Answer: meperidine (Demerol) 60 mg = 0.6 mL
        Atropine 0.4 mg = 1 mL

Procedure: Mix two drugs in a syringe for IM injection:
1. Remove 1 mL of atropine solution from the vial.
2. Withdraw 0.6 mL of meperidine (Demerol) from the ampule into the syringe containing atropine solution.
3. Syringe contains atropine 1 mL and meperidine 0.6 mL = total 1.6 mL.

PROBLEM 2: Order: meperidine 25 mg, Vistaril 25 mg, and Robinul 0.1 mg, IM. All three drugs are compatible.
Drugs available: meperidine (Demerol) is in a 2-mL Tubex cartridge labeled 50 mg/mL. Hydroxyzine (Vistaril) is in a 50-mg/mL ampule. Glycopyrrolate (Robinul) is available in a 0.2-mg/mL vial.

How many milliliters of each drug would you give?
Explain how the drugs could be mixed together.
Methods:
a. meperidine 25 mg. Label: 50 mg/mL.

$$\text{BF:}\frac{D}{H} \times V = \frac{25 \text{ mg}}{50 \text{ mg}} \times 1 \text{ mL} = 0.5 \text{ mL}$$

or
RP: H : V :: D : X
       50 mg : 1 mL :: 25 mg : X mL
            50 X = 25
                X = ½ mL or 0.5 mL

or
FE: $\frac{H}{V} = \frac{D}{X} = \frac{50 \text{ mg}}{1 \text{ mL}} = \frac{25 \text{ mg}}{X}$
   (Cross multiply) 50 X = 25
                X = 0.5 mL

or
DA: $\text{mL} = \dfrac{1 \text{ mL} \times \overset{1}{25 \text{ mg}}}{\underset{2}{50 \text{ mg}} \times 1} = \dfrac{1}{2}$ mL or 0.5 mL meperidine

b. Vistaril 25 mg. Label: 50 mg/mL ampule.

$$\text{BF:}\frac{D}{H} \times V = \frac{25 \text{ mg}}{50 \text{ mg}} \times 1 \text{ mL} = 0.5 \text{ mL}$$

or

RP: H : V :: D : X
50 mg : 1 mL :: 25 mg : X mL
50 X = 25
X = ½ mL or 0.5 mL

or

FE: $\dfrac{H}{V} = \dfrac{D}{X} = \dfrac{50 \text{ mg}}{1 \text{ mL}} = \dfrac{25 \text{ mg}}{X}$

50 X = 25
X = 0.5 mL

c. Robinul 0.1 mg. Label: 0.2 mg/mL.

BF: $\dfrac{D}{H} \times V = \dfrac{0.1 \text{ mg}}{0.2 \text{ mg}} \times 1 \text{ mL} = 0.5 \text{ mL Robinul}$

or

FE: $\dfrac{H}{V} = \dfrac{D}{X} = \dfrac{0.2 \text{ mg}}{1 \text{ mL}} = \dfrac{0.1 \text{ mg}}{X}$

0.2 X = 0.1
X = 0.5 mL

or

RP: H : V :: D : X
0.2 mg : 1 mL :: 0.1 mg : X mL
0.2 X = 0.1
X = 0.5 mL

or

DA: $mL = \dfrac{1 \text{ mL} \times 0.1 \text{ mg}}{0.2 \text{ mg} \times 1} = \dfrac{0.1}{0.2} = \dfrac{1}{2} \text{ or } 0.5 \text{ mL}$

Answer: meperidine (Demerol) 25 mg = 0.5 mL; Vistaril 25 mg = 0.5 mL; Robinul 0.1 mg = 0.5 mL

Procedure: Mix three drugs in the cartridge:
1. Check drug dose and volume on pre-filled cartridge. Expel 0.5 mL of meperidine and any excess of drug solution from cartridge.
2. Draw 0.5 mL of air into the cartridge and inject into the vial containing the Robinul.
3. Withdraw 0.5 mL of Robinul from the vial into the pre-filled cartridge containing meperidine.
4. Withdraw 0.5 mL of Vistaril from the ampule into the cartridge.

PRACTICE PROBLEMS ▶ III INTRAMUSCULAR INJECTIONS

Answers can be found on pages 193 to 199.

Round off to the nearest tenths.

1. Order: tobramycin (Nebcin) 50 mg, IM, q8h.
   Drug available:

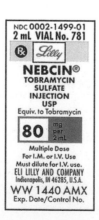

How many milliliters of tobramycin would you give?_____

2. Order: methylprednisolone (Solu-Medrol) 75 mg, IM, daily.
   Drug available: 125 mg/2 mL in vial.

   How many milliliters would you give?_____

3. Order: vitamin B$_{12}$ (cyanocobalamin) 300 mcg, IM, daily.
   Drug available:

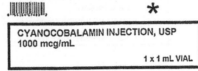

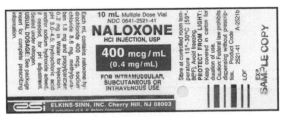

   CYANOCOBALAMIN INJECTION, USP
   1000 mcg/mL
                                                    1 x 1 mL VIAL

   FOR INTRAMUSCULAR OR SUBCUTANEOUS USE ONLY

   Each mL contains: Cyanocobalamin 1000 mcg, Sodium
   Chloride 0.9%, Benzyl Alcohol 1.5%, Water for Injection q.s.
   pH (range 4.5 - 7.0) adjusted with Hydrochloric Acid and/or
   Sodium Hydroxide.

   Directions for Use: See product insert for prescribing
   information, precautions and warnings.

   STORAGE: Store at 20 - 25 C (68 - 77 F); excursions
   permitted to 15 - 30 C (59 - 86 F) (See USP Controlled
   Room Temperature).

   WARNING: PROTECT FROM LIGHT.

   RX ONLY

   Bulk NDC 0517-0031-25

   How many milliliters of cyanocobalamin would you give?_____

4. Order: naloxone 0.2 mg, IM, STAT.
   Drug available:

   How many milliliters would you give?_____

5. Order: diazepam 4 mg, IM, q6h.
   Drug available:

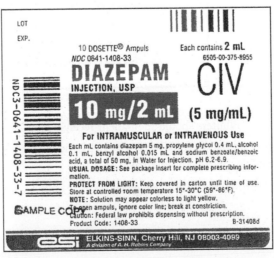

   How many milliliters would you give?_____

6. Order: cefepime HCl (Maxipime) 500 mg, IM, q12h.
   Drug available:

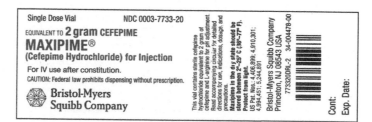

a. Which single-dose vial of Maxipime would you select?_____

   Explain_____

b. How many milliliters (mL) of diluent should you use for reconstitution of the drug?

   _____

   Note: The drug label does not indicate the amount of diluent to use. This may be found in the drug information insert. Usually, if you inject 2.6 mL of diluent, the amount of drug solutio may be 3.0 mL. If you inject 3.4 or 3.5 mL of diluent, the amount of drug solution shoul be 4.0 mL.

c. How many milliliters of drug solution should the patient receive?_____

7. Order: prochlorperazine (Compazine) 4 mg, IM, q8h, as needed.
   Drug available:

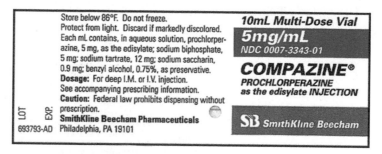

   How many milliliters should the patient receive?_____

8. Order: secobarbital (Seconal) 125 mg, IM, 1 hour before surgery.
   Drug available: Seconal 50 mg/mL.

   How many milliliters would you give?_____

9. Order: thiamine HCl 75 mg, IM, daily.
   Drug available: 100- and 200-mg/mL vials.

   a. Which vial would you use?_____

   b. How many milliliters would you give?_____

10. Order: hydroxyzine (Vistaril) 25 mg, deep IM, STAT.
    Drug available: Vistaril 100 mg/2 mL in a vial.

    How many milliliters would you give?_____

11. Order: loxapine HCl (Loxitane) 25 mg, IM, q6h until desired response and then 50 mg.
    Drug available:

    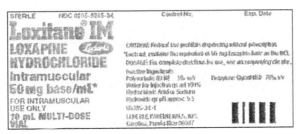

    How many milliliters would you administer intramuscularly for the initial dose?_____

12. Order: penicillin G potassium (Pfizerpen) 250,000 units, IM, q6h.
    Drug available:

    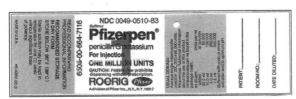

    a. Select the appropriate dilution for the ordered dose. How many milliliters of diluent would you add?_____

    b. How many milliliters should the patient receive per dose?_____

13. Order: cefonicid (Monocid) 750 mg, IM, daily.
    Drug available:

    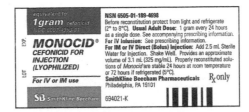

    Change grams to milligrams (3 spaces to the right) or milligrams to gram (3 spaces to the left).

    1.000 g = 1000 mg or 1000 mg = 1 g

    a. How many gram(s) is 750 mg, IM, daily?_____

    b. How many milliliters of diluent should be injected into the vial (see drug label)?_____

    c. How many milliliters of cefonicid (Monocid) should the patient receive per day?_____

14. Order: meperidine (Demerol) 35 mg and promethazine (Phenergan) 10 mg, IM.
Drugs available: meperidine 50 mg/mL in an ampule; promethazine 25 mg/mL in an ampule.

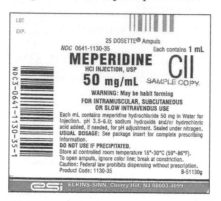

a. How many milliliters of meperidine would you give?_____

b. How many milliliters of promethazine would you give?_____

c. Explain how the two drugs should be mixed

_____

15. Order: meperidine (Demerol) 50 mg and atropine sulfate 0.3 mg, IM.
Drugs available:

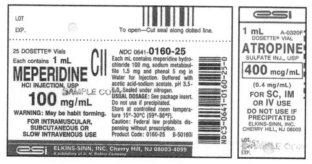

a. How many milliliters of meperidine would you give?_____

b. How many milliliters of atropine would you give?_____

c. Explain how the two drugs should be mixed.

_____

16. Order: codeine phosphate 20 mg IM × 1 dose.
Drug available:

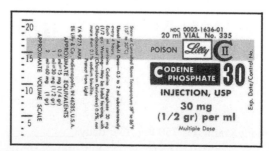

How many milliliters would the patient receive?_____

17. Order: Butorphanol tartrate 1.5 mg, IM.
Drug available:

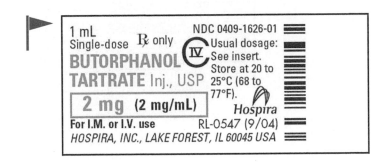

How many milliliters would you give?_____

18. Order: chlordiazepoxide HCl (Librium) 50 mg, IM, STAT.
Drug available: Librium (100 mg) powder in ampule.

Add 2 mL of special intramuscular diluent to the ampule. When diluted, the powder content may increase the volume.

How many milliliters would be equivalent to 50 mg?_____

Explain_____

19. Order: cefamandole (Mandol) 500 mg, IM, q6h.
Drug available:

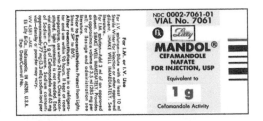

a. Change milligrams to grams (see Chapter 1).

_____

b. How many milliliters of diluent would you add (see drug label)? _____

c. What size syringe would you use?_____

d. How many milliliters should the patient receive? _____

20. Order: ticarcillin (Ticar), 400 mg, IM, q6h.
Drug available:

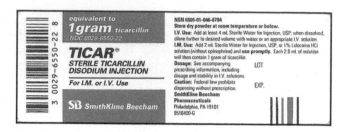

    a. Drug label reads to add 2 mL of diluent. Total volume of solution is _____

    b. How many milliliters of ticarcillin should be withdrawn? _____

21. Order: morphine 10 mg IM, STAT.
Drug available:

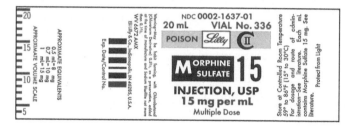

How many milliliters of morphine would you give? _____

22. Order: hydroxyzine (Vistaril) 25 mg, deep IM, q4-6h, PRN for nausea.
Drug available:

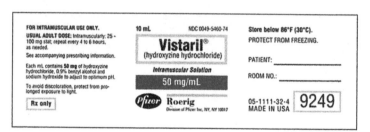

How many milliliters should the patient receive per dose? _____

23. Order: Decadron (dexamethasone) 2 mg, IM, q6h.
Adult parameters: 0.75-9 mg/day in 2 to 4 divided doses.
Drug available:

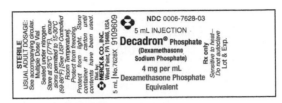

 a. Is the dose according to adult parameters? _____

 b. How many milliliters would you give? _____

 c. What type of syringe could be used? _____

 d. Can the Decadron vial be used again? Explain_____

24. Order: ceftazidime (Fortaz) 500 mg, IM, q8h.
Add 2 mL of diluent = 2.6 mL drug solution. Check the drug information insert.
Drug available:

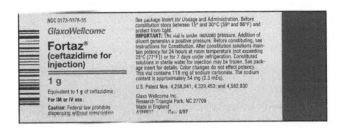

 a. How many gram(s) of ceftazidime (Fortaz) should the patient receive per day?

_____

 b. How many milliliters of ceftazidime would you give per dose?

_____

25. Order: streptomycin sulfate 750 mg IM × 1 dose.
Drug available:

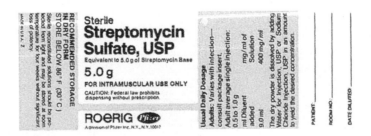

 a. How many milliliters of diluent would you add to the vial? _____

 b. How many milliliters would the patient receive? _____

26. Order: diazepam 8 mg, IM, STAT and repeat in 4 hours if necessary.
Drug available:

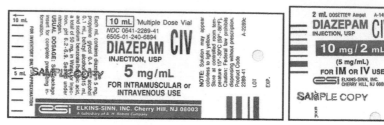

    a. Which ampule or vial of diazepam would you select? _____

    b. How many milliliters (mL) of diazepam should the patient receive? _____

27. Order: benztropine mesylate (Cogentin) 1.5 mg, IM, daily.
Drug available:

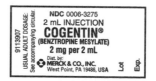

How many milliliters (mL) of Cogentin should the patient receive? _____

28. Order: cefotaxime Na (Claforan) 750 mg, IM, bid.
Drug available: Pamphlet states to add 3 mL of diluent equal to 3.4 mL.

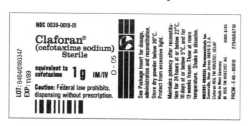

    a. 1 g = _____ mg
    b. How many milligrams should the patient receive per day? _____
    c. How many milliliters would you give per dose? _____

29. Order: diphenhydramine HCl 30 mg, IM, STAT.
Drug available:

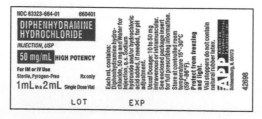

How many milliliters should the patient receive? _____

30. Order: interferon alfa-2b (Intron A) 10 million international units IM 3 × week.
   Drug available: interferon alfa-2b (Intron A) 25 million international units/5-mL vials.

   How many milliliters would you give per dose? _____

31. Order: vitamin K (AquaMEPHYTON) 2.5 mg IM × 1.
   Drug available:

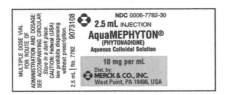

   How many milliliters would you give? _____

32. Order: ampicillin/sulbactam (Unasyn) 1 g, IM, q8h.
   Drug available:
   (Add 3.6 mL of diluent to the vial; drug and diluent equals 4 mL.)

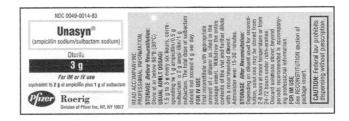

   a. Unasyn 3-g vial equals _____
   b. How many milliliters of Unasyn would you give every 8 hours? _____

Questions 33 through 38 relate to additional dimensional analysis. Refer to Chapter 6.

33. Order: droperidol 2 mg, IM, STAT.
   Drug available: droperidol 5 mg/2 mL.
   Factors: 5 mg/2 mL; 2 mg/1
   Conversion factor: *None;* order and drug are both available in milligrams.

   How many milliliters of droperidol should be given? _____

34. Order: dexamethasone 5 mg, IM, daily.
   Drug available:

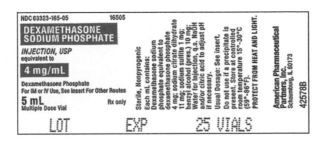

   How many milliliters should be administered daily? _____

35. Order: levothyroxine (Synthroid) 100 mcg, IM, STAT then 0.025 mg, po, daily.
Drugs available: levothyroxine 200 mcg/mL for IM; levothyroxine 12.5 mcg/tablet, po

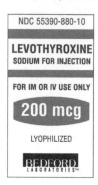

a. How many milliliters would you give IM? _____

b. How many tablets would you give per dose? _____

36. Order: cefobid 500 mg, IM, q6h.
Add 2 mL of diluent to equal 2.4-mL solution.
Drug available:

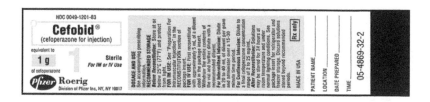

a. Cefobid 1 g = _____ mL; 500 mg = _____ mL
Conversion factor: 1 g = 1000 mg

b. How many milliliters of Cefobid would you give? _____

37. Order: ceftriaxone 1000 mg, IM, daily.
Drug available:

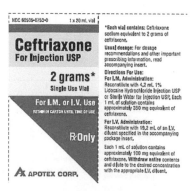

a. How many milliliters diluent would you add to the vial? _____

b. What is the reconstituted concentration for IM use? _____

c. How many milliliters of ceftriaxone would you give? _____

38. Order: cefazolin (Ancef) 0.25 g, IM, q12h.
Drug available: 2.0 mL of diluent = 2.2 mL

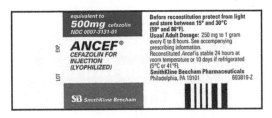

Note: change grams to milligrams; drug label is in milligrams.

How many milliliters of Ancef would you give? _____

Questions 39 through 42 relate to drug dosage per body weight.

39. Order: amikacin (Amikin) 15 mg/kg/day, q8h, IM.
Drug available:

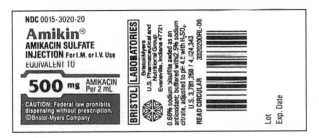

Patient weighs 140 pounds.
a. How many kilograms does the patient weigh? _____
b. How many milligrams should the patient receive daily? _____
c. How many milligrams should the patient receive q8h (three divided doses)?

_____

d. How many milliliters should the patient receive q8h? _____

40. Order: netilmicin sulfate (Netromycin) 2 mg/kg, q8h, IM.
Patient weighs 174 pounds.
Drug available: netilmicin 100 mg/mL.

a. How many kilograms does the patient weigh? _____
b. How many milligrams should the patient receive daily? _____
c. How many milligrams should the patient receive q8h? _____
d. How many milliliters should the patient receive q8h? _____

41. Order: midazolam HCl (Versed) 0.07 mg/kg, IM before general anesthesia.
Patient weighs: 156 pounds.
Drug available:

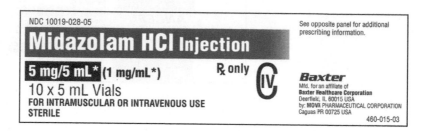

a. How many kilograms does the patient weigh? _____

b. How many milligrams should the patient receive? _____

c. How should midazolam be administered? _____

42. Order: Robinul 4 mcg/kg, IM × 1 dose.
Drug available:

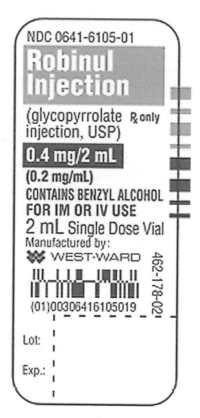

Patient weighs 72 kilograms.

a. How many milligrams should the patient receive? _____

b. How many milliliters should the patient receive? _____

43. Order: Lasix 0.5 mg/kg, IM, bid.
Drug available:

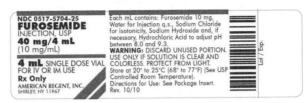

Patient weighs 130 pounds.

a. How many kilograms does the patient weigh? _____

b. How many milligrams should the patient receive per day? _____

c. How many milligrams should the patient receive every 12 hours? _____

d. How many milliliters per dose should the patient receive? _____

ANSWERS

I Needles

1. The 21-gauge needle because it is the smaller gauge number.
2. The 26-gauge needle because it is the larger gauge number.
3. The 20-gauge needle because it has the larger lumen (smaller gauge). A needle with a 20-gauge and 1½-inch length is used for IM injection.
4. The 25-gauge needle, because it has the smaller lumen (larger gauge). It is used for subcutaneous injections. The needle is not long enough for an IM injection.
5. The 21-gauge needle with 1½-inch length (21 g/1½ inch). Muscle is under subcutaneous or fatty tissue, so a longer needle is needed.

II Subcutaneous Injections

1. *Both* needle gauge and length combinations could be used.
2. **a.** 0.75 mL
   b. 45 to 90-degree angle. The angle depends on the amount of fatty tissue in the patient.
3. 0.5 mL
4. **BF:** $\dfrac{D}{H} \times V = \dfrac{13,000}{20,000} \times 2 = 1.3$ units

   FE: $\dfrac{H}{V} = \dfrac{D}{X} = \dfrac{20,000}{2} = \dfrac{13,000}{X} =$

   (Cross multiply) $20,000\,X = 26,000$

   $X = 1.3$ units

   RP:
   $$H : V :: \quad D \ : X$$
   $$20,000 : 2 :: 13,000 : X$$
   $$20,000\,X = 26,000$$
   $$X = 1.3 \text{ units}$$

   DA:
   $$V = \dfrac{V}{H} \times \dfrac{D}{1} = \dfrac{2}{20,000} \times \dfrac{13,000}{1} = 1.3 \text{ units}$$

5. BF: $\dfrac{D}{H} \times V = \dfrac{0.6 \text{ mg}}{0.4 \text{ mg}} \times 1 \text{ mL} = \dfrac{0.6}{0.4} = 1.5 \text{ mL}$

or

RP: H : V :: D : X
0.4 mg : 1 mL :: 0.6 mg : X mL
0.4 X = 0.6

$X = \dfrac{0.6}{0.4} = 1.5 \text{ mL}$

or

DA: mL $= \dfrac{1 \text{ mL} \times 0.6 \text{ mg}}{0.4 \text{ mg} \times 1} = \dfrac{0.6}{0.4} = 1.5 \text{ mL}$

6. BF: $\dfrac{D}{H} \cdot V = \dfrac{8}{12}$ $0.6 = 0.4 \text{ mL}$

RP: H : V :: D : X
12 : 0.6 :: 8 : X
12 X = 4.8
X = 0.4 mL

7. **a.** 198 lbs ÷ 2.2 kg = 90 kg
   b. 90 kg × 6 mcg/kg = 540 mcg

   c. $\dfrac{D}{H} \times V = \dfrac{540 \text{ mcg}}{300 \text{ mcg}} \times 1 \text{ mL} = 1.8 \text{ mL}$

   Answer: Neupogen 540 mcg = 1.8 mL

   d. Drug can be prepared in two syringes, one with 1 mL, and the other with 0.8 mL. With subcutaneous injections, one (1) mL is given per site unless the person weighs more than 200 lbs or the dose has been approved by the health care provider.

8. BF: $\dfrac{D}{H} \times V = \dfrac{0.3}{1} \times 1 = 0.3 \text{ mL}$

   FE: $\dfrac{H}{V} = \dfrac{D}{X} = \dfrac{1}{1} = \dfrac{0.3}{X} =$

   (Cross multiply) 1 X = 0.3
   X = 0.3 mL

   RP: H : V :: D : X
   1 : 1 :: 0.3 : X
   1 X = 0.3
   X = 0.3 mL

   DA : V $= \dfrac{V}{H} \times \dfrac{D}{1} = \dfrac{1}{1} \times \dfrac{0.3}{1} = 0.3 \text{ mL}$

9. BF: $\dfrac{D}{H} \times V = \dfrac{8 \text{ mg}}{15 \text{ mg}} \times 1 \text{ mL} = 0.53 \text{ mL or } 0.5 \text{ mL}$

   or

   FE: $\dfrac{H}{V} = \dfrac{D}{X} = \dfrac{15 \text{ mg}}{1 \text{ mL}} = \dfrac{8 \text{ mg}}{X}$

   (Cross multiply) 15 X = 8
   X = 0.53 mL or 0.5 mL

   or

   RP: H : V :: D : X
   15 mg : 1 mL :: 8 mg : X
   15 X = 8
   X = 0.53 mL or 0.5 mL

10. **a.** 120 units × 65 kilograms = 7800 units

    b. BF: $\dfrac{D}{H} \times V = \dfrac{7800 \text{ Iunits}}{10,000 \text{ Iunits}} \times 0.4 \text{ mL} = \dfrac{3120}{10,000} = 0.3 \text{ mL subcut}$

    or

    RP: H : V :: D : X
    10,000 Iunits : 0.4 mL :: 7800 Iunits : X
    10,000 X = 3120
    X = 0.3 mL

III Intramuscular Injections (Round off in tenths)

1. BF: $\dfrac{D}{H} \times V = \dfrac{50 \text{ mg}}{80 \text{ mg}} \times 2 \text{ mL} = \dfrac{100}{80} = 1.25 \text{ mL or } 1.3 \text{ mL}$

or
RP: H : V :: D : X
  80 mg : 2 mL :: 50 mg : X mL
    80 X = 100
      $X = \dfrac{100}{80} = 1.25 \text{ mL or } 1.3 \text{ mL}$

or
FE: $\dfrac{H}{V} = \dfrac{D}{X} = \dfrac{80 \text{ mg}}{2 \text{ mL}} = \dfrac{50 \text{ mg}}{X} =$
(Cross multiply) 80 X = 100
      X = 1.25 or 1.3 mL

or
DA: no conversion factor

$$mL = \dfrac{2 \text{ mL} \times \overset{5}{\cancel{50 \text{ mg}}}}{\underset{8}{\cancel{80 \text{ mg}}} \times 1} = \dfrac{10}{8} = 1.25 \text{ mL or } 1.3 \text{ mL}$$

Answer: tobramycin 50 mg = 1.25 mL or 1.3 mL

2. BF: $\dfrac{D}{H} \times V = \dfrac{\overset{3}{\cancel{75}} \text{ mg}}{\underset{5}{\cancel{125}} \text{ mg}} \times 2 \text{ mL} = \dfrac{6}{5} = 1.2 \text{ mL}$

or
RP: H : V :: D : X
   125 mg : 2 mL :: 75 mg : X mL
      125 X = 150
        X = 1.2 mL

Answer: methylprednisolone 75 mg = 1.2 mL
3. 0.3 mL of vitamin B_{12} (cyanocobalamin)
4. 0.5 mL of naloxone (Narcan)

5. BF: $\dfrac{D}{H} \times V = \dfrac{4 \text{ mg}}{10 \text{ mg}} \times 2 \text{ mL} = \dfrac{8}{10} = 0.8 \text{ mL diazepam}$

RP: H : V :: D : X
  10 mg : 2 mL :: 4 mg : X
    10 X = 8
      X = 0.8 mL of diazepam

or
FE: $\dfrac{H}{V} = \dfrac{D}{X} = \dfrac{10 \text{ mg}}{2 \text{ mL}} = \dfrac{4 \text{ mg}}{X}$
(Cross multiply) 10 X = 8
      X = 0.8 mL of diazepam

or
DA: no conversion factor

$$mL = \dfrac{2 \text{ mL} \times \overset{2}{\cancel{4 \text{ mg}}}}{\underset{5}{\cancel{10 \text{ mg}}} \times 1} = \dfrac{4}{5} = 0.8 \text{ mL of diazepam}$$

6. a. Select the Maxipime 1-g vial. The Maxipime 2-g vial is for intravenous use according to the drug label and cannot be used for intramuscular injection.
  b. Using 2.6 mL diluent = 3.0 mL of solution
  c. Change 500 mg to 0.5 g or 1 g to 1000 mg

  BF: $\dfrac{D}{H} \times V = \dfrac{0.5 \text{ g}}{1 \text{ g}} \times 3 \text{ mL} = 1.5 \text{ mL of cefepime twice a day}$

7. BF: $\dfrac{D}{H} \times V = \dfrac{4 \text{ mg}}{5 \text{ mg}} \times 1 \text{ mL} = \dfrac{4}{5} = 0.8 \text{ mL of compazine}$

or
RP: H : V :: D : X
  5 mg : 1 mL :: 4 mg : X
    5 X = 4
      X = 0.8 mL

or
FE: $\dfrac{H}{V} = \dfrac{D}{X} = \dfrac{5 \text{ mg}}{1 \text{ mL}} = \dfrac{4 \text{ mg}}{X} = 5 X = 4$
(Cross multiply) X = 0.8 mL

or
DA: $mL = \dfrac{1 \text{ mL} \times 4 \cancel{\text{ mg}}}{5 \cancel{\text{ mg}} \times 1} = \dfrac{4}{5} = 0.8 \text{ mL}$

8. 2.5 mL of secobarbital
9. **a.** 100-mg vial
   b. 0.75 mL of thiamine
10. ½ or 0.5 mL of hydroxyzine
11. 0.5 mL (½ mL) of Loxitane
12. **a.** 4.0 mL of diluent = 1,000,000 units (drug label)

   b. BF: $\dfrac{D}{H} \times V = \dfrac{\overset{1}{\cancel{250,000}\ \text{units}}}{\underset{4}{\cancel{1,000,000}\ \text{units}}} \times 4\ \text{mL} = \dfrac{4}{4} = 1\ \text{mL Pfizerpen}$

   DA: 1 million units = 1,000,000 units

   $\text{mL} = \dfrac{4\ \text{mL} \quad \times\ \overset{1}{\cancel{250,000}\ \text{units}}}{\underset{4}{\cancel{1,000,000}\ \text{units}} \times \quad 1} = \dfrac{4}{4} = 1\ \text{mL of Pfizerpen}$

13. **a.** 750 mg of cefonicid (Monocid) is equivalent to 0.75 g.
    b. Drug label indicates that 2.5 mL of diluent should be added to the drug powder, which yields 3.1 mL of drug solution.

    c. BF: $\dfrac{D}{H} \times V = \dfrac{0.75\ \text{g}}{1\ \text{g}} \times 3.1\ \text{mL}$

    $= 2.33\ \text{mL or } 2.3\ \text{mL of cefonicid solution}$

14. **a.** meperidine 35 mg = 0.7 mL
    b. promethazine 10 mg = 0.4 mL
    c. Procedure: 1. Obtain 0.7 mL of meperidine from the ampule and 0.4 mL of promethazine from the ampule.
    2. Discard the remaining solutions within the ampules.
15. **a.** meperidine 50 mg = ½ or 0.5 mL
    b. atropine 0.3 mg = 0.75 or 0.8 mL (Round off in tenths)
    Atropine

    BF: $\dfrac{D}{H} \times V = \dfrac{0.3\ \text{mg}}{0.4\ \text{mg}} \times 1\ \text{mL} = 0.75 \text{ or } 0.8\ \text{mL}$

    or

    Atropine
    RP: H : V :: D : X
    0.4 mg : 1 mL :: 0.3 mg : X mL
    0.4 X = 0.3
    $X = \dfrac{0.3}{0.4} = 0.75 \text{ or } 0.8\ \text{mL}$

    or

    Atropine
    FE: $\dfrac{H}{V} = \dfrac{D}{X} = \dfrac{0.4\ \text{mg}}{1\ \text{mL}} = \dfrac{0.3\ \text{mg}}{X} =$
    0.4 X = 0.3
    X = 0.75 or 0.8 mL

    Meperidine
    DA: mL $= \dfrac{1\ \text{mL} \quad \times\ \overset{1}{\cancel{50}\ \text{mg}}}{\underset{2}{\cancel{100}\ \text{mg}} \times \quad 1} = \dfrac{1}{2}$ or 0.5 mL

c. 1. The two drugs are compatible.

2. Inject 0.75 (0.8) mL of air into the atropine vial.

3. Inject 0.5 mL of air into the meperidine vial and withdraw 0.5 mL of meperidine.

4. Withdraw 0.8 mL of atropine from the atropine vial. Discard both vials.

16. BF: $\dfrac{D}{H} \times V = \dfrac{20 \text{ mg}}{30 \text{ mg}} \times 1 \text{ mL} = 0.66 \text{ or } 0.7 \text{ mL}$

or

RP: H : V :: D : X

30 mg : 1 mL :: 20 mg : X

30 X = 20

X = 0.66 or 0.7 mL

17. BF: $\dfrac{D}{H} \times V = \dfrac{1.5}{2} \times 1 = 0.75 \text{ mL}$

RP: H : V :: D : X

2 : 1 :: 1.5 : X

2 X = 1.5

X = 0.75 mL

18. Librium 50 mg = 1 mL (100 mg = 2 mL)

After adding 2 mL of diluent, withdraw the entire drug solution to determine the total volume of drug solution. Expel half of the solution; the remaining drug solution is equivalent to chlordiazepoxide (Librium) 50 mg.

19. a. Change milligrams to grams by moving the decimal point three spaces to the *left:* 500. mg = 0.5 g.

Because the drug weight on the label is in grams, the conversion is to grams. However, the drug can be converted to milligrams by changing grams to milligrams (moving the decimal point three spaces to the *right*): 1 g = 1.000 mg = 1000 mg.

b. Drug label states to add 3 mL of diluent and, after it is reconstituted, the drug solution will be 3.5 mL. Mandol 1 g = 3.5 mL.

c. A 5-mL syringe is preferred: however, a 3-mL syringe can be used because less than 3 mL of the drug solution is needed.

d. BF: $\dfrac{D}{H} \times V = \dfrac{0.5 \text{ g}}{1 \text{ g}} \times 3.5 \text{ mL} = 1.75 \text{ or } 1.8 \text{ mL}$

or

RP: H : V :: D : X

1000 mg : 3.5 mL :: 500 mg : X mL

1000 X = 1750

X = 1.75 or 1.8 mL

or

DA: $\text{mL} = \dfrac{3.5 \text{ mL} \times 0.5 \text{ g}}{1 \text{ g} \times 1} = 1.75 \text{ or } 1.8 \text{ mL}$

Answer: cefamandole (Mandol) 500 mg = 1.8 mL

20. Change 400 milligrams to grams.

400 mg = 0.400 g or 0.4 g

a. Total volume of drug solution is 2.6 mL; see drug label.

b. BF: $\dfrac{D}{H} \times V = \dfrac{0.4 \text{ g}}{1 \text{ g}} \times 2.6 = 1 \text{ mL}$

or

RP: H : V :: D : X

1 g : 2.6 mL :: 0.4 g : X mL

X = 2.6 × 0.4

X = 1 mL

ticarcillin 400 mg or 0.4 g = 1 mL

or

FE: $\dfrac{H}{V} = \dfrac{D}{X} = \dfrac{1 \text{ g}}{2.6 \text{ mL}} = \dfrac{0.4 \text{ g}}{X} =$

(Cross multiply) X = 1.04 mL or 1 mL

or

DA $= \dfrac{2.6 \text{ mL} \times 0.4 \text{ g}}{1 \text{ g} \times 1} = 1.04 \text{ mL or } 1 \text{ mL}$

21. $\text{BF: } \dfrac{D}{H} \times V = \dfrac{\overset{2}{\cancel{10}} \text{ mg}}{\underset{3}{\cancel{15}} \text{ mg}} \times 1 \text{ mL} = \dfrac{2}{3} = 0.66 \text{ or } 0.7 \text{ mL}$

or

$\text{RP: } \quad H \; : \; V \; :: \; D \; : \; X$
$\quad\quad 15 \text{ mg} : 1 \text{ mL} :: 10 \text{ mg} : X \text{ mL}$
$\quad\quad\quad\quad\quad 15\,X = 10$
$\quad\quad\quad\quad\quad\quad X = 0.66 \text{ or } 0.7 \text{ mL}$

22. 0.5 mL of Vistaril

23. **a.** Yes, 8 mg per day

b. $\text{BF: } \dfrac{D}{H} \times V = \dfrac{\overset{1}{\cancel{2}} \text{ mg}}{\underset{2}{\cancel{4}} \text{ mg}} \times 1 \text{ mL} = \frac{1}{2} \text{ or } 0.5 \text{ mL}$
$\qquad\qquad$ or
$\qquad\qquad \text{DA: } \text{mL} = \dfrac{1 \text{ mL} \times \overset{1}{\cancel{2}} \text{ mg}}{\underset{2}{\cancel{4}} \text{ mg} \times 1} = \frac{1}{2} \text{ or } 0.5 \text{ mL}$

c. 3-mL syringe

d. Yes, the vial has a rubber top that is self-sealing.

24. **a.** Change milligrams to grams; move the decimal point three spaces to the *left:* 500. mg = 0.5 g.

$\quad$ 0.5 g $\times$ 3 (q8h) = 1.5 g per day

b. Add 2 mL of diluent to yield 2.6 mL (check drug information insert):

$\text{BF: } \dfrac{D}{H} \times V = \dfrac{0.5 \text{ g}}{1 \text{ g}} \times 2.6 \text{ mL} = 1.3 \text{ mL per dose}$

25. **a.** Add 9 mL of diluent to yield 400 mg/mL

b. **BF:** D/H $\times$ V = 750 mg/400 mg $\times$ 1 mL = 1.9 mL

$\quad$ **FE:** H/V = D/X
$\quad\quad$ 400 mg/1 mL = 750 mg/X
$\quad\quad\quad\quad$ X = 1.9 mL

$\quad$ **RP:** H : V :: D : X
$\quad\quad$ 400 mg : 1 mL :: 750 mg : X

$\quad\quad\quad\quad$ X = 1.9 mL

$\quad$ **DA:** mL = 1 mL $\times$ 750 mg/400 mg $\times$ 1 = 1.9 mL

26. **a.** Either the ampule or the vial could be used. The diazepam 5 mg/mL is a multiple-dose vial that contains 10 mL of drug solution.

b. **BF:** Ampule: $\dfrac{8 \text{ mg}}{10 \text{ mg}} \times 2 \text{ mL} = 1.6 \text{ mL of diazepam}$ $\qquad$ **BF:** Vial: $\dfrac{8 \text{ mg}}{5 \text{ mg}} \times 1 \text{ mL} = 1.6 \text{ mL of diazepam}$

$\quad$ or $\qquad\qquad\qquad\qquad\qquad\qquad\qquad\qquad\qquad$ or

$\quad$ **DA:** Ampule: mL $= \dfrac{2 \text{ mL} \times \overset{4}{\cancel{8}} \text{ mg}}{\underset{5}{\cancel{10}} \text{ mg} \times 1} = \dfrac{8}{5} = 1.6 \text{ mL}$ $\qquad$ **DA:** Vial: mL $= \dfrac{1 \text{ mL} \times 8 \text{ mg}}{5 \text{ mg} \times 1} = \dfrac{8}{5} = 1.6 \text{ mL}$

27. $\text{BF: } \dfrac{D}{H} \times V = \dfrac{1.5 \text{ mg}}{\underset{1}{\cancel{2}} \text{ mg}} \times \overset{1}{\cancel{2}} \text{ mL} = 1.5 \text{ mL of Cogentin}$

28. a. $1 \text{ g} = 1000 \text{ mg}$

   b. $750 \text{ mg} \times 2 = 1500 \text{ mg}$ of cefotaxime Na per day

   c. BF: $\dfrac{D}{H} \times V = \dfrac{\overset{3}{\cancel{750} \text{ mg}}}{\underset{4}{\cancel{1000} \text{ mg}}} \times 3.4 \text{ mL} = \dfrac{10.2}{4} = 2.55 \text{ mL}$ or 2.6 mL of cefotazime Na (rounded off in tenths)

         DA: $\text{mL} = \dfrac{3.4 \text{ mL} \times \overset{3}{\cancel{750} \text{ mg}}}{\underset{4}{\cancel{1000} \text{ mg}} \times 1} = \dfrac{10.2}{4} = 2.55 \text{ mL}$ or 2.6 mL of cefotazime Na (rounded off in tenths)

29. RP: H : V :: D : X

      $50 \text{ mg} : 1 \text{ mL} :: 30 \text{ mg} : X$

          $50 X = 30$

            $X = 0.6 \text{ mL}$ of diphenhydramine HCl

  FE: $\dfrac{H}{V} = \dfrac{D}{X} = \dfrac{50 \text{ mg}}{1 \text{ mL}} = \dfrac{30 \text{ mg}}{X}$

    (Cross multiply) $50 X = 30$

            $X = 0.6 \text{ mL}$ of diphenhydramine HCl

30. BF: $\dfrac{D}{H} \times V = \dfrac{10}{25} \times 5 = \dfrac{50}{25} = 2 \text{ mL}$

                or

               RP: H : V :: D : X

                $25 \text{ million units} : 5 \text{ mL} :: 10 \text{ million units} : X \text{ mL}$

                       $25 X = 50$

                         $X = 2 \text{ mL}$

Answer: Intron A 2 mL three times a week

31. BF: $\dfrac{D}{H} \times V = \dfrac{2.5 \text{ mg}}{10 \text{ mg}} \times 1 \text{ mL} = 0.25 \text{ mL}$ or 0.3 mL

  or

  RP: H : V :: D : X

      $10 \text{ mg} : 1 \text{ mL} :: 2.5 \text{ mg} : X$

         $10 X = 2.5$

           $X = 0.25 \text{ mL}$ or 0.3 mL

                              or

                               FE: $\dfrac{H}{V} = \dfrac{D}{X} = \dfrac{10 \text{ mg}}{1 \text{ mL}} = \dfrac{2.5 \text{ mg}}{X} =$

                                      $10 X = 2.5$

                                        $X = 0.25 \text{ mL}$ or 0.3 mL

  or

  DA: no conversion factor

  $\text{mL} = \dfrac{1 \text{ mL} \times \overset{1}{\cancel{2.5} \text{ mg}}}{\underset{4}{\cancel{10} \text{ mg}} \times 1} = \dfrac{1}{4}$ or 0.25 mL

Answer: AquaMEPHYTON 2.5 mg = 0.25 mL or 0.3 mL

32. a. $4 \text{ mL} = 3 \text{ g}$

                                          or

   b. BF: $\dfrac{D}{H} \times V = \dfrac{1 \text{ g}}{3 \text{ g}} \times 4 \text{ mL} = \dfrac{4}{3} = 1.3 \text{ mL}$ of Unasyn   **RP:** H : V :: D : X

                                                        $3 \text{ g} : 4 \text{ mL} :: 1 \text{ g} : X \text{ mL}$

                                                           $3 X = 4$

                                                           $X = 1.3 \text{ mL}$ of Unasyn

33. DA: $\text{mL} = \dfrac{2 \text{ mL} \times 2 \text{ mg}}{5 \text{ mg} \times 1} = \dfrac{4}{5} = 0.8 \text{ mL}$ of droperidol

34. DA: $\text{mL} = \dfrac{1 \text{ mL} \times 5 \text{ mg}}{4 \text{ mg} \times 1} = \dfrac{5}{4} = 1.25 \text{ mL}$ or 1.3 mL of dexamethasone (rounded off in tenths)

35. DA: a: $\text{mL} = \dfrac{1 \text{ mL} \times \overset{1}{\cancel{100} \text{ mcg}}}{\underset{2}{\cancel{200} \text{ mcg}} \times 1} = 0.5$ or $\frac{1}{2} \text{ mL}$ of levothyroxine

  DA: b: Conversion factor: $1 \text{ mg} = 1000 \text{ mcg}$

$$\text{Tablet} = \frac{1 \text{ tablet} \times \overset{80}{\cancel{1000}} \cancel{\text{mcg}} \times 0.025 \cancel{\text{mg}}}{\underset{1}{\cancel{12.5}} \cancel{\text{mcg}} \times 1 \cancel{\text{mg}} \times 1} = 80 \times 0.025 = 2 \text{ tablets of levothyroxine}$$

36. a. 1 g = 2.4; 500 mg = 1.2 mL

   b. DA: $\text{mL} = \dfrac{2.4 \text{ mL} \times 1 \cancel{g} \times \overset{1}{\cancel{500}} \cancel{\text{mg}}}{1 \cancel{g} \times \underset{2}{\cancel{1000}} \cancel{\text{mg}} \times 1} = \dfrac{2.4}{2} = 1.2 \text{ mL}$

   Give 1.2 mL of Cefobid.

37. a. 4.2 mL

   b. 350 mg/mL

   c. BF: $\dfrac{D}{H} \times V = \dfrac{1000 \text{ mg}}{350 \text{ mg}} \times 1 \text{ mL} = 2.85 \text{ mL or } 2.9 \text{ mL}$ **or**
          RP: H   :   V   ::   D   : X

                                                350 mg : 1 mL :: 1000 mg : X

                                                  350 X = 1000

                                                      X = 2.85 mL or 2.9 mL

   or
   FE: $\dfrac{H}{V} = \dfrac{D}{X} = \dfrac{350 \text{ mg}}{1 \text{ mL}} = \dfrac{1000 \text{ mg}}{X}$ **or**
                                                 DA: $\text{mL} = \dfrac{1 \text{ mL} \times 1000 \text{ mg}}{350 \text{ mg} \times 1} = 2.85 \text{ mL or } 2.9 \text{ mL}$

   (Cross multiply) 350 X = 1000

                      X = 2.85 mL or 2.9 mL

38. 0.25 g = 0.250 mg (250 mg)

   a. Give 1.1 mL of Ancef.

39. a. 140 ÷ 2.2 = 63.6 kg

   b. 15 mg × 63.6 × 1 = 954 mg daily

   c. 954 ÷ 3 = 318 mg of amikacin q8h

   d. BF: $\dfrac{D}{H} \times V = \dfrac{318 \text{ mg}}{500 \text{ mg}} \times 2 = \dfrac{636}{500} = 1.27 \text{ or } 1.3 \text{ mL}$ **or**
                                              FE: $\dfrac{H}{V} = \dfrac{D}{X} = \dfrac{500 \text{ mg}}{2 \text{ mL}} = \dfrac{318 \text{ mg}}{X \text{ mL}} =$

   or
                                         (Cross multiply) 500 X = 636
   RP: H   :   V   ::   D   : X

                                                       X = 1.27 or 1.3 mL
      500 mg : 2 mL :: 318 mg : X mL

               500 X = 636

                     X = 1.27 or 1.3 mL (tenths)

   or

   DA: $\text{mL} = \dfrac{2 \text{ mL} \times 318 \cancel{\text{mg}}}{500 \cancel{\text{mg}} \times 1} = \dfrac{636}{500} = 1.3 \text{ mL per dose}$

   Answer: Give 1.27 or 1.3 mL of amikacin q8h (three times a day).

40. a. 174 ÷ 2.2 = 79.1 kg

   b. 2 mg × 79.1 = 158.2 or 158 mg daily

   c. 158 ÷ 3 = 52.6 mg or 50 mg q8h (Round off to a number that can be administered; check with your institution.)

   d. BF: $\dfrac{D}{H} \times V = \dfrac{\overset{5}{\cancel{50}} \text{ mg}}{\underset{10}{\cancel{100}} \text{ mg}} \times 1 \text{ mL} = \dfrac{5}{10} = 0.5 \text{ mL}$

   or
   RP: H   :   V   ::   D   : X   **or**
                                                    FE: $\dfrac{H}{V} = \dfrac{D}{X} = \dfrac{100 \text{ mg}}{1 \text{ mL}} = \dfrac{50 \text{ mg}}{X \text{ mL}} =$
      100 mg : 1 mL :: 50 mg : X mL

              100 X = 50   100 X = 50

                 X = 0.5 mL   X = 0.5 mL or

$$DA: mL = \frac{1\ mL \times \overset{1}{\cancel{50}}\ mg}{\underset{2}{\cancel{100}}\ mg \times 1} = \frac{1}{2} \text{ or } 0.5\ mL$$

Answer: netilmicin 50 mg = 0.5 mL

41. **a.** 156 pounds = 70.9 or 71 kg
 b. 0.07 mg × 71 kg = 4.97 mg or 5 mg (rounded off)
 c. Administered IM in two syringes at two sites, 2.5 mL in each syringe unless otherwise instructed

42. **a.** 4 mcg × 72 kg = 288 mcg or 0.288 mg or 0.3 mg
 Move the decimal place three places to the left to convert mcg to mg.

 b. BF: $\dfrac{D}{H} \times V = \dfrac{0.3\ mg}{0.4\ mg} \times 2\ mL = \dfrac{0.6}{0.4} = 1.5\ mL$ of Robinul

 or
 FE: $\dfrac{H}{V} = \dfrac{D}{X} = \dfrac{0.4\ mg}{2\ mL} = \dfrac{0.3\ mg}{X}$
 (Cross multiply) 0.4 X = 0.6
 X = 1.5 mL

43. **a.** 130 lbs = 59 kg
 b. 59 milligrams per day
 c. 29.5 milligrams per dose

 d. BF: $\dfrac{D}{H} \times V = \dfrac{29.5\ mg}{40\ mg} \times 4\ mL = 2.95\ mL$ or 3 mL

 or
 RP: H : V :: D : X
 350 mg : 4 mL :: 29.5 mg : X
 40 X = 118
 X = 2.95 mL or 3 mL

 or
 FE: $\dfrac{H}{V} = \dfrac{D}{X} = \dfrac{40\ mg}{4\ mL} = \dfrac{29.5\ mg}{X}$
 (Cross multiply) 40 X = 118
 X = 2.95 mL or 3 mL

 or
 DA: $mL - \dfrac{4\ mL \times 29.5\ mg}{40\ mg \times 1} = 2.95\ mL$ or 3 mL

NGN® PREP

1. A 45-year-old female clinic patient was recently diagnosed with severe anemia, and the healthcare provider ordered an intramuscular injection of cyanocobalamin 1000mcg. Drug available: Cyanocobalamin 2000mcg in a 5mL multidose vial.

 The correct amount of drug to administer is __A__. When preparing the medication, it is important to __B__.

 Choose the best answer.

Option A	Option B
1mL	Add air to vial to facilitate medication removal
2mL	Use a tuberculin syringe for an accurate measurement
0.5mL	Add sterile water to flush medication from vial
2.5mL	Change needle after withdrawing medication

2. A 15-year-old male seen in ER for severe tonsilitis, positive for group A Streptococcus, headache, difficulty swallowing, and swollen lymph nodes in his neck. Patient says his throat has been sore for 4 days. Vital signs are Temp 102.4, B/P 110/65, RR 16, HR 78, and SaO2 97%. HCP orders Penicillin G Benzathine injectable suspension 1,200,000units IM.

Drug available: Penicillin G. Benzathine injectable suspension 2,400,000Units per 4mL. The patient should receive _A_ and the maximum volume that should be given at any one site is _B_.

Option A	Option B
3mL	4mL
2.5mL	3mL
1.5mL	2mL
2mL	1mL

ANSWERS - NGN® PREP

1. $\dfrac{D}{H} = \dfrac{1000mcg}{2000mcg} \times 1mL = 0.5mL$

When preparing medication for injection, add air to vial to facilitate medication removal.

2. $\dfrac{D}{H} \times V = \dfrac{1,200,000units}{2,400,000units} \times 4mL = 2mL$

Average volume of solution for IM injection is 1-2mL and the maximum is 3mL.

For additional practice problems, refer to the parenteral dosages section of the Elsevier's Interactive drug calculation application, Version 1 on evolve.

CHAPTER 10

Antidiabetic Medications

Objectives • Identify the different types of oral antidiabetic medications.
• Identify the different types of insulin.
• Determine prescribed insulin dosage in units using an insulin syringe.
• Describe the sites and angle for administering insulin.
• Explain the methods for mixing two insulin solutions in one insulin syringe.
• Explain the various methods of insulin administration, such as insulin pens, insulin pump.

Outline **BLOOD GLUCOSE MONITORING**
ORAL ANTIDIABETIC MEDICATIONS
INSULIN SYRINGES
INSULIN BOTTLES
SITES AND ANGLES FOR INSULIN INJECTIONS
TYPES OF INSULIN
MIXING INSULINS
INSULIN PEN DEVICES
INSULIN PUMPS

Diabetes mellitus (DM) is a complex and chronic metabolic disorder associated with high blood glucose levels also known as hyperglycemia, which occurs from deficiencies in insulin secretion, action of insulin, or both. The chronic metabolic imbalances caused by hyperglycemia puts patients at high risk for long- term microvascular and macrovascular complications which may include: stroke, myocardial infarction, vision loss, neuropathy, sexual dysfunction, loss of limb, kidney failure, and premature death.

DM is characterized as type 1 or type 2. Type 1 DM indicates a complete lack of insulin production by the pancreas. Insulin must be used with type 1 DM and must be injected or inhaled. Type 2 DM indicates inadequate insulin production and/or insulin resistance at the cellular level. While insulin alone is used to treat type 1 DM, oral antidiabetic agents alone or in conjunction with insulin may be used to treat type 2 DM. Oral antidiabetic agents work in a variety of ways. Treatment includes agents that increase the sensitivity of target organs to insulin, agents that decrease the rate at which glucose is absorbed from the gastrointestinal tract, and agents that increase the amount of insulin secreted by the pancreas.

According to the national diabetes statistics report from the Centers for Disease Control and Prevention (CDC), in 2017, 30.3 million people had diabetes. Of that number, an estimated 7.2 million were undiagnosed. Type 2 DM accounts for 90%-95% of all diabetes cases.

BLOOD GLUCOSE MONITORING

Testing is essential for maintaining glucose control. The oldest method is the fingerstick and the use of a glucometer. Newer methods such as continuous glucose monitoring which use patches that measure glucose in the interstitial fluid between the cells right under the skin are now available. Close monitoring of glucose levels will give improved control by determining the dosages of antidiabetic agents.

ORAL ANTIDIABETIC MEDICATIONS

Oral antidiabetic medications, which are used to treat type 2 DM, can be taken alone or used in conjunction with insulin. There are several classes of oral antidiabetic drugs that target glucose metabolism in various ways. Examples are listed in Table 10.1

TABLE 10.1 Classes of Oral Antidiabetic Medications

Class	Generic Name (Brand Name)	Action	When to Take
Alpha-glucosidase inhibitors	Acarbose (Precose) Miglitol (Glyset)	Slows absorption of carbohydrates	With first bite of food
Biguanides	Glucophage (Metformin)	Reduces production of glucose by the liver	During meals or at dinner
Dipeptidylpeptidase-4 inhibitors	Sitagliptine (Januvia) Alogliptin (Nestina)	Intensifies effect of incretines (intestinal hormones) involved in glucose control	Same time of day, with or without food
Meglitinides	Nateglinide (Starlix) Repaglinide (Prandix)	Stimulates the pancreas to produce more insulin	15 minutes before meals, do not take at bedtime
Sodium glucose cotransporter 2 inhibitors	Empagliflozin (Jardiance) Canagliflozin (Ivokana)	Helps eliminate glucose in the urine; prevents glucose being reabsorbed in kidneys	Before the first meal of the day
Sulfonylurea	Glimepride (Amaryl) Glyburide (Diabeta)	Stimulates the pancreas to produce more insulin	30 minutes before meals, do not take at bedtime
Thiazolidinedones	Pioglitazone (Actose) Rosiglitazone (Avandia)	Increases cellular insulin sensitivity; reduces production of glucose by liver	Same time of day, with or without food

EXAMPLE PROBLEM: Order: glucophage (Metformin) 1000 mg, daily.

Drug available:

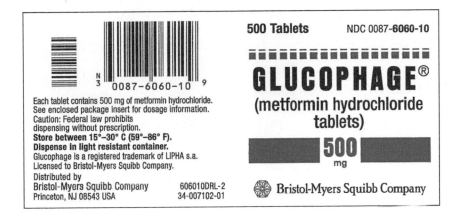

Methods: **BF** : $\dfrac{D}{H} \times V = \dfrac{1000 \text{ mg}}{500} \times \text{tab} = 2 \text{ tablets}$

or

RP ; H: V :: D : X

500 mg: 1 tab :: 1000 mg: X

$$500 \, X = 1000$$

$$X = 2$$

INSULIN SYRINGES

Insulin syringes are used for the subcutaneous administration of insulin. They have a capacity of 0.3 to 1 mL. Insulin is measured in *units* and must NOT be calculated in milliliters. Each calibration in the syringe represents 1 unit. Insulin syringes arc available in 3 sizes: 30 unit (0.3 mL), 50 unit (0.5 mL), and 100 unit (1 mL) (Figure 10.1). The insulin syringe is usually marked on one side in even units (10, 20, 30) and on the other side in odd units (5, 15, 25) (Figure 10.2). The 30-unit and 50-unit syringes are referred to as low-dose insulin syringes. They are designed to deliver lower doses of insulin with greater accuracy. The 100-unit syringe is referred to as the "standard" insulin syringe and is the one most commonly utilized.

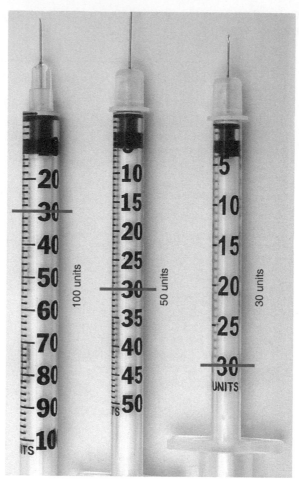

Figure 10.1 Three types of insulin syringes. From left to right: 30 units are measured on a 100-unit, 50-unit, and 30-unit syringe, respectively. (From Macklin D, Chernecky C, Infortuna H: *Math for clinical practice,* ed 2, St Louis, 2011, Mosby.)

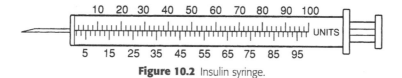

Figure 10.2 Insulin syringe.

INSULIN BOTTLES

Insulin is prescribed and measured according to U.S. Pharmacopeia (USP) units. Most insulins are produced in concentrations of 100 units/mL. Insulin should be administered with an insulin syringe that is calibrated to correspond with the 100 units of insulin bottle. DO NOT use a tuberculin syringe. The insulin bottle and syringe are color-coded "orange" to avoid medication errors.

Insulin is ordered in units. For example, if the prescribed insulin dosage is 30 units, withdraw 30 units from the bottle of 100 units of insulin using a 100-unit calibrated insulin syringe (Figure 10.3).

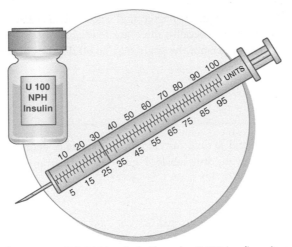

Figure 10.3 Unit-100 insulin bottle and unit-100 insulin syringe.

SITES AND ANGLES FOR INSULIN INJECTIONS

Insulin is a protein that can be given only by injection. Gastrointestinal (GI) secretions destroy the insulin structure. Figure 10.4 indicates the sites for insulin injection. People who inject their insulin usually use sites 3, 4, 5, or 6. Caregivers or health care workers who administer insulin usually use sites 1 or 2 (upper arm or the deltoid area).

> **! CAUTION**
>
> • DO NOT administer insulin with a tuberculin syringe.

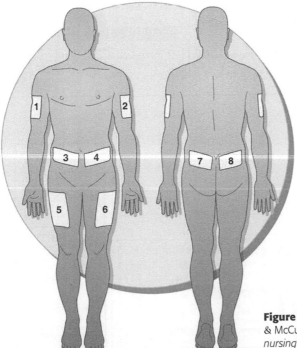

Figure 10.4 Sites for insulin injection. (From Kee, J. L., Hayes, E. R., & McCuistion, L. E. [2015]. *Pharmacology: a patient-centered nursing process approach.* 8th ed., Philadelphia: Elsevier.)

Insulin is administered at a 45-or 90-degree angle into the subcutaneous tissue. The subcutaneous absorption rate of insulin is slower because there are fewer blood vessels in the fatty tissue than in the muscular tissue. For an obese person, the angle may be 90 degrees, and for a very thin person the angle may be 45 degrees.

TYPES OF INSULIN

Insulin is categorized as rapid-acting, fast-acting, intermediate-acting, long-acting, and as commercial premixed insulin. The following drug labels (Figure 10.5) are arranged according to insulin action.

Rapid-Acting Insulins

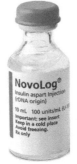
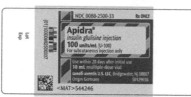
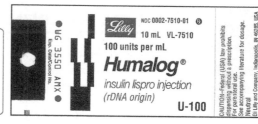

(From Novo Nordisk, Inc., Princeton, N.J.)

(Product images and trademarks are the property of and used with the permission of sanofi-aventis U.S. LLC, Bridgewater, N.J. as of September, 2015.)

Fast-Acting Insulins

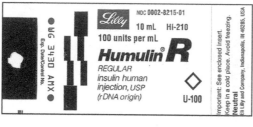
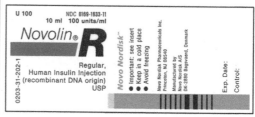

Intermediate-Acting Insulins

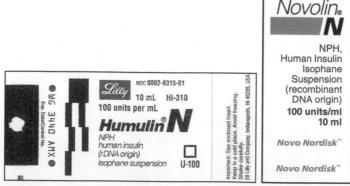

Figure 10.5 Types of insulins. (From Novo Nordisk Inc., Princeton, N.J.)

Long-Acting Insulins

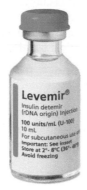

(From Novo
Nordisk, Inc.,
Princeton, N.J.)

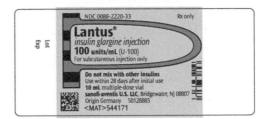

(Product images and trademarks are the property
of and used with the permission of sanofi-aventis
U.S. LLC, Bridgewater, N.J. as of September, 2015.)

Combinations: Rapid- and Intermediate-Acting Insulins

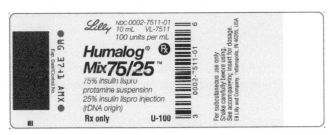

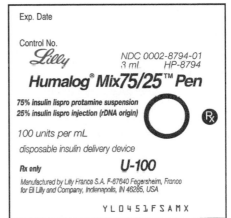

Fast- and Intermediate-Acting Insulins

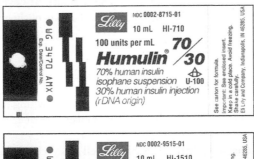

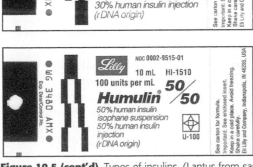

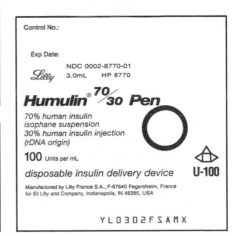

Figure 10.5 (cont'd) Types of insulins. (Lantus from sanofi-aventis U.S. Inc., Bridgewater, N.J.)

Insulins have various descriptions including color, action, and source. They are either clear (regular) or cloudy (NPH). Only clear insulin can be given intravenously as well as subcutaneously.

Insulin action is broken down into onset, peak, and duration. *Onset* is how long it takes the insulin to begin working. *Peak* is when the insulin is working most effectively, and *duration* is how long the insulin remains effective. *Human insulin* is synthetic (manufactured) while *analog insulin* is grown in a laboratory but genetically altered to give it desirable properties.

Insulin is categorized as rapid-acting, fast-acting, intermediate-acting, long-acting, and commercial premixed insulin (see Figure 10.5 and Table 10.2). Insulin that controls blood glucose between meals and during sleep is referred to as basal insulin. Insulin that controls blood glucose when someone eats is referred to as bolus or mealtime insulin. Intermediate-acting and long-acting insulins are basal insulins while rapid- and fast-acting insulins are bolus insulins.

Rapid-Acting Insulin

Rapid-acting insulin becomes effective within 5-15 minutes of injection and lasts 3-5 hours. Rapid- acting insulin covers insulin needs for meals eaten at the same time as the injection. Rapid-acting insulin is clear in color.

Fast-Acting Insulin

Fast-acting insulin (regular insulin) is administered 30 minutes before meals and is effective for 6-8 hours. It covers insulin needs for meals eaten within 30-60 minutes. If given during or after a meal, the patient may experience hypoglycemia. It is also clear in color.

Intermediate-Acting Insulin

Intermediate-acting insulin is administered 30 minutes before meals and becomes effective in 1-2 hours and is effective for 12-18 hours. It covers insulin needs for about half the day or overnight. It is cloudy in color and can only be given subcutaneously.

Long-Acting Insulin

Long-acting insulin acts within 1-2 hours and is effective for 18-24 hours. It covers insulin needs for about 1 full day. It is clear in color but must only be administered subcutaneously and cannot be mixed with other insulins.

Premixed Combination Insulin

Premixed insulins combine specific amounts of fast-acting and intermediate-acting insulins in one bottle or insulin pen. The numbers following the brand name indicate the percentage of each type of insulin (see Table 10-2). They are generally taken before mealtime.

Rapid- and fast-acting insulins can be given intravenously as well as subcutaneously. Intermediate- and long-acting insulins can ONLY be administered subcutaneously.

The onset, peak, and duration times are given in Table 10.2 for four groups of insulins: rapid-acting, fast-acting, intermediate-acting, and long-acting. The table includes the peak and return times after the insulins are administered.

TABLE 10.2 Types of Insulin

Generic (Brand)	Route	Color	Pregnancy Category	Time to Administer	ACTION		
					Onset	Peak	Duration (Dose-Related)
Rapid-Acting Insulin (Short Duration)							
aspart (NovoLog)	A: subcut, IV	Clear	B	5-15 min before meals	5-15 min	1-3 h	3-5 h
glulisine (Apidra)	A: subcut, IV	Clear	B	5-15 min before meals	5-15 min	1-2 h	3-4.5 h
lispro (Humalog)	A: subcut, IV	Clear	B	5-15 min before meals	5-15 min	0.5-2 h	3-5 h
Fast-Acting Insulin (Slower Duration)							
regular insulin (Humulin R, Novolin R)	A,C: subcut, IV	Clear	B	15-30 min before meals	0.5-1 h	2-4 h	6-8 h
Intermediate-Acting Insulin							
NPH Insulin, Humulin N, Novolin N	A,C: subcut	Cloudy	B	30 min before meals	1-2 h	6-12 h	12-18 h
Long-Acting Insulin							
determir (Levemir)	A: subcut	Clear	C	Dinner or bedtime	1-2 h	6-8 h	14-24h(dose-related)
glargine (Lantus)	A: subcut	Clear	C	bedtime	1.5-2 h	No peak	24 h
COMBINATIONS							
Rapid- and Intermediate-Acting Insulin							
70% aspart protamine/ 30% aspart insulin (NovoLog mix 70/30)	A: subcut	Cloudy	B	15 min before meals	15 min	1-4 h	12-18 h
75% lispro protamine/ 25% lispro insulin (Humalog mix 75/25)	A: subcut	Cloudy	B	15 min before meals	15 min-2 h	2-6 h	14-18 h
Fast- and Intermediate-Acting Insulin							
70% NPH/30% regular insulin (Humulin 70/ 30, Novolin 70/30)	A: subcut	Cloudy	B	15 min before meals	30-60 min	2-8 h	10-18 h
50% NPH/50% regular insulin (Humulin 50/50)	A: subcut	Cloudy	B	15 min before meals	15-60 min	2-6 h	10-18 h

A, Adult; *C*, child; *h*, hour; *min*, minute; *subcut*, subcutaneous; *IV*, intravenous.
CAUTION: Levemir and Lantus should NOT be mixed with other Insulins and should NEVER be given Intravenously.

U-500 Insulin

With severe hypoglycemia, U-500 insulin may be ordered. This unit type is of high potency and not for ordinary use. U-100 insulin indicates 100 units per mL (this is the most common concentration of insulin). U-500 insulin is 500 units per mL and is five times more potent than U-100 insulin. It is considered a highrisk drug and should be used with caution. U-500 insulin should always be measured in a 1-mL syringe.

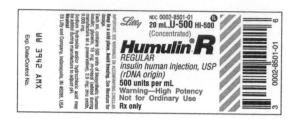

Sliding Scale

Sliding scale, or sliding scale insulin coverage, is a term used to describe how insulin dosages are adjusted to lower hyperglycemia. Rapid-acting or fast-acting is given to treat the range of elevated blood glucose levels. Sliding scale is used two ways, the first is for diabetics who need insulin coverage for the carbohydrates they eat for meals and the second is for hyperglycemia that occurs with an acute illness or surgery. Health care provider orders the coverage depending on the patient's insulin sensitivity.

TABLE 10.3 Example of Sliding Scale Insulin Coverage	
Blood glucose (mg/dL)	**Lispro subcutaneous coverage**
Less than 140	No coverage
140 to 180	2 units
181-220	3 units
221-240	4 units
241-300	5 units

Intravenous Insulin

Continuous intravenous (IV) insulin is used in the hospital setting to manage acute hyperglycemia. IV insulin delivery offers some advantages over SQ insulin delivery. It eliminates the need for multiple injections, allows for more accurate dose administration, and provides a quick response to rapidly changing glucose levels. The concentration is usually 1 unit per mL in a 0.9% NaCl solution. Insulin should always be in its own IV tubing and not mixed with other IV infusions.

Hypoglycemia

If a patient experiences severe hypoglycemia (blood glucose less than 40 mg/mL) and/or becomes unconscious, a glucagon or 50% dextrose injection may be given. Many diabetic patients have glucagon emergency kits in their homes for use if this occurs (Figure 10.6).

Figure 10.7 compares the action-time and rapid-acting, fast-acting, intermediate-acting, and long-acting insulins.

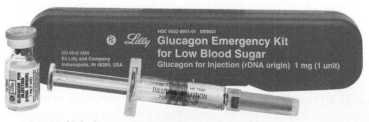

Figure 10.6 Glucagon emergency kit for home use. (From Eli Lilly and Company. All rights reserved. Used with permission.)

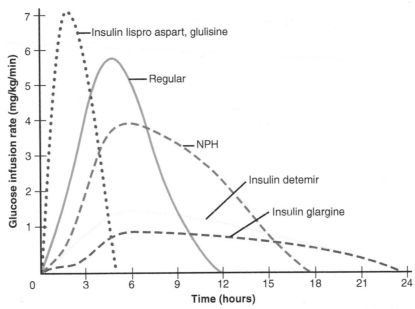

Figure 10.7 Activity profiles of different types of insulin. *NPH*, Neutral protamine Hagedorn. (Adapted from Rosenstock, J., Wyne, K. [2003]. Insulin treatment in type 2 diabetes. In Goldstein BJ, Muller-Wieland D, editors: *Textbook of type 2 diabetes,* London, Martin Dunitz, Ltd.; Plank J., Bodenlenz, M., Sinner, F., et al. [2005]. A double-blind, randomized, dose-response study investigating the pharmacodynamic and pharmacokinetic properties of the long-acting insulin analog detemir, *Diabetes Care* 28:1107-1112. Rave, K., Bott, S., Heinemann, L., et al. [2005]. Time-action profile of inhaled insulin in comparison with sub-cutaneously injected insulin lispro and regular human insulin, *Diabetes Care* 28:1077-1082.)

MIXING INSULINS

Regular insulin is frequently mixed with insulins containing protamine, such as Humulin N. REMEMBER: Insulin is prescribed in units and administered in units. Long-acting insulins can **NOT** be mixed with rapid- or fast-acting insulins.

EXAMPLE Problem and method for mixing insulin.

PROBLEM: Order: Humulin R insulin 10 units and Humulin N insulin 40 units, subcut.
Drug available: Humulin R insulin labeled U-100 and Humulin N insulin labeled U-100, both in multi-dose vials. The insulin syringe is marked 100 units.

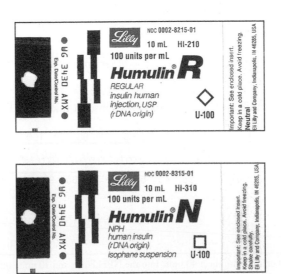

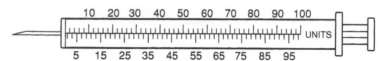

Method:

1. Gently roll insulin bottles between palms to evenly distribute the insulin solution. DO NOT shake insulin. Cleanse the rubber tops with alcohol.
2. Draw up 40 units of air* and inject into the Humulin N insulin bottle. Do not allow the needle to come into contact with the Humulin N insulin solution. Withdraw the needle.
3. Draw up 10 units of air and inject into the Humulin R insulin bottle.
4. Withdraw 10 units of Humulin R insulin. **Humulin R insulin is withdrawn before Humulin N insulin.**
5. Withdraw 40 units of Humulin N insulin.
6. Administer the two insulins immediately after mixing. Do not allow the insulin mixture to stand, because unpredicted physical changes might occur.

PRACTICE PROBLEMS ▶ I INSULIN

Answers can be found on pages 217 to 218.

1. Order: Humulin N insulin 35 units, subcut.
   Drug available: Humulin N insulin labeled U-100. The insulin syringe is marked 100 units. Indicate on the insulin syringe the amount of insulin that should be withdrawn.

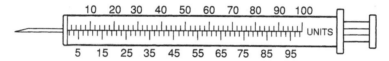

2. Order: Apidra (insulin glulisine) 10 units, subcut, STAT.
   Drug available: The insulin syringe is marked 100 units.

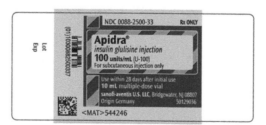

(Product images and trademarks are the property of and used with the permission of sanofi-aventis U.S. LLC, Bridgewater, N.J. as of September, 2015.)

Indicate on the insulin syringe the amount of insulin that should be withdrawn.

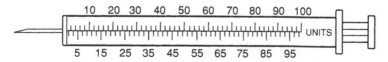

---

*You may draw up 50 units of air; inject 40 units into the NPH bottle and 10 units into the regular insulin bottle.

3. Order: Humalog insulin 8 units and Humulin N insulin 52 units.
Drug available: Humalog insulin labeled U-100 and Humulin N insulin labeled U-100. The insulin syringe is marked 100 units.
Explain the method for mixing the two insulins.

_____

Indicate on the U-100 insulin syringe how much Humalog insulin should be withdrawn and how much Humulin N insulin should be withdrawn.

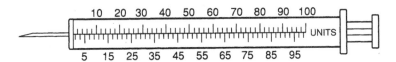

4. Order: Humulin R insulin 15 units and Humulin N 45 units.
Drug available: Humulin R insulin labeled U-100 and Humulin N insulin labeled U-100. The insulin syringe is marked 100 units.
Explain the method for mixing the two insulins.

_____

Indicate on the U-100 insulin syringe how much Humulin R insulin and how much Humulin N insulin should be withdrawn.

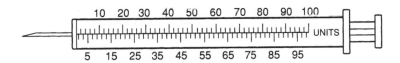

5. Order: Insulin detemir (Levemir) 40 units, subcut, at bedtime/hour of sleep.
Drug available: The insulin syringe is marked 100 units.

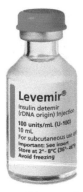

(From Norvo Nordisk, Inc., Princeton, N.J.)

Indicate on the insulin syringe the amount of insulin that should be given.

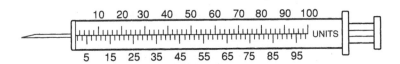

a. Can Levemir be mixed with regular insulin?_____

6. Order: Novolin N insulin, 38 units, subcut, 30 minutes before breakfast.
Drug available: The insulin syringe is marked 100 units.

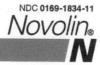

NDC 0169-1834-11

Novolin®
N

NPH,
Human Insulin
Isophane
Suspension
(recombinant
DNA origin)
100 units/ml
10 ml

Novo Nordisk™

Novo Nordisk™

Indicate on the insulin syringe the amount of Novolin N insulin that should be given.

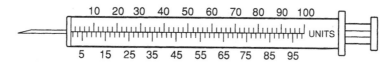

7. Order: Lantus insulin, 35 units, subcut, at bedtime.
Drug available: The insulin syringe is marked 100 units.

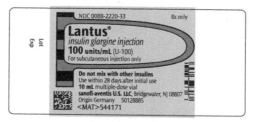

(Product images and trademarks are the property
of and used with the permission of sanofi-aventis
U.S. LLC, Bridgewater, N.J. as of September, 2015.)

Indicate on the insulin syringe the amount of Lantus insulin that should be given.

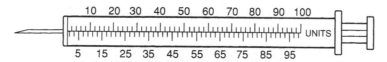

INSULIN PEN DEVICES

Insulin pens are devices that look like a pen or a marker and are used to deliver a dialed amount of insulin. Some patients prefer this method of administration especially if they have difficulty manipulating a vial and syringe. There are 2 types of insulin pen devices: pre-filled and reusable. The pens include an insulin cartridge, a dial to measure dosage, and a disposable needle. A pre-filled insulin pen contains a pre-filled insulin cartridge with 300 units (3 mL) of insulin. Once used, the entire pen unit is discarded (Figure 10.8). A reusable pen contains a replaceable insulin cartridge with 150 units (1.5 mL) or 300 units (3 mL) of insulin. Once empty, the cartridge is discarded and replaced with a new one.

Insulin administration is the same for pre-filled and reusable insulin pens. As the dose is dialed in, the plunger comes out. After the dose is dialed, the needle is placed subcutaneously and the plunger pushed down. The needle is then discarded. Following the insulin delivery, the dose indicator returns to zero.

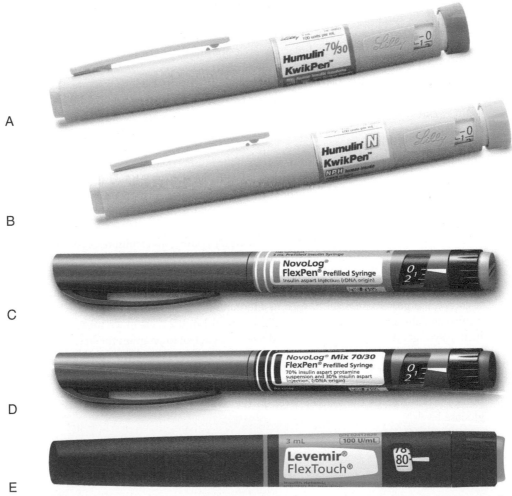

Figure 10.8 Prefilled insulin pens. **A,** Humulin 70/30 short- and intermediate-acting. **B,** Humulin N intermediate-acting. **C,** NovoLog® rapid-acting. **D,** NovoLog® 70/30 short- and intermediate-acting. **E,** Levemir® long-acting. (**A** and **B,** Copyright Eli Lilly and Co. All rights reserved. Used with permission. **C** to **E,** Used with permission of Novo Nordisk Inc.; © 2019 Novo Nordisk, all rights reserved.)

Answers can be found on page 219.

1. Your patient receives 25 units of U-100 Levemir insulin by FlexPen twice a day. The pen holds 300 units. How many days will one pen last?

_____

2. Lantus SoloStar Pens are dispensed in boxes of five pens. Each pen holds 300 units. If your patient receives 75 units of U-100 Lantus insulin once a day at bedtime, how many doses can the patient get from the box of five pens?

_____

INSULIN PUMPS

There are two types of insulin pumps—the implantable and the external (portable). The implantable insulin pump is surgically implanted in the abdomen and delivers a basal insulin infusion and bolus doses with meals either intravenously or intraperitoneally. With implantable insulin pumps, there are fewer hypoglycemic reactions, and blood glucose levels are mostly controlled.

External (portable) insulin pumps, also called *continuous subcutaneous insulin infusion* or CSII, have been available since 1983. CSII mimics the body's normal delivery of insulin. The external insulin pump keeps blood glucose (sugar) levels as close to normal as possible. The continuous delivery of insulin is called the *basal rate* and the larger pre-meal doses are called *bolus doses*. The insulin delivery setting is programmed by a diabetes expert and adjusted by the patient. Before the patient eats, the pump is programmed to dispense a large dose through the catheter. The patient then (1) programs insulin infusion at a basal rate of units per hour (a rate that can be adjusted), (2) delivers bolus infusions to cover meals (the patient pushes a button to deliver a bolus dose during meals), (3) changes delivery rates at specific times of the day (e.g., from 3 AM to 9 AM) to avoid early-morning hyperglycemia, and (4) overrides the set basal rate to allow for unexpected changes in activity such as early-morning exercise.

Most insulin pump systems consist of the insulin pump, an insulin reservoir, plastic tubing, and insertion set. The insulin reservoir holds 150 to 300 units of rapid- or fast-acting insulin, which is held in the insulin pump. The plastic tubing is attached to a metal or plastic needle and placed subcutaneously by the patient. The needle can be inserted into the abdomen, upper thigh, or upper arm. Only regular insulin is used because protamine insulin, such as Humulin N, can cause unpredictable blood glucose levels. The pump can deliver small amounts of insulin such as 0.1 or 0.2 units much more accurately than a traditional insulin syringe. Again, these pumps used a remote control to program the basal rates and bolus doses. The patient usually changes the insertion site every 3 days.

A glucose sensor device is available to check the fluid glucose level. The sensor is separate from the insulin pump and is attached to the body surface area. Radio-like wave sounds are transmitted to the pump, which records the glucose level on the pump every 5 minutes. An alarm warns of low or high glucose levels.

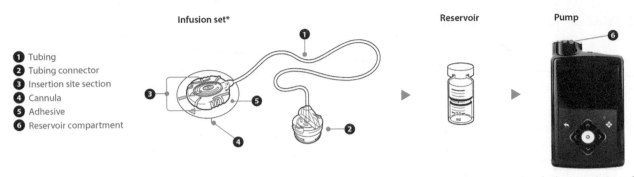

Figure 10.9 Medtronic MiniMed™ insulin pump (©2021 Medtronic. All Rights Reserved. Used with the permission of Medtronic). (From Medtronic, Inc., Minneapolis, Minn.)

The use of the insulin pump helps to decrease the risk of severe hypoglycemic reactions and maintains glucose control. However, glucose levels should still be monitored at least daily with or without an insulin pump. The person with type 1 diabetes mellitus has the greatest benefit from use of an insulin pump. This method should reduce the number of long-term diabetic complications compared with the use of multiple injections of regular and modified types of insulins. Figure 10.9 shows an example of an insulin pump.

PRACTICE PROBLEMS ▶ III INSULIN PUMP

Answers can be found on page 219.

1. Your patient receives 50 units of basal insulin in a 24-hour period. His basal rate is the same for all 24 hours. How much insulin does your patient receive each hour?

    _____unit/hour/24 hours

2. Your patient's pump settings are:

    | Midnight to 3 AM | 1.4 units/hr = _____ units for 3 hours |
    | 3 AM to 7 AM | 2.6 units/hr = _____ units for 4 hours |
    | 7 AM to 5 PM | 1.2 units/hr = _____ units for 10 hours |
    | 5 PM to midnight | 1.4 units/hr = _____ units for 7 hours |

    How much basal insulin would your patient receive in 24 hours? _____

3. Your patient's insulin reservoir holds 180 units of insulin. The patient uses 2.5 units per hour. How often does the patient need to refill the insulin reservoir? _____

ANSWERS

I Insulin

1. Withdraw 35 units of Humulin N insulin to the 35 mark on the insulin syringe. Both the insulin and the syringe have the same concentration: units 100.

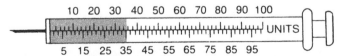

2. Withdraw 10 units of Apidra insulin.

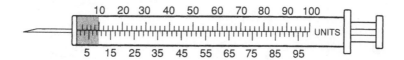

3. Inject 52 units of air into the Humulin N insulin bottle. Do not allow the needle to touch the insulin solution. Inject 8 units of air into the Humalog insulin bottle and withdraw 8 units of Humalog insulin. Withdraw 52 units of Humulin N insulin. Total amount of insulin should be 60 units. Do *not* allow the insulin mixture to stand. Administer immediately because Humulin N contains protamine, and unpredicted physical changes could occur with a delay in administration.

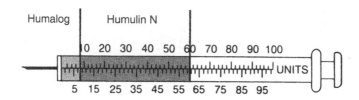

4. Inject 45 units of air into the Humulin N insulin bottle. Inject 15 units of air into the Humulin R insulin bottle and withdraw 15 units of Humulin R insulin. Withdraw 45 units of Humulin N insulin. Total amount of insulin should be 60 units.

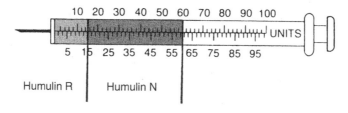

5. Withdraw 40 units of Levemir insulin.

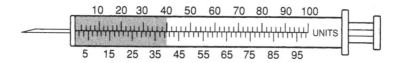

a. No. CANNOT BE MIXED WITH REGULAR INSULIN.

6. Withdraw 38 units of Novolin N insulin.

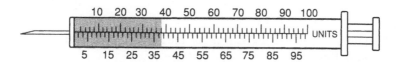

7. Withdraw 35 units of Lantus insulin.

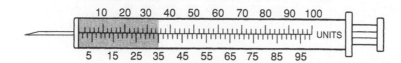

II Insulin Pen Devices

1. 300 units per pen ÷ 25 units = 12 doses per pen
   12 ÷ 2 doses per day = 6 days
2. 300 units per pen × 5 pens = 1500 units per box
   1500 units (5 pens) ÷ 75 units per day = 20 doses per box

III Insulin Pumps

1. 50 units per 24 hours ÷ 24 hours per day = 2.08 units of basal insulin per hour
2. Patient receives 36.4 units of insulin (basal) in 24 hours

   Midnight to 3 AM: 1.4 units/hr, 3 hours × 1.4 units = 4.2 units in 3 hours
   3 AM to 7 AM: 2.6 units/hr, 4 hours × 2.6 units = 10.4 units in 4 hours
   7 AM to 5 PM: 1.2 units/hr, 10 hours × 1.2 units = 12.0 units in 10 hours
   5 PM to midnight: 1.4 units/hr, 7 hours × 1.4 units = 9.8 units in 7 hours

3. 2.5 units per hours × 24 hours = 60 units per 24 hours or per day
   180 units per reservoir ÷ 60 units per day = 3 days
   Patient must refill insulin reservoir every 3 days.

NEXT-GENERATION NCLEX® EXAMINATION-STYLE QUESTIONS

A patient with a history of type II diabetes is admitted to the hospital for a biopsy to rule out colon cancer. The patient has an order for blood glucose checks 3 times daily before meals, at bedtime, and prn. The MAR for this patient includes the following medication orders:

1. Lantus 10 units at bedtime (2200)
2. Lispro insulin 4 units 5-15 min before meals.
3. Sliding scale to be administered if glucose is greater than 140 mg/dL: Lispro Regular insulin.
4. Glucagon 50% dextrose injection
5. Tylenol 650mg PO q8h prn
6. Atorvastatin 20 mg PO daily
7. Heparin 5000 units SQ Q8h

The RN checks the patient's glucose level at 5:45 pm, and it is 110. Immediately after having her glucose checked, the patient refused to eat dinner.

Choose the most likely options for the information missing from the statements below by selecting from the list of options provided.

The RN understands that the <u>A</u> and <u>B</u> insulin doses should be held and that the <u>C</u> dose should be given. An hour later the patient becomes complains of feeling warm and dizzy. The RN notes that the patient is pale, confused, and diaphoretic.

Choose the most likely options for the information missing from the statements below by selecting from the list of options provided.

The RN understands that she should <u>D</u> and administer <u>E</u> if the patient is <u>F</u>.

Option A	Option B	Option C
Lispro	Lispro	Lispro
Take the patient's blood pressure	Take the patient's blood pressure	Take the patient's blood pressure
Lantus	Lantus	Lantus

Option A	Option B	Option C
Take the patient's temperature	Take the patient's temperature	Take the patient's temperature
Hypoglycemic	Hypoglycemic	Hypoglycemic
Check the patient's glucose	Check the patient's glucose	Check the patient's glucose
Tylenol	Tylenol	Tylenol
Tachypneic	Tachypneic	Tachypneic
Atorvastatin	Atorvastatin	Atorvastatin
Glucagon 50% dextrose injection	Glucagon 50% dextrose injection	Glucagon 50% dextrose injection
Sliding scale insulin	Sliding scale insulin	Sliding scale insulin
Check the patient's heart rate	Check the patient's heart rate	Check the patient's heart rate

Option D	Option E	Option F
Lispro	Lispro	Lispro
Take the patient's blood pressure	Take the patient's blood pressure	Take the patient's blood pressure
Lantus	Lantus	Lantus
Take the patient's temperature	Take the patient's temperature	Take the patient's temperature
Hypoglycemic	Hypoglycemic	Hypoglycemic
Check the patient's glucose	Check the patient's glucose	Check the patient's glucose
Tylenol	Tylenol	Tylenol
Tachypneic	Tachypneic	Tachypneic
Atorvastatin	Atorvastatin	Atorvastatin
Glucagon 50% dextrose injection	Glucagon 50% dextrose injection	Glucagon 50% dextrose injection
Sliding scale insulin	Sliding scale insulin	Sliding scale insulin
Check the patient's heart rate	Check the patient's heart rate	Check the patient's heart rate

ANSWERS – NEXT-GENERATION NCLEX® EXAMINATION-STYLE QUESTIONS

Option A	Option B	Option C
Lispro	**Lispro**	Lispro
Take the patient's blood pressure	Take the patient's blood pressure	Take the patient's blood pressure
Lantus	Lantus	**Lantus**
Take the patient's temperature	Take the patient's temperature	Take the patient's temperature
Hypoglycemic	Hypoglycemic	Hypoglycemic
Check the patient's glucose	Check the patient's glucose	Check the patient's glucose

Option A	Option B	Option C
Tylenol	Tylenol	Tylenol
Tachypneic	Tachypneic	Tachypneic
Atorvastatin	Atorvastatin	Atorvastatin
Glucagon 50% dextrose injection	Glucagon 50% dextrose injection	Glucagon 50% dextrose injection
Sliding scale insulin	**Sliding scale insulin**	Sliding scale insulin
Check the patient's heart rate	Check the patient's heart rate	Check the patient's heart rate

Option D	Option E	Option F
Lispro	Lispro	Lispro
Take the patient's blood pressure	Take the patient's blood pressure	Take the patient's blood pressure
Lantus	Lantus	Lantus
Take the patient's temperature	Take the patient's temperature	Take the patient's temperature
Hypoglycemic	Hypoglycemic	**Hypoglycemic**
Check the patient's glucose	Check the patient's glucose	Check the patient's glucose
Tylenol	Tylenol	Tylenol
Tachypneic	Tachypneic	Tachypneic
Atorvastatin	Atorvastatin	Atorvastatin
Glucagon 50% dextrose injection	**Glucagon 50% dextrose injection**	Glucagon 50% dextrose injection
Sliding scale insulin	Sliding scale insulin	Sliding scale insulin
Check the patient's heart rate	Check the patient's heart rate	Check the patient's heart rate

Rationale:

The Lispro should only be given prior to meals, and the sliding scale should be held since the glucose was not over 140. Lantus is a long acting insulin and is not meal or glucose dependent and should be given despite the patient skipping a meal and having a hypoglycemic episode. The patient is exhibiting signs of hypoglycemia and should have their blood glucose checked. The Glucagon should be given because it is much faster acting than an infusion of D5%W.

For additional practice problems, refer to the Dosages Measured in Units section of the Elsevier's Interactive Drug Calculation Application, Version 1 on Evolve.

CHAPTER 11

Intravenous Preparations With Clinical Applications

Objectives
- Identify different catheter types and sites for intravenous (IV) access.
- Examine the three methods for calculating IV flow rates.
- Calculate drops per minute of prescribed IV solutions for IV therapy.
- Determine the drop factor according to the manufacturer's product specification.
- Calculate the drug dosage for IV medications.
- Calculate the flow rate for IV drugs being administered in a prescribed amount of solution.
- Explain the types and uses of electronic IV infusion devices.
- Calculate the rate of direct IV injection.

Outline
INTRAVENOUS SITES AND DEVICES
DIRECT INTRAVENOUS INJECTIONS
CONTINUOUS INTRAVENOUS ADMINISTRATION
CALCULATION OF INTRAVENOUS FLOW RATE
INTERMITTENT INTRAVENOUS ADMINISTRATION
FLOW RATES FOR INFUSION PUMPS AND SECONDARY SETS

Intravenous (IV) therapy is used for administering fluids containing water, dextrose, fat emulsions, vitamins, electrolytes, and drugs. Approximately 90% of all hospitalized patients, some outpatients, and some home-care patients receive IV therapy. Many drugs cannot be absorbed through the gastrointestinal tract and must be administered intravenously to provide bioavailability with direct absorption and fast action. Certain drugs that need to be absorbed immediately are administered by direct IV injection, sometimes over several minutes. However, many drugs administered intravenously are irritating to the veins because of the drug's pH or osmolality and must be diluted and administered slowly.

Advantages of IV drug therapy are (1) rapid drug distribution into the bloodstream, (2) rapid onset of action, and (3) no drug loss to tissues. There are many complications of IV therapy, some of which are sepsis, thrombosis, phlebitis, air emboli, infiltration, and extravasation. The nurse must monitor for signs of these complications during the course of IV therapy.

Three methods are used to administer IV fluid and drugs: (1) direct IV drug injection, (2) continuous IV infusion, and (3) intermittent IV infusion. Continuous IV administration replaces fluid loss, maintains fluid balance, and is a vehicle for drug administration. Intermittent IV administration is primarily used for giving IV drugs at prescribed intervals.

Nurses play an important role in preparing and administering IV solutions and drugs. Nursing functions and responsibilities include (1) knowledge of IV sets and their drop factors, (2) calculating IV flow rates, (3) verifying compatibility of the IV solution and the drug, (4) mixing and diluting drugs in IV solution, (5) regulating IV infusion devices, (6) maintaining patency of IV accesses, and (7) monitoring for signs and symptoms of infiltration or other potential complications.

INTRAVENOUS SITES AND DEVICES

The successful administration of IV drugs and fluids depends on patent vascular access. The most common site for short-term (less than 1 week) IV therapy is the peripheral short site, which uses the dorsal and ventral surfaces of the upper extremities. Catheter length is normally 1 to 3 inches (Figure 11.1, *A* and *B*).

The peripheral midline site for IV therapy uses the veins in the area of the antecubital fossa—the basilic, brachial, cephalic, cubital, or medial. Midline peripheral catheters are between 3 and 8 inches in length and can stay in place 2 to 4 weeks.

The peripherally inserted central catheter (PICC) (Figure 11.2) can be used for IV therapy for up to 1 year. The catheter length is 21 inches. The insertion site is the region of the antecubital fossa that uses the same veins as the peripheral midline. The catheter is advanced through the vein in the upper arm until the tip rests in the lower third of the superior vena cava. Because the tip of the PICC line rests in the superior vena cava, it is considered a central line. Compared to other types of access, the multilumen PICC is more dependable and cost-effective. It is also versatile because it can be used for IV medications, IV fluids, blood products, total parenteral nutrition (TPN), and blood sampling. Infection rates are also very low with PICC lines. Another benefit of the PICC line is that it can be maintained on an outpatient basis, therefore patients can be discharged earlier from the hospital. In some states, registered nurses certified in IV therapy can insert PICC lines.

Central venous access is used for patients who need long-term continuous infusions of fluids, medication, or nutritional support that cannot be sustained with a peripheral site. Central venous access is also used for patients who have poor peripheral veins, require a large amount of IV fluid or blood products in a short amount of time, or are receiving medication that is known to be too caustic for peripheral vessels. Central venous catheters (CVC) provide access to the superior vena cava and the inferior vena cava. A CVC placed in the internal jugular vein or the right or left subclavian vein is commonly used to access the superior vena cava. The inferior vena cava can be accessed through the femoral vein (Figure 11.3). Length of the CVC can vary from 6 to 28 inches. Insertion requires a competent provider to perform a sterile procedure involving the cannulation of the selected percutaneous vein with a single- or multi- lumen catheter. An x-ray is taken at the end of the procedure to confirm placement of the tip of the catheter in the superior vena cava just above the right atrium.

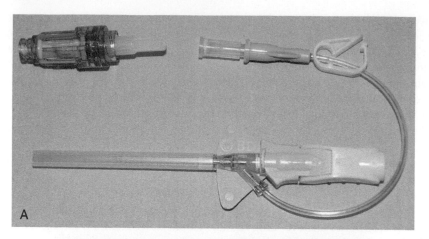

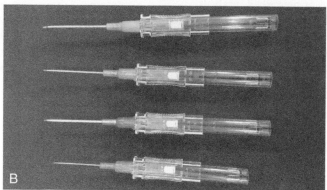

Figure 11.1 A, BD Nexiva IV catheter system has a single port with cap adapter. **B,** Various types of Becton Dickinson (BD) catheters.

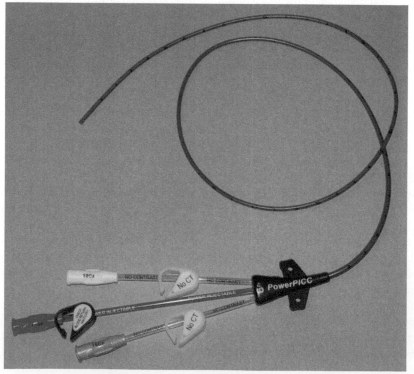

Figure 11.2 Bard PowerPICC triple-lumen catheter.

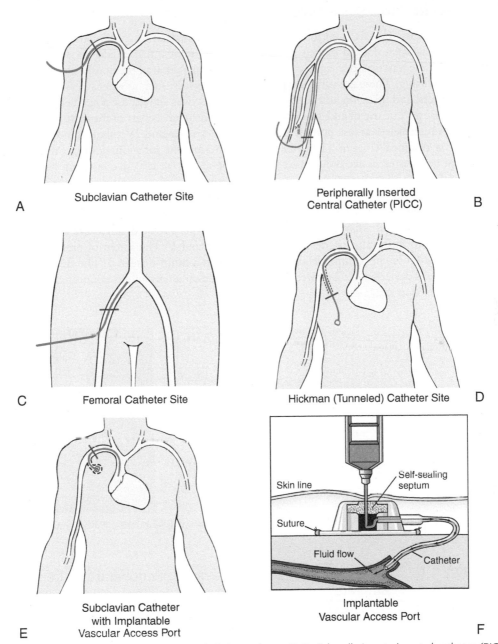

A Subclavian Catheter Site

B Peripherally Inserted
Central Catheter (PICC)

C Femoral Catheter Site

D Hickman (Tunneled) Catheter Site

E Subclavian Catheter
with Implantable
Vascular Access Port

F Implantable
Vascular Access Port

Skin line

Self-sealing
septum

Suture

Fluid flow

Catheter

Figure 11.3 Central venous access sites. **A,** Subclavian catheter. **B,** Peripherally inserted central catheter (PICC). **C,** Femoral catheter. **D,** Hickman (tunneled) catheter. **E,** Subclavian catheter with implantable vascular access port. **F,** Implantable vascular access port. (**F,** From Perry AG, Potter PA, Ostendorf WR: *Clinical nursing skills and techniques,* ed 9, St Louis, 2018, Mosby.)

Patients who need vascular access for long-term use, such as chemotherapy, antibiotic therapy, or nutritional support, are given much longer catheters, which are tunneled under the skin after the vein is cannulated. The catheter and its drug infusion port exit from the subcutaneous tissue to a site on the chest. Examples of these devices are the Hickman, Groshong, NeoStar, and Cook catheters.

Another type of catheter for long-term use has an implantable infusion port that is inserted in the subcutaneous tissue under the skin. These devices are called *vascular access ports,* also known as Port-a-caths, and they have a larger drug port or septum than other catheters. Care must be taken to use a non-coring needle that slices the port instead of making holes, so that the septum will close instead of leaking after the needle has been removed (see Figure 11.3).

Intermittent Infusion Add-On Devices

When IV access sites are used for intermittent therapy instead of continuous infusions, it is sometimes referred to as saline locked or hep-locked. An intermittent infusion add-on device can be attached to the end of the vascular device to close the connection that was previously attached to the IV tubing that was infusing. There are various types of add-on devices, such as extension loops and sets, stopcocks, manifold sets, and injection access ports. All add-on devices should use a needleless luer-lock design as a safety measure. The use of add-on devices should be included as part of the institution's policies. Add-on devices are needleless access ports (stoppers) where syringes and IV tubing can be attached when drug therapy is resumed (Figure 11.4). The use of intermittent infusion devices promote greater patient mobility, reduces excessive fluid intake, and can be more cost effective by using less IV tubing supplies and regulating equipment.

IV sites should be assessed frequently and flushed every 8 to 12 hours or before and after each drug infusion, depending on your institution's policy, to maintain patency. Table 11.1 offers suggested IV flushing intervals and volumes based on the catheter type. Prefilled single-use syringes of normal saline are available to flush infusion devices (Figure 11.5, *A* and *B*).The intent of prefilled single-use syringes is to prevent cross-contamination that can occur with a multi-dose vial. The flush volume used for the vascular access device should be twice the volume of the catheter plus any connected devices such as a stopcock or extension set.

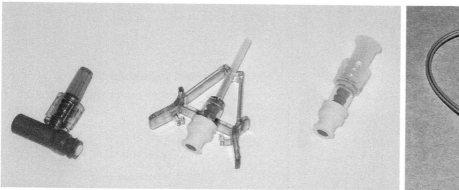
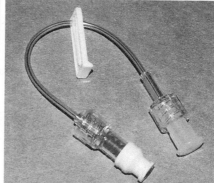

Figure 11.4 A variety of needless add-on connectors. IV tubing and syringes can easily attach to the access port on the infusion device.

TABLE 11.1 Venous Access Devices: Flushing for Peripheral and Central Venous Catheters*

Catheter Type	Length (inches)	Flush Before Drug Use	Flush After Drug Use	Volume/mL
Peripheral	1-2	NS	NS	1-3
Central venous				
Single-lumen	8	NS	HS	1-3
Multilumen	8	NS	HS	1-3
External tunneled	35	NS	HS or NS	10
Hickman, Cook,			Flush q12h if not used	
or Groshong				
Peripherally inserted	20	NS	NS	10
central catheter (PICC)			Flush q12h if not used	
Implanted vascular	35	NS	HS or NS	10
access device			Flush q12h if not used	

*If the adapter/cap is pressurized, then normal saline is used, not a heparin solution. Follow the institution policy procedure and manufacturer's guidelines.
HS, Heparinized saline; *NS,* normal saline.

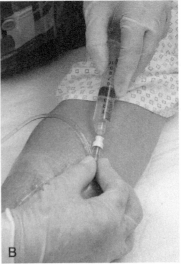

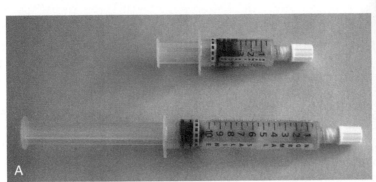

Figure 11.5 A, BD 3-mL and 10-mL prefilled, single-use syringes of normal saline. **B,** The prefilled single-use syringe is attached to the IV tubing's needleless luer-lock port and used to flush the IV catheter. (**B,** From Perry AG, Potter PA, Ostendorf WR: *Clinical nursing skills and techniques,* ed 9, St Louis, 2018, Mosby.)

DIRECT INTRAVENOUS INJECTIONS

Medications that are given by direct IV injection are often referred to as *IV push*. This route uses the patient's intravenous line to administer a small volume of medication directly into the blood stream. Direct IV injections have the fastest rate of absorption and thus the quickest onset of action. Medications ordered to be given IV push might need to be diluted with a compatible solution to avoid a concentration that may irritate the vein and IV site. Clinically, IV injection is the preferred route of administration for patients with poor muscle mass, decreased circulation, or for drugs that are poorly absorbed from the tissues. Drug information inserts must be read carefully and attention must be paid to the amount of drug that can be given per minute. Calculation errors can result in serious, even fatal, consequences. Additionally, if a medication is administered at a faster rate than specified, adverse reactions can occur. Calculating the amount of time needed to deliver a drug by direct IV infusion is the same method used for administering intramuscular (IM) injections and it can be done by using the ratio and proportion **(RP)** method.

 YOU MUST REMEMBER

When giving drugs by direct IV infusion, always verify the compatibility of the IV solution and the drug, or precipitation may result. Precipitation is a crystallization or suspension of particles in a solution, causing an occlusion of the intravenous line. Incompatibility can be avoided if the IV tubing is flushed with a compatible solution such as normal saline before and after administration.

EXAMPLES Set up a ratio and proportion using the recommended amount of drug per minute on one side of the equation; these are the known variables. On the other side of the equation are the desired amount of the drug and the unknown desired minutes: For each order, determine the amount of the medication to administer in milliliters (mL) and the duration in minutes that the medication should be given over.

PROBLEM 1: Order: Dilantin 200 mg, IV, STAT.

Drug available: Dilantin 250 mg/5 mL. IV infusion not to exceed 50 mg/min.

a. $\mathbf{BF:} \dfrac{D}{H} \times V = \dfrac{\overset{4}{\cancel{200}}\,mg}{\underset{5}{\cancel{250}}\,mg} \times 5\,mL = \dfrac{20}{5} = 4\,mL$

or

$\mathbf{RP:}$ H : V :: D : X

250 mg : 5 mL :: 200 mg : X mL

250 X = 1000

X = 4 mL

or

$\mathbf{FE:} \dfrac{H}{V} = \dfrac{D}{X} = \dfrac{250\,mg}{5\,mL} = \dfrac{200\,mg}{X}$

(Cross multiply)   250 X = 1000

X = 4 mL

or

$\mathbf{DA:} mL = \dfrac{5\,mL \times \overset{4}{\cancel{200}}\,\cancel{mg}}{\underset{5}{\cancel{250}}\,\cancel{mg} \times 1} = \dfrac{20}{5} = 4\,mL$

200 mg = 4 mL (discard 1 mL of the 5 mL)

b. known drug : known minutes :: desired drug : desired minutes

50 mg : 1 min :: 200 mg : X min

50 X = 200

X = 4 min

PROBLEM 2: Order: Lasix 120 mg, IV, STAT.

Drug available: Lasix 10 mg/mL. IV infusion not to exceed 40 mg/min.

a. $\mathbf{RP:}$ H : V :: D : X

10 mg : 1 mL :: 120 mg : X mL

10 X = 120

X = 12 mL of Lasix

or

$\mathbf{DA:} mL = \dfrac{1\,mL \times \overset{12}{\cancel{120}}\,\cancel{mg}}{\underset{1}{\cancel{10}}\,\cancel{mg} \times 1} = 12\,mL\ of\ Lasix$

b. known drug : known minutes :: desired drug : desired minutes

40 mg : 1 min :: 120 mg : X min

40 X = 120

X = 3 min

NOTE

When dosing instructions give the amount of drug and specify infusion time, the amount of drug can be divided by the number of minutes to attain the per-minute amount to be infused.

PROBLEM 3: Order: inamrinone (Inocor) 65 mg, IV bolus over 3 minutes.

Drug available: Inocor 100 mg/20 mL.

a. $\mathbf{RP:}$ H : V :: D : X

100 mg : 20 mL :: 65 mg : X mL

100 X = 1300

X = 13 mL

or

$\mathbf{DA:} mL = \dfrac{\overset{1}{\cancel{20}}\,mL \times 65\,\cancel{mg}}{\underset{5}{\cancel{100}}\,\cancel{mg} \times 1} = \dfrac{65}{5} = 13\,mL$

b. $\dfrac{13\,mL}{3\,min} = 4.3\,mL/min$

PRACTICE PROBLEMS ▶ I DIRECT IV INJECTION

Answers can be found on pages 256 to 257.

For each practice problem, determine the amount of drug to deliver in milliliters (mL) and the duration of administration in minutes for each direct IV drug dose.

1. Order: protamine sulfate 50 mg, IV, STAT.
   Drug available:

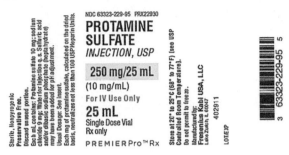

   IV infusion not to exceed 5 mg/min.

   a. Amount in milliliters _____

   b. Number of minutes_____

2. Order: dextrose 50% in 50 mL, IV, STAT.
   Drug available: dextrose 50% in 50 mL.
   IV infusion not to exceed 10 mL/min.

   Number of minutes to administer 50% of 50 mL _____

3. Order: protonix 40 mg, IV, STAT.
   Drug available:

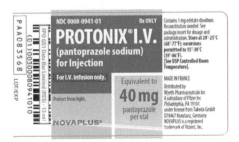

   Drug Insert: Add 10 mL of normal saline to reconstitute to 4 mg/mL. IV Infusion not to exceed 2.7 mg/min.

   a. Amount in milliliters _____

   b. Number of minutes _____

4. Order: fentanyl 12.5 mcg, IV, q4h, PRN for pain.
   Drug available: entanyl 100 mcg in 2 mL.
   IV infusion not to exceed 10 mcg/min.

   a. Amount in milliliters _____

   b. Number of minutes _____

5. Order: morphine sulfate 6 mg, IV, q3h, PRN.
Drug available:

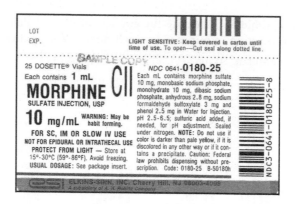

IV infusion not to exceed 10 mg/4 min.

a. Amount in milliliters _____

b. Number of minutes _____

6. Order: digoxin 0.25 mg, IV, daily.
Drug available:

Infuse slowly over 5 minutes.

a. Amount in milliliters _____

b. How many mL/min should be infused? _____

7. Order: Haldol 2 mg, IV, q4h, PRN.
Drug available: Haldol 5 mg/mL.
IV infusion not to exceed 1 mg/min.

a. Amount in milliliters _____

b. Number of minutes _____

8. Order: Ativan 6 mg, IV, q6h, PRN.
Drug available: Ativan 4 mg/mL.
IV infusion not to exceed 2 mg/min.

a. Amount in milliliters _____

b. Number of minutes _____

9. Order: diltiazem (Cardizem) 20 mg IV over 2 minutes.
   Drug available:

   > NDC 0088-1790-32
   >
   > **CARDIZEM® Injectable**
   > (diltiazem HCl Injection)
   > **25 mg (5 mg/mL)**   FOR DIRECT INTRAVENOUS BOLUS
   > INJECTION AND CONTINUOUS
   > INTRAVENOUS INFUSION
   >
   > Sterile 5-mL Vial
   > SINGLE-USE CONTAINER. DISCARD UNUSED PORTION.   Mfd. for
   > Date Removed From Refrigeration _____   Hoechst Marion Roussel, Inc.
   > Kansas City, MO 64137 USA
   > Date To Be Discarded _____   50007742   C6

   a. How many milliliters would you give? _____

   b. How many milliliters would you infuse per minute? _____

10. Order: granisetron (Kytril) 10 mcg/kg, 30 minutes before chemotherapy.
    Infuse 1 mg over 60 seconds.
    Patient weighs 140 pounds.
    Drug available:

    > *Each 1 mL contains, in sterile aqueous solution,
    > granisetron hydrochloride, 1.12 mg, equivalent to
    > granisetron, 1 mg; sodium chloride, 9 mg; citric acid,
    > 2 mg; benzyl alcohol, 10 mg, as a preservative.
    > **Store between 20° and 25°C (68° and 77°F)**
    > **[see USP]. Do not freeze.** Protect from light.
    > **Usual Dosage:** 10 mcg/kg administered intra-
    > venously either undiluted over 30 seconds, or diluted
    > with 0.9% Sodium Chloride or 5% Dextrose and
    > given over 5 minutes. See accompanying prescribing
    > information. **Caution:** Federal law prohibits
    > dispensing without prescription.
    > LOT   EXP.
    > 670759-B **SmithKline Beecham Pharmaceuticals**
    > Philadelphia, PA 19101
    >
    > *4mL Multi-Dose Vial*
    > **1mg/mL**
    > NDC 0029-4152-01
    > **KYTRIL®**
    > **GRANISETRON HCl**
    > **INJECTION**
    > **SB** SmithKline Beecham

    a. How many kilograms (kg) does the patient weigh? _____

    b. How many milligrams (mg) should the patient receive? _____

    c. For how many seconds should the drug dose be infused? _____

YOU MUST REMEMBER

Consider the length of the injection port on the tubing from the patient's IV site. If the IV rate is very low, (e.g., 30 mL/hr), the IV medication may take a long time to reach the patient. The drug dose is not complete until all of the drug has entered the patient. Therefore, the tubing will have to be flushed to ensure that the dose reaches the patient in a timely manner.

CONTINUOUS INTRAVENOUS ADMINISTRATION

When IV fluids are required, the health care provider orders the amount of solution per liter or milliliter to be administered for a specific time, such as 24 hours. The nurse calculates the IV flow rate according to the drop factor, the amount of fluid to be administered, and the infusion time.

Intravenous Infusion Sets

All infusion sets have the same components: a sterile spike for entry into the IV bag or bottle, a drip chamber for counting drops and managing flow, a roller clamp that controls flow through the tubing, tubing length from drip chamber to IV site, Y-site injection port for adding a secondary set or administering IV drugs, and the needleless adapter (which attaches to the IV catheter in the vessel) (Figure 11.6). Often a filter is added to the IV line to remove bacteria, particles, and air. Figure 11.7 shows two types of IV containers.

IV sets are either vented or unvented. Vented sets are used for IV bottles that have no vents and need a vent for air to enter the bottle so that the fluid will flow out. Unvented sets are for bottles or bags that either have their own venting system or do not need a venting system. Glass bottles are primarily used when the medication is not compatible with plastic because the drug either adheres to the plastic or is absorbed by the plastic.

If the IV infusion is not placed on a flow control device but instead is delivered by gravity, then the hourly rate will have to be adjusted manually. It is necessary to know the drop factor of the IV set to calculate the hourly infusion rate. The drop factor, or the number of drops per milliliter (mL), is printed on the package of the infusion set and found on top of the drip chamber. Sets that deliver large drops per milliliter (10, 15, or 20 gtt/mL) are referred to as *macrodrip sets,* and those that deliver small drops per milliliter (60 gtt/mL) are called *microdrip* or *minidrip* sets (Figure 11.8).

Drip rates are adjusted by counting the drops coming into the drip chamber. While looking at the second hand of your watch, adjust the roller clamp to determine the correct number of drops in one minute. It is more difficult to count when the drops are smaller and the drop rate is faster. One advantage of the microdrip set is that the number of milliliters per hour is the same as the drops per minute (e.g., if the infusion rate is 50 mL/hr, the drip rate is 50 gtt/min). When the IV rate is 100 mL/hr or higher, the macrodrip set generally is used. Slow drip rates (less than 100 mL/hr) make macrodrip adjustments too difficult (e.g., at 50 mL/hr, the macrodrip rate would be 8 gtt/min). Therefore if the IV rate is 100 mL/ hr or lower, the microdrip is preferred.

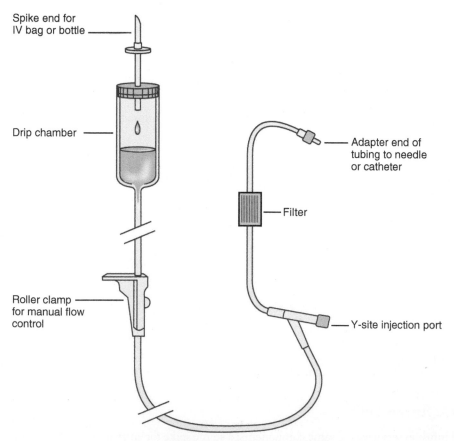

Figure 11.6 Intravenous tubing set.

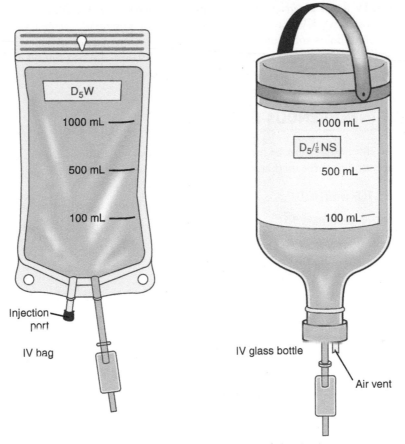

Figure 11.7 Intravenous bag and glass bottle.

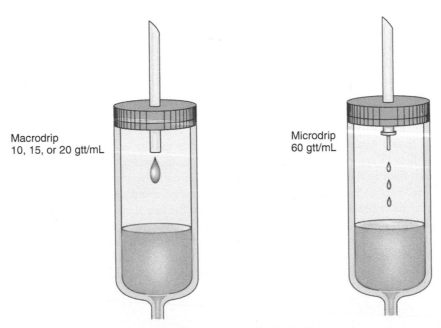

Figure 11.8 Macrodrip and microdrip sizes.

At times, IV fluids are given at a slow rate to *keep vein open* (KVO), also called *to keep open* (TKO). Reasons for ordering KVO include (1) a suspected or potential emergency situation requiring rapid administration of fluids and drugs, and (2) the need to maintain an open line to give IV drugs at specified hours. For KVO, a microdrip set (60 gtt/mL) and a 250-mL IV bag can be used. KVO should have a specific infusion rate, such as 10 to 20 mL/hr, or should be given according to the institution's protocol.

CALCULATION OF INTRAVENOUS FLOW RATE

Three different methods can be used to calculate IV flow rate (drops per minute or gtt/min). The nurse should select one of these methods, memorize it, and use it to calculate dosages.*

▶ THREE-STEP METHOD

a. $\dfrac{\text{Amount of solution}}{\text{Hours to administer}} = \text{mL/hr}$

b. $\dfrac{\text{mL per hour}}{60 \text{ minutes}} = \text{mL/min}$

c. mL per minute × gtt per mL of IV set = gtt/min

▶ TWO-STEP METHOD

a. Amount of fluid ÷ Hours to administer = mL/hr

b. $\dfrac{\text{mL per hour} \times \text{gtt/mL(IV set)}}{60 \text{ minutes}} = \text{gtt/min}$

▶ ONE-STEP METHOD

$\dfrac{\text{Amount of fluid} \times \text{gtt/mL(IV set)}}{\text{Hours to administer} \times \text{Minutes per hour(60)}} = \text{gtt/min}$

Safety Considerations

All IV infusions should be checked every half-hour or hour, according to the policy of the institution, to ensure the appropriate rate of infusion and to assess for potential problems, especially when manual flow control is used. Common problems associated with IV infusions are kinked tubing, infiltration, and "free-flow" IV rates. If IV tubing kinks and the flow is interrupted, the prescribed amount of fluid will not be given, and the access site can clot. When IV infiltration occurs, fluid leaks into the tissues around the IV site, causing redness, swelling, and discomfort. A more serious complication is extravasation, which occurs when the infiltrated medication damages the tissues at the IV site, resulting in sloughing and necrosis of exposed tissue. Again, in this situation the prescribed amount of IV fluid is not infused.

Free-flow IV rate refers to a rapid infusion of IV fluids, faster than prescribed, causing fluid overload, or too much fluid in the intravascular space, which can cause hypertension, pulmonary edema, and/or dyspnea. Medications that are administered faster than prescribed also can result in toxicity. A free-flow IV rate is the most prevalent drug error and has led to the use of electronic infusion devices.

Electronic infusion devices are not without flaws; mechanical problems occur and these devices can be incorrectly programmed, resulting in the wrong infusion rate. Fluid overload, thrombus formation, infiltration, and extravasation are complications of IV therapy that can be avoided with frequent monitoring of IV infusions. See *Appendix A* for more detailed information on safe practice for IV drug administration.

---

*The two-step method is the most commonly used method of calculating IV flow rate.

Adding Drugs Used for Continuous Intravenous Administration

Nurses may need to prepare medications from vials and add the medication into the patient's IV solution bag for some continuous infusions. This process of mixing or compounding an IV solution should be completed before the IV bag or bottle is hung. The medication is prepared using sterile technique and is added through the injection port to the bag or bottle where it then needs to be rotated, or gently agitated, to ensure that the drug is evenly dispersed. Failure to adequately disperse the medication can result in a higher concentration of medication close to the bottom of the bag or bottle. Thus, a higher concentration of the added medication could be delivered, potentially causing harm to the patient. Medication labels must be placed on the IV bag or bottle, clearly stating the patient's name and any other identifiers as specified by policy, such as name of the drug, amount, concentration, and strength of all ingredients without abbreviation. Also, the date, time, nurse's initials, and the time the IV should be completed should be provided. It is important to follow institutional policies and procedures when adding medication to continuous IV fluid.

NOTE

DO NOT add the drug while the infusion is running unless the bag is rotated. A drug solution injected into an upright infusing IV solution causes the drug to concentrate into the lower portion of the IV bag and not be dispersed. The patient will receive a concentrated drug solution, and this can be harmful (e.g., if the drug is potassium chloride).

Types of Solutions

All IV solutions contain various solutes and electrolytes that are added for specific therapies. Common solutes include dextrose (D) and sodium chloride (NaCl). The strength of the solution is expressed in percent (%), such as 0.45%, which means 0.45 g in 100 mL. Common commercially prepared IV solutions are dextrose in water (D_5W), dextrose with one-half normal saline solution (D_5 0.45%), normal saline solution (0.9% NaCl), one-half normal saline solution (0.45% NaCl), and lactated ringer's solution (LR). Lactated ringer's solution contains sodium, chloride, potassium, calcium, and lactate.

Tonicity of IV Solutions

The term *tonicity* and *osmolality* have been used interchangeably, but *tonicity* refers to the concentration of solute particles (osmoles) in IV solutions, and *osmolality* is the total concentration of solutes in body fluids (e.g., blood, serum). IV solutions produce tonicity in the cells of the body, which causes the movement of water molecules into and out of the cells based on their surrounding aqueous environment. Based on their tonicity, IV solutions are divided into three categories: hypertonic, hypotonic, and isotonic. The range of tonicity is measured in milliosmoles, (mOsm) and the normal range is 240 to 340 mOsm: +50 mOsm and/or −50 mOsm of 290 mOsm. IV fluids, such as lactated ringers (LR) and 0.9% normal saline (NS), that have an osmolality that approximates blood plasma (290 mOsm/L) are considered isotonic. Isotonic solutions maintain the same concentration of water molecules on both sides of the cell, thus no net movement occurs. The osmolality of isotonic solutions ranges from 240 to 340 mOsm/L. Hypertonic solutions have an osmolality of >340 mOsm. These solutions have a higher concentration of solutes causing water molecules to diffuse out of the cells and into the surrounding extracellular fluid (ECF). This shift of fluid out of cells can cause cells to shrink. An example of a hypertonic solution is D_5 0.9% normal saline (NS) with an osmolarity of 560 mOsm/L. Hypotonic solutions have an osmolality <240 mOsm. These solutions have a lower concentration of solutes compared to blood plasma causing water molecules from the ECF to diffuse into the cell. The movement of fluid into the cells can hydrate the cell or even cause it to swell. An example of a hypotonic solution is 0.45% normal saline (NS) with an osmolarity of 154 mOsm/L. D_5W is an isotonic solution with an osmolality of 250 mOsm/L; however, the solution's dextrose is metabolized quickly, leaving only water, thus making the solution hypotonic. Table 11.2 lists the names of selected IV solutions, as well as their abbreviations, tonicity, and osmolarity (mOsm).

TABLE 11.2 Abbreviations for IV Solutions with Tonicity and Osmolarity

IV Solution	Tonicity	mOsm	Abbreviation(s)
5% dextrose in water	Iso	250	D_5W, 5% D/W
10% dextrose in water	Hyper	500	$D_{10}W$, 10% D/W
0.9% sodium chloride, normal saline solution	Iso	310	0.9% NaCl, NS
0.45% sodium chloride, ½ normal saline solution	Hypo	154	0.45% NaCl, ½ NS
5% dextrose in 0.9% sodium chloride	Hyper	560	D_5NS, 5% D/NS, 5% D/0.9% NaCl, D_5 PSS
Dextrose 5%/0.2% sodium chloride	Iso	326	D_5/0.2% NaCl
5% dextrose in 0.45% sodium chloride, 5% dextrose in ½ normal saline solution	Hyper	410	D_5½ NS, 5% D½, NSS
Lactated Ringer's solution	Iso	274	LR

Osmolarity and osmolality are both terms used to describe the solute concentration of a solution and are often used interchangeably since 1 liter of water is understood to weigh 1 kilogram (kg). Osmolality is the quantity of solutes (osmoles) in 1 kilogram of solution (mOsm/kg), whereas osmolarity is the quantity of solutes (osmoles) in 1 liter of solution (mOsm/L).

EXAMPLES Two problems in determining IV flow rate are provided. Each problem is solved with each of the three methods for calculating IV flow rate. For the purpose of avoiding errors, the use of a hand calculator is strongly suggested.

PROBLEM 1: Order: 1000 mL of D_5½ NS (5% dextrose in ½ normal saline solution) in 6 hours.
Available: 1 L (1000 mL) of D_5½ NS solution bag: IV set labeled 10 gtt/mL.
How many drops per minute (gtt/min) should the patient receive?

Three-Step Method: **a.** $\dfrac{1000 \text{ mL}}{6 \text{ hr}} = 166.6$ or 167 mL/hr

b. $\dfrac{167 \text{ mL}}{60 \text{ min}} = 2.7$ or 2.8 mL/min

c. 2.8 mL/min × 10 gtt/mL = 28 gtt/min

Two-Step Method: **a.** 1000 mL ÷ 6 hr = 167 mL/hr

b. $\dfrac{167 \text{ mL/hr} \times \overset{1}{\cancel{10}} \text{ gtt/mL}}{\underset{6}{\cancel{60}} \text{ min}} = \dfrac{167}{6} = 28$ gtt/min

10 and 60 cancel to 1 and 6.

If mL/hr is given, use only part b of the two-step method for calculating IV flow rate.

One-Step Method: $\dfrac{1000 \text{ mL} \times \overset{1}{\cancel{10}} \text{ gtt/mL}}{6 \text{ hr} \quad \times \quad \underset{6}{\cancel{60}} \text{ min}} = \dfrac{1000}{36} = 28$ gtt/min

10 and 60 cancel to 1 and 6.

Answer: 28 gtt/min

PROBLEM 2: Order: 1000 mL of D_5W (5% dextrose in water), 1 vial of MVI (multiple vitamin), and 20 mEq of KCl (potassium chloride) every 8 hours.

Available: 1000 mL D_5W solution bag
1 vial of MVI = 5 mL
40 mEq/20 mL of KCl in an ampule
IV set labeled 15 gtt/mL

How many milliliters (mL) of KCl would you withdraw as equivalent to 20 mEq of KCl?
How would you mix KCl in the IV bag?
How many drops per minute should the patient receive?

Procedure: MVI: Inject 5 mL of MVI into the rubber stopper on the IV bag.
KCl: Calculate the prescribed dosage for KCl by using the basic formula **(BF)**, ratio and proportion **(RP)**, fractional equation **(FE)** method, or dimensional analysis **(DA)**.

$$\textbf{BF:}\ \frac{D}{H} \times V = \frac{20\ \text{mEq}}{40\ \text{mEq}} \times 20\ \text{mL} = \frac{400}{40} = 10\ \text{mL}$$

or

RP:
$$H \ :\ V \ ::\ D \ :\ X$$
$$40\ \text{mEq}:20\ \text{mL}::20\ \text{mEq}:X\ \text{mL}$$
$$40\,X = 400$$
$$X = 10\ \text{mL}$$

or

$$\textbf{FE:}\ \frac{H}{V} = \frac{D}{X} = \frac{40\ \text{mEq}}{20\ \text{mL}} = \frac{20\ \text{mEq}}{X}$$
(Cross multiply) $40\,X = 400$
$$X = 10\ \text{mL}$$

or

$$\textbf{DA:}\ \text{mL} = \frac{V \times D}{H \times 1}$$

$$\text{mL} = \frac{20\ \text{mL} \times \overset{1}{\cancel{20\ \text{mEq}}}}{\underset{2}{\cancel{40\ \text{mEq}}} \times 1} = \frac{20}{2} = 10\ \text{mL}$$

Withdraw 10 mL of KCl and inject it into the rubber stopper on the IV bag. Make sure the KCl solution and MVI additives are dispersed throughout the IV solution by rotating the IV bag.

Three-Step Method: **a.** $\dfrac{1000\ \text{mL}}{8\ \text{hr}} = 125\ \text{mL/hr}$

b. $\dfrac{125\ \text{mL}}{60\ \text{min}} = 2.0\ \text{or}\ 2.1\ \text{mL/min}$

c. $2.1 \times 15 = 31\ (31.25\ \text{gtt/min})$

Two-Step Method: **a.** $1000 \div 8 = 125\ \text{mL/hr}$

b. $\dfrac{125\ \text{mL/hr} \times \overset{1}{\cancel{15}}\ \text{gtt/mL}}{\underset{4}{\cancel{60}}\ \text{min}} = \dfrac{125}{4} = 31\ (31.25\ \text{gtt/min})$

15 and 60 cancel to 1 and 4.

One-Step Method: $\dfrac{1000\ \text{mL} \times \overset{1}{\cancel{15}}\ \text{gtt/mL}}{8\ \text{hr} \times \underset{4}{\cancel{60}}\ \text{min}} = \dfrac{1000}{32} = 31\ \text{gtt/min}\ (31.25\ \text{gtt/min})$

15 and 60 cancel to 1 and 4.

Answer: 31 gtt/min

NOTE

Medication volume can be added to the total volume if strict intake and output are recorded. In general, an IV bag contains more fluid than is labeled on the bag; some estimates are as high as 50 mL. Count all volume added to bag, 1 mL or greater. If an electronic infusion device is used, the patient will receive the amount programmed into the device.

PRACTICE PROBLEMS ▶ II CONTINUOUS INTRAVENOUS ADMINISTRATION

Answers can be found on pages 257 to 258.

Select *one* of the three methods for calculating IV flow rate. The two-step method is preferred by most nurses.

1. Order: 1000 mL of D$_5$W to run for 12 hours.

  a. Would you use a macrodrip or microdrip IV set?_____

  b. Calculate the drops per minute (gtt/min).

  _____

2. Order: 3 L of IV solutions for 24 hours: 2 L of 5% D/½ NS and 1 L of D$_5$W.

  a. One liter is equal to_____mL.

  b. Each liter should run for_____hours.

  c. The institution uses an IV set with a drop factor of 15 gtt/mL. How many drops per minute (gtt/min) should the patient receive? _____

3. Order: 250 mL of D$_5$W for KVO.

  a. What type of IV set would you use? _____
  Why? _____

  b. How many drops per minute (gtt/min) should the patient receive? _____

4. Order: 1000 mL of 5% D/0.2% NaCl with 10 mEq of KCl for 10 hours.
  Available: Macrodrip IV set with a drop factor of 20 gtt/mL and microdrip set;
  KCl 20 mEq/20 mL vial.

  a. How many milliliters (mL) of KCl should be injected into the IV bag?

  _____

  b. How is KCl mixed in the IV solution? _____

  c. How many drops per minute (gtt/min) should the patient receive with both the macrodrip set and the microdrip set? _____

5. A liter (1000 mL) of IV fluid was started at 9 AM and was to run for 8 hours. The IV set delivers 15 gtt/mL. Four hours later, only 300 mL has been infused.

  a. How much IV fluid is left? _____

  b. Recalculate the flow rate for the remaining IV fluids._____

6. The patient is to receive D₅W, 100 mL/hr.
Available: Microdrip set (60 gtt/mL).
How many drops per minute (gtt/min) should the patient receive? _____

7. Order: 1000 D₅W with 40 mEq KCl at 125 mL/hr.
Drug available:

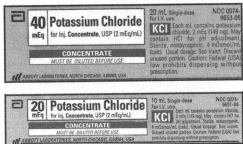

a. Which concentration of KCl would you choose? _____

b. How many milliliters (mL) of KCl should be injected into the IV bag? _____

c. How many hours will the IV infusion last? _____

8. Order: 1000 D₅/½ NS with 20 mEq KCl at 100 mL/hr.
Available: Macrodrip set (10 gtt/mL).
Drug available:

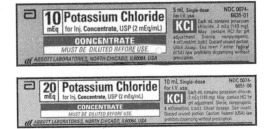

a. Which concentration of KCl would you choose? _____

b. How many milliliters (mL) of KCl should be injected into the IV bag? _____

c. How many hours will the IV infusion last? _____

d. How many drops per minute (gtt/min) should the patient receive? _____

INTERMITTENT INTRAVENOUS ADMINISTRATION

Giving drugs via the intermittent IV route has many advantages. The IV route allows for rapid therapeutic concentration of the drug and control over the onset of action and peak concentrations. Blood serum concentrations can be achieved via the IV route if the oral route is unavailable because of the patient's condition, such as gastrointestinal malabsorption or neurological deficits that prevent swallowing. The intermittent IV route can be used on an outpatient basis and can ensure compliance with drug therapy. The IV route also allows for the rapid correction of electrolyte imbalances. IV medications can be given at intervals within a 24-hour period for days or weeks. These medications are administered in a small volume of fluid (50 to 250 mL of D₅W or saline solution). The drug solution is usually delivered to the patient over 15 minutes to 2 hours, depending on the medication. A separate delivery set or secondary set is used for intermittent therapy if the patient is also receiving a continuous infusion through the same IV site.

Secondary Intravenous Sets

Secondary IV sets are used to infuse small fluid volumes such as, 50, 100, 250, and 500 mL in bags or bottles. Three types of tubing can be used. The first is similar to a regular IV set but with shorter tubing that is inserted or piggybacked into the primary IV line port. The second is a calibrated cylinder or chamber, which holds 150 mL, with brand names such as Buretrol, Volutrol, and SoluSet, also inserted into the primary set port. The third type is the regular set used with the infusion pump and piggybacked into the primary set at a port closer to the patient (Figure 11.9).

Medication is prepared and injected into a bag or a cylinder. If the cylinder is used, the drug is diluted with a measured amount of IV solution. After infusion, the cylinder is rinsed with 15 to 30 mL of the IV solution to clear the medication from the tubing. If the bag is used, the infusion runs until the bag is emptied.

If the fluid is delivered by gravity flow, the medication bag or cylinder needs to be raised higher than the primary set for the medication to infuse. Be aware that the drip chamber of the primary set must be observed to see that the medication is infusing properly from the secondary set and is not flowing into the primary set instead of the patient. If the secondary set is not flowing properly, then the IV site must be checked for patency.

Adding Drugs Used for Intermittent Intravenous Administration

Drugs that are given by intermittent infusion must be diluted and infused over a specific period of time. The pH and the osmolarity determine the dilution. A slower infusion time allows for the medication to be diluted in the blood vessel, thereby preventing phlebitis and high concentrations in the plasma and tissues,

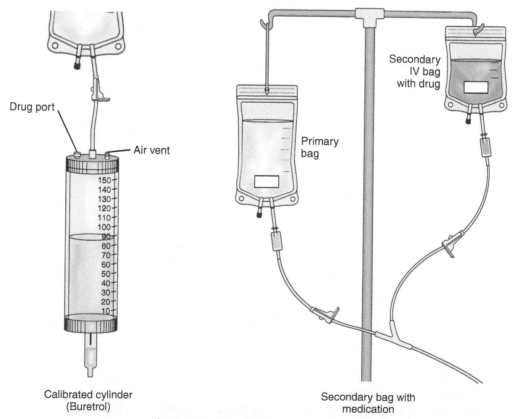

Figure 11.9 Equipment for secondary intravenous sets.

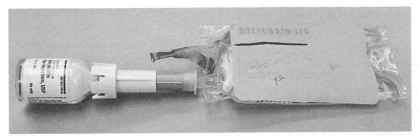

Figure 11.10 Medication mixed and attached to an IV bag.

which might cause time-related overdose, toxic effects, or allergic reactions. Drug-dosing instructions indicate the amount and type of solution and the length of infusion time. If the medication is not premixed from the pharmacy, the nurse must calculate the drug dose from the physician's order, then calculate the flow rate from the drug-dosing information.

Clinical agencies frequently have their own protocols for dilutions; if not, the drug information insert should provide infusion guidelines. If the information is not available, the hospital's pharmacy should be contacted. It is recommended that one set be used for the same drug to prevent admixture. Every set should be dated and labeled because one set can be used multiple times for the same drug in a 24-hour period. Guidelines and protocols help prevent drug and fluid incompatibilities.

Drugs administered by Buretrol, Volutrol, or SoluSet may be prepared by the nurse. Powdered drugs must be reconstituted with sterile water or normal saline solution following manufacturers' guidelines. Once the medication is added to the Buretrol, then the appropriate amount and type of IV fluid is added to the medication, and the infusion rate is adjusted. For medication diluted in bags or bottles, the powdered drug can be reconstituted the same way, or a spike adaptor can be used that can be attached to the vial and the bag. Fluid from the IV bag is flushed into the vial, reconstituting the powder, and then is flushed back into the bag. This process decreases contamination and is cost-effective. Mixing may be done by either the pharmacy or by the nurse (Figure 11.10).

The current trend in IV administration is the use of premixed or "ready to use" IV drugs in 50 mL to 1000 mL bags. These premixed IV medications can be prepared by the manufacturer or by the hospital's pharmacy. Problems of contamination and drug errors are decreased with the use of premixed IV medication. Each IV drug bag has separate tubing to prevent admixture. The actual cost of premixed medication is lower because there is less risk and less waste; it also saves nurses time. Because not all hospitals have admixture pharmacy systems in place, nurses will continue to prepare some drugs for IV administration.

NOTE

Sometimes the medication volume that is added to a bag or bottle adds a significant amount of volume. In those situations the 10% guideline applies. If the volume of medication for IV infusion exceeds 10% of the IV solution volume in the bag or bottle, then the amount of the medication volume should be withdrawn from the IV bag/bottle and replaced with the medication. For example, if the medication volume is 10 mL and a 100 mL bag is used, 10 mL should be aspirated from the IV bag injection port and replaced with the medication so that the total volume will still be 100 mL. If the medication's volume is less than 10%, then add the volume of medication to the volume of the bag or bottle. For example, 7 mL of medication is less than 10% of a 100 mL bag, so the total volume will be 107 mL. Follow your institution's protocol.

ADD-Vantage System

This system is similar to a secondary IV infusion or a piggyback system in which the nurse or pharmacist prepares the IV drugs. Figure 11.11 shows steps that the nurse takes in preparing the ADD-Vantage drug for IV administration.

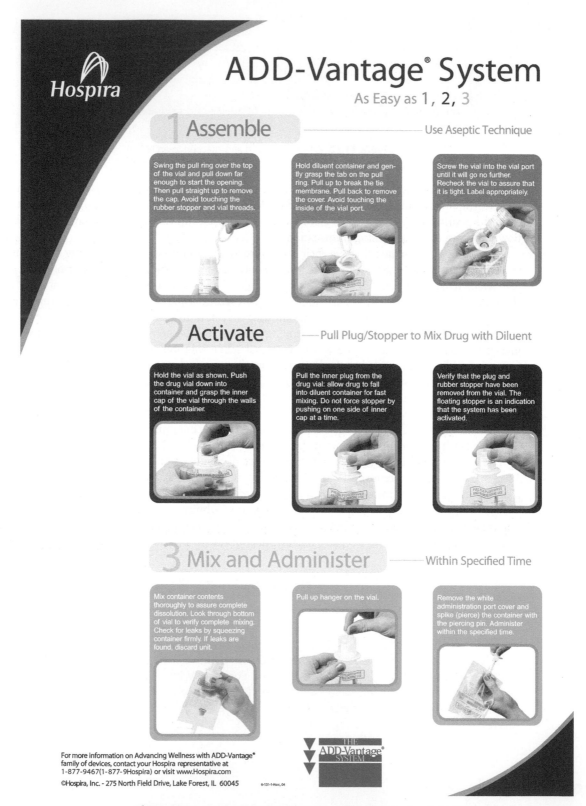

Figure 11.11 Hospira ADD-Vantage system. (From Hospira, Inc., Lake Forest, Ill.)

Electronic Intravenous Infusion Pumps

Infusion pumps are used for accurate fluid and drug administration (Figure 11.12). The peristaltic, volumetric, and syringe are three basic types of infusion pumps and all use a motor mechanism to create positive pressure to infuse fluid. The first is the linear peristaltic pump that uses a specially designed IV administration set that when placed in the pump, allows for ridges in the pump to move in a wavelike motion against the tubing to propel fluid along. The volumetric pump also has a specifically designed administration set with a reservoir that fills and empties every cycle to deliver the programmed fluid rate. The increments of fluid delivered with volumetric pumps can be as small as one tenth to one hundredth of a milliliter. The volumetric pump is considered more accurate than the peristaltic pump and the volumetric design is more widely manufactured.

The syringe pump uses a gear and screw mechanism to push fluid through IV tubing. One advantage of the syringe pump is that it does not require special tubing. A major disadvantage of the syringe pump is that it can only hold 2 mL to 100 mL syringes. The syringe pump is ideal for infusion of very small increments and some brands of pumps can infuse in nanograms. Syringe pumps are commonly used in pediatrics, oncology, obstetrics, and anesthesia (Figure 11.13, *A*).

The general-purpose pumps have safety features such as air-in-line, occlusion and infusion-complete alarms, as well as low-battery or low-power alerts (Figure 11.13, *B* and *C*). Pumps deliver a specific volume of fluid at a specific rate, measured in milliliters per hour (mL/hr). The general-purpose pump delivers at the rate of 0.1 to 999.9 mL/hr. The tubing for infusion pumps includes a safety feature called a flow regulator to prevent "free flow" when the tubing is removed from the pump. These regulators can be adjusted similarly to the roller clamp but are to be used only temporarily until the tubing can be placed back in the pump. Sensors in the pumps detect full or partial occlusion, especially at low flow rates. Another design feature is an alarm that notifies the nurse of an empty fluid container or any upstream occlusion, such as a clamp, that has not been released.

Programmable infusion pumps now offer important safety features that help in preventing IV drug errors. Programmable pumps, often referred to as "smart" pumps, have customized software that contains a library of medications and the maximum and minimum rates, known as guardrail limit, at which the medications should safely infuse (Figure 11.13, *E*). Hospitals can develop dosing parameters for each IV drug used in each patient area and update as needed. Once the IV medication solution is prepared, the nurse chooses the drug from the pump's library, then selects the dose to be given, the amount of solution in which the drug is diluted, and the duration of the infusion. The pump calculates the infusion rate and will infuse the drug at the correct rate. If the software recognizes an incorrect concentration or infusion time, the pump will alarm to alert the nurse so that the problem can be evaluated and corrected.

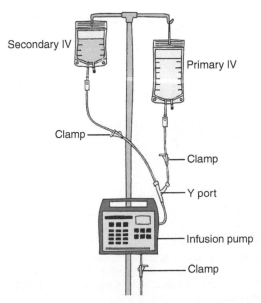

Figure 11.12 Typical IV setup with infusion pump.

Multichannel Pumps

Multichannel smart pumps have a main software module or platform that houses the drug library. The infusion channel where the IV tubing is placed is docked or added to the platform. The platform controls infusion rates through the channel, and extra channels (up to four) can be added to handle multiple drug infusions at different infusion rates (Figure 11.13, *F*).

Ambulatory Pumps

Ambulatory pumps are volumetric and used primarily for outpatients because of their small size and light weight. This type of programmable pump is used for intermittent and continuous infusion or demand dosing. Ambulatory pumps can accommodate high volume rates, such as 125 mL/hr, and low dosing rates, such as 0.02 to 1 mL.

Patient-Controlled Analgesia

Patient-controlled analgesia (PCA) pumps are computerized devices that are programmed so patients can self-administer IV analgesics (Figure 11.13, *D*). These battery-operated infuser pumps latch onto a cassette or bag of a narcotic that can be infused into a patient with the use of PCA-compatible tubing. A continuous rate, demand dose, and frequency of administration can be programmed into the pump. These set limits are ordered by the prescriber and prevent overdosage. The patient is able to administer a dose of pain medication using a control button attached to the PCA pump. The pump keeps a record of how much pain medication was delivered and how frequently the pain button was used. Each patient's

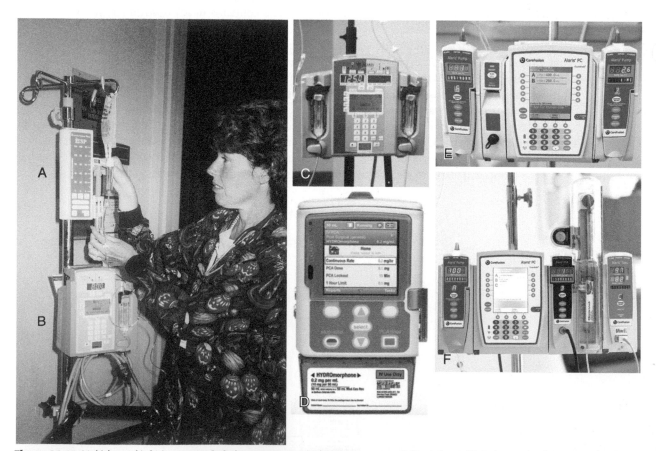

Figure 11.13 Multichannel infusion pump. **A,** Syringe pump. **B,** Single-infusion pump. **C,** Dual-channel infusion pump. **D,** CADD Solis Patient-controlled analgesia (PCA) pump. **E,** Alaris System Large Volume Pump with PCA. **F,** Example of the Medley pump module attached to the Medley programming module. (**A, B,** and **C,** From ALARIS Medical Systems, Inc., San Diego, Calif. **D,** From Smiths Medical, Dublin, OH. **E** and **F,** Courtesy and © Becton, Dickinson and Company)

pain score should be assessed and PCA therapy should be documented per your institution's policy. Commonly used narcotics administered on a PCA pump are morphine, fentanyl, and hydromorphone.

The use of infusion pumps is becoming the standard of care for IV medication delivery. IV pumps with programmable software allow for the precise and accurate delivery of medication, especially compared to the roller clamp adjustment and visual drop counting method. Remember, every model of pump has different features and capabilities. It is essential that the nurse has a working knowledge and understanding of the equipment to deliver safe patient care.

FLOW RATES FOR INFUSION PUMPS AND SECONDARY SETS

When medication is given via the infusion pump, the primary IV flow is halted while the medication is infused. Once the secondary infusion is complete, the primary IV fluid can be restarted (see Figure 11.12). If a smart pump is used, the drug is selected from the library with the prescribed concentration, and the rate per hour is determined by the calculations from the pump. However, if a general-purpose pump is used, the nurse must calculate the rate per hour. If pumps are not available for infusion, then the nurse must calculate the secondary set IV rate in drops per minute (gtt/min).

▶ ONE-STEP METHOD FOR IV DRUG CALCULATION WITH SECONDARY SET

$$\frac{\text{Amount of solution} \times \text{gtt/mL of the set}}{\text{Minutes to administer}} = \text{gtt/minute}$$

$$\text{Amount of solution} \div \frac{\text{Minutes to administer}}{60 \text{ minutes/hour}} = \text{mL/hour}$$

NOTE

Medication volume that exceeds 1 mL should be added to the dilution volume in intermittent drug therapy. Because smaller volumes of fluid are used for IV infusion, the drug dosage may be decreased if the volume of medication is not included in the dilution volume. The amount of solution in the formula should include both volumes.

EXAMPLES Determine the volume of medication to be added to the total volume and the flow rate using a calibrated cylinder (Buretrol), a secondary set, or an infusion pump, as indicated in each qustion.

PROBLEM 1: Order: Tagamet 200 mg, IV, q6h.
Drug available:

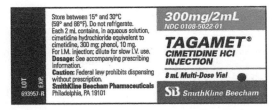

Set and solution: Buretrol set with drop factor of 60 gtt/mL; 500 mL of D$_5$W.
Instructions: Dilute drug in 100 mL of D$_5$W and infuse over 20 minutes.

Drug calculation:

$$\textbf{BF:} \frac{\text{D}}{\text{H}} \times \text{V} = \frac{200 \text{ mg}}{300 \text{ mg}} \times 2 \text{ mL} = \frac{400}{300} = 1.3 \text{ mL of Tagamet}$$

or
RP: H   :   V   ::   D   :   X

     300 mg : 2 mL :: 200 mg : X mL

        300 X = 400

$$X = \frac{400}{300}$$

$$X = 1.3 \text{ mL of Tagamet}$$

or
FE: $\dfrac{H}{V} = \dfrac{D}{X} = \dfrac{300 \text{ mg}}{2 \text{ mL}} = \dfrac{200 \text{ mg}}{X} =$

(Cross multiply) 300 X = 400

            X = 1.3 mL of Tagamet

or
DA: $mL = \dfrac{2 \text{ mL} \times \overset{2}{\cancel{200} \text{ mg}}}{\underset{3}{\cancel{300} \text{ mg}} \times 1} = \dfrac{4}{3} = 1.3$ mL of Tagamet

Flow rate calculation: 100 mL + 1.3 mL = 101.3 mL or 101 mL

$$\frac{\text{Amount of solution} \times \text{gtt/mL}}{\text{Minutes to administer}} = \frac{101 \text{ mL} \times \overset{3}{\cancel{60}} \text{ gtt}}{\underset{1}{\cancel{20}} \text{ min}} = 303 \text{ gtt/min}$$

Answer: Inject 1.3 mL of Tagamet into 100 mL of D₅W in the Buretrol chamber.
Regulate IV flow rate to 303 gtt/min.
It would be impossible to count 303 gtt/min. Instead of using the Buretrol, the nurse could use a secondary set with a larger drop factor or a regulator.

PROBLEM 2: Order: Mandol 500 mg, IV, q6h.
Drug available:

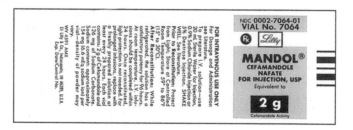

Label: Add 20 mL of diluent.
Set and solution: Secondary set with 100 mL D₅W and a drop factor of 15 gtt/mL.

Instructions: Dilute in 100 mL of D₅W and infuse over 30 minutes.

Drug calculation: (2.0 g = 2.000 mg).

BF: $\dfrac{D}{H} \times V = \dfrac{500 \text{ mg}}{2000 \text{ mg}} \times 20 \text{ mL} = \dfrac{10,000}{2000} = 5$ mL of Mandol

or
RP: H   :   V   ::   D   :   X

   2000 mg : 20 mL :: 500 mg : X mL

     2000 X = 10,000

       X = 5 mL of Mandol

or
FE: $\dfrac{H}{V} = \dfrac{D}{X} = \dfrac{2000 \text{ mg}}{20 \text{ mL}} = \dfrac{500 \text{ mg}}{X} =$

(Cross multiply) 2000 X = 10,000

        X = 5 mL of Mandol

or
DA: $mL = \dfrac{\overset{10}{\cancel{20} \text{ mL}} \times 1 \text{ g} \times \overset{1}{\cancel{500} \text{ mg}}}{\underset{1}{\cancel{2} \text{ g}} \times \underset{2}{\cancel{1000} \text{ mg}} \times 1} = \dfrac{10}{2} = 5$ mL of Mandol

Flow rate calculation: 100 mL + 5 mL = 105 mL

$$\frac{\text{Amount of solution} \times \text{gtt/mL}}{\text{Minutes to administer}} = \frac{105 \text{ mL} \times \overset{1}{\cancel{15}} \text{ gtt/mL}}{\underset{2}{\cancel{30}} \text{ min}} = \frac{105}{2} = 52.5 \text{ or } 53 \text{ gtt/min}$$

Answer: Inject 5 mL of Mandol into the 100 mL D$_5$W bag.
Regulate IV flow rate to 53 gtt/min.

PROBLEM 3: Order: Zithromax 500 mg IV daily for 2 days.
Drug available:

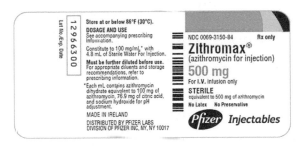

Label: Add 4.8 mL of sterile water to reconstitute to 100 mg/mL = 5 mL.
Set and solution: Use an infusion pump.

Instructions: Dilute in 250 mL D$_5$W and infuse over 3 hours.

Flow rate calculation: 250 mL D$_5$W + 5 mL of medication = 255 mL

$$\text{Amount of solution} \div \frac{\text{Minutes to administer}}{60 \text{ minutes/hr}} = 255 \text{ mL} \div \frac{\overset{3}{\cancel{180}} \text{ min}}{\underset{1}{\cancel{60}} \text{ min/hr}} = 255 \times \frac{1}{3} = 85 \text{ mL/hr}$$

Answer: Infusion rate should be set at 85 mL/hr.

PROBLEM 4: Order: albumin 25 g, IV, now.
Available: albumin 25 g in 50 mL.
Set: Use an infusion pump.

Instructions: Administer over 25 minutes, or 2 mL/min.

Drug calculation: Not applicable.

Infusion pump rate:

$$50 \text{ mL} \div \frac{25 \text{ min}}{60 \text{ min}} = 50 \times \frac{60}{25} = \frac{3000}{25} = 120 \text{ mL/hr}$$

Answer: Infusion rate should be set at 120 mL/hr.

PROBLEM 5: Order: potassium phosphate 10 mM IV in 100 mL NS over 90 minutes.
Drug available:

POTASSIUM PHOSPHATES	NDC 0517-2305-25
INJECTION, USP	Each mL provides 285 mg (3 mM) of Phosphate and 170 mg (4.4 mEq) of Potassium.
15 mM/5 mL Phosphate	7.4 mOsm/mL Sterile, nonpyrogenic.
22 mEq/5 mL Potassium	CAUTION: Federal (USA) law prohibits dispensing without prescription.
5 mL SINGLE DOSE VIAL FOR IV USE AFTER DILUTION	WARNING: DISCARD UNUSED PORTION. USE ONLY IF SOLUTION IS CLEAR. Store at 15°-30°C (59°-86°F).
AMERICAN REGENT LABORATORIES, INC. SHIRLEY, NY 11967	Usual Dosage: See package insert. REV. 3/92

Set: Use an infusion pump.

Drug calculation:

$$\textbf{BF:}\ \frac{D}{H} \times V = \frac{10\ mM}{15\ mM} \times 5\ mL = \frac{50}{15} = 3.3\ mL\ of\ potassium\ phosphate$$

or
$$\textbf{RP:}\quad H\ :\ V\ ::\ D\ :\ X$$
$$15\ mM : 5\ mL :: 10\ mM : X\ mL$$
$$15\ X = 50$$
$$X = 3.3\ mL\ of\ potassium\ phosphate$$

or
$$\textbf{FE:}\ \frac{H}{V} = \frac{D}{X} = \frac{15\ mM}{5\ mL} = \frac{10\ mM}{X\ mL}$$
$$(\text{Cross multiply})\ 15\ X = 50$$
$$X = 3.3\ mL\ of$$
$$potassium$$
$$phosphate$$

or
$$\textbf{DA:}\ mL = \frac{5\ mL \times \overset{2}{\cancel{10}}\ mM}{\underset{3}{\cancel{15}}\ mM \times 1} = \frac{10}{3} = 3.3\ mL$$

Infusion pump rate: $Amount\ of\ solution \div \dfrac{Minutes\ to\ administer}{60\ minutes} = mL/hr$

$$103\ mL \div \frac{90\ min}{60\ min} = 103 \times \frac{60}{90} = 68.6\ or\ 69\ mL/hr$$

Answer: Rate on the infusion pump should be 69 mL/hr to deliver potassium phosphate 10 mM in 90 minutes.

NOTE

When the electrolyte potassium is administered peripherally, the maximum infusion rate is 10 mEq/hr.

PRACTICE PROBLEMS ▶ III INTERMITTENT INTRAVENOUS ADMINISTRATION

Answers can be found on pages 258 to 262.

Calculate the fluid rate by using a calibrated cylinder (Buretrol), a secondary set, or an infusion pump, as indicated in each question.

1. Order: Cefazolin 250 mg, IV, q6h.
   Drug available: Cefazolin 1 g vial to be diluted with 2.5 mL.

   Set solution: Set Buretrol for a drop factor of 60 gtt/mL.

   Instructions: Dilute drug in 75 mL of NS and infuse over 30 minutes in Buretrol.
   a. 250 mg = _____ grams

   b. *Drug calculation:* _____

   c. *Flow rate calculation (gtt/min):* _____

2. Order: acetaminophen 500 mg, IV, q6h PRN for a temperature >38° C.
Patient's temperature is currently 38.5° C.
Drug available: Ofirmev 1000 mg/100 mL.

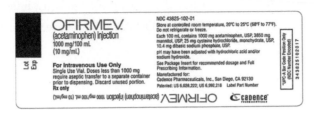

Set: Secondary set with a drop factor of 6 gtt/mL.

Instructions: Infuse over 15 minutes.

a. *Drug calculation:*

_____

b. *Flow rate calculation (gtt/min):*

_____

3. Order: ticarcillin (Ticar) 500 mg, IV, q6h.
Drug available:

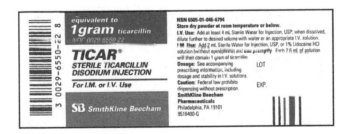

Set and solution: Buretrol set with a drop factor of 60 gtt/mL; infusion pump; 500 mL of D$_5$W.
Instructions: Dilute drug in 75 mL of D$_5$W and infuse over 40 minutes.

a. *Drug calculation:* Add_____ mL to ticarcillin vial (see drug label).

_____

b. *Flow rate calculation (gtt/min):*
How many drops per minute should the patient receive with use of the Buretrol set?

_____

c. *Infusion pump rate calculation (mL/hr):*
With an infusion pump, how many mL/hr should be administered?

_____

4. Order: piperacillin 2.5 g, IV, q6h.

Drug available: piperacillin 4-g vial in powdered form; add 7.8 mL of diluent to yield 10 mL of drug solution (4 g = 10 mL).

Set and solution: Buretrol set with a drop factor of 60 gtt/mL; infusion pump; 500 mL of D₅W.

Instructions: Dilute drug in 100 mL of D₅W and infuse over 30 minutes.

a. *Drug calculation:*

_____

b. *Flow rate calculation (gtt/min):*
How many drops per minute should the patient receive with use of the Buretrol set?

_____

c. *Infusion pump rate calculation (mL/hr):*
With an infusion pump, how many mL/hr should be administered?

_____

5. Order: methicillin (Staphcillin) 1 g, IV, q6h.

Drug available: Staphcillin 4 g in powdered form in vial; add 5.7 mL of diluent to yield 8 mL (1 g = 2 mL).

Set and solution: Secondary set with a drop factor of 15 gtt/mL; 100 mL bag of D₅W; infusion pump.

Instructions: Dilute drug in 100 mL of D₅W and infuse over 40 minutes.

a. *Drug calculation:* _____
Explain the procedure for diluting the drug and adding it to the IV bag.

_____

b. *Flow rate calculation (gtt/min):*
How many drops per minute should the patient receive with use of a secondary set?

_____

c. *Infusion pump rate calculation (mL/hr):*
With an infusion pump, how many mL/hr should be administered?

_____

6. Order: ciprofloxacin 250 mg, IV, q12h.
   Drug available:

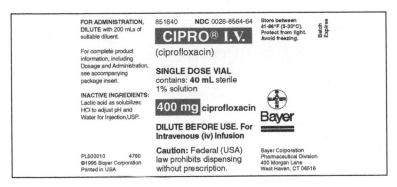

Set and solution: Secondary set with drop factor 15 gtt/mL; 250 mL of D₅W.

Instructions: Add ciprofloxin 250 mg to 250 mL D₅W and infuse over 60 minutes.

   a. *Drug calculation:*

_____

   b. *Flow rate calculation (gtt/min):*
   How many drops per minute should the patient receive?

_____

7. Order: doxycycline (Vibramycin), 100 mg, IV, q12h.
   Drug available:

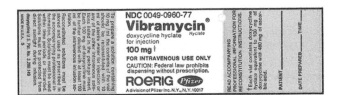

Set and solution: 100 mL of D₅W; secondary set with drop factor 15 gtt/mL; infusion pump.

Instructions: Mix Vibramycin vial with 10 mL of diluent; dilute in 100 mL of D₅W and infuse in 40 minutes.

   a. *Flow rate calculation (gtt/min):*

_____

   b. *Infusion pump rate calculation (mL/hr):*

_____

8. Order: ranitidine (Zantac) 50 mg, IV, q6h.
Set: infusion pump.
Drug available: premixed drug in bag (Zantac 50 mg in 0.45% NaCl).

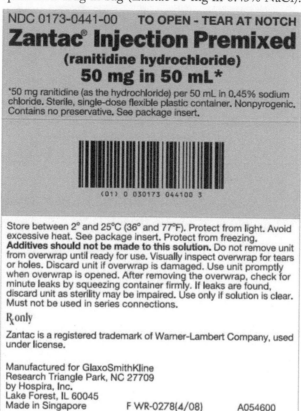

Instructions: Infuse over 15 minutes.

a. *Infusion pump rate calculation (mL/hr):* _____

9. Order: cefepime (Maxipime) 750 mg, IV, q12h.
Set and solution: infusion pump; 100 mL D₅W.
Drug available:

Instructions: Add 8.7 mL of diluent to Maxipime to yield 10 mL of drug solution. Dilute in 100 mL of D₅W; infuse over 30 minutes.

a. *Drug calculation:*

_____

b. *Infusion pump rate calculation (mL/hr):* _____

10. Order: rifampin (Rifadin) 600 mg, IV, daily.
Set and solution: infusion pump; 500 mL D₅W.
Drug available: Rifadin, 600 mg sterile powder.

Instructions: Add 10 mL of diluent to the rifampin vial. Dilute rifampin in 500 mL of D₅W; infuse over 3 hours.

a. *Infusion pump rate calculation (mL/hr):* _____

11. Order: cefoxitin (Mefoxin) 2 g, IV, q8h.
Drug available: ADD-Vantage vial.

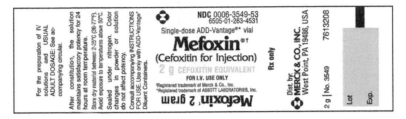

Set and solution: 100 mL of 0.9% NaCl diluent bag for ADD-Vantage; Mefoxin vial for ADD-Vantage.

Instructions: Dilute Mefoxin in 100 mL of NS (0.9% NaCl) and infuse in 30 minutes.

a. How would you prepare Mefoxin 2-g powdered vial with the diluent bag? (See page 231 as needed.) _____

b. *Infusion pump rate calculation (mL/hr):* _____

12. Order: Hycamtin (topotecan HCl) 1.5 mg/m²/day, IV, daily for 5 days.
Adult weight and height: 140 lbs, 66 inches.
Drug available:

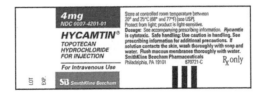

Set and solution: 100 mL of D₅W; infusion pump.

Instructions: Mix Hycamtin with 5.6 mL of diluent, equals 6 mL of Hycamtin; dilute in 100 mL of D₅W and infuse over 30 minutes.

a. What is the patient's m² (BSA)? (See Figure 7.1.) _____

b. *Drug calculation:* _____

c. *Infusion pump rate calculation (mL/hr):* _____

13. Order: Velban (vinblastine): initially 3.7 mg/m^2 as a single dose.
    Adult weight and height: 180 lbs, 70 inches.
    Drug available:

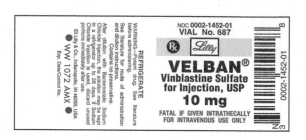

Set and solution: 250 mL of D$_5$W; infusion pump.
Instructions: Mix vinblastine powdered vial with 10 mL of diluent and inject solution into 250 mL of D$_5$W. Infuse over 1 hour.

a. What is the patient's m^2 (BSA)? _____

b. *Drug calculation:* _____

c. *Infusion pump rate calculation (mL/hr)* _____

14. Order: Cleocin Phosphate 600 mg, IV, q8h.
    Drug available:

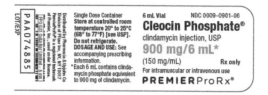

Set and solution: 50 mL D$_5$W; infusion pump.
Instructions: Dilute Cleocin in 50 mL of D$_5$W and infuse over 90 minutes.

a. *Drug calculation:* _____

b. *Infusion pump rate calculation (mL/h):* _____

15. Order: magnesium sulfate 5 g in 100 mL D5W infused over 3 hours.

Drug available:

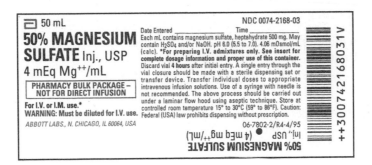

Set and solution: Secondary set with drip factor of 15 gtt/mL; 100-mL bag D₅W; infusion pump.

Drug calculation:

a. 1 mL = _____ mg (see drug label)

b. 5 g = _____ mL

c. *Infusion pump rate calculation (mL/hr):* _____

16. Order: calcium gluconate 10%, 16 mEq in 100 mL D5W, infused over 30 minutes.

Drug available:

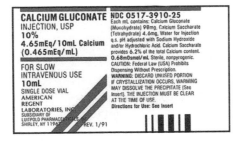

Set and solution: Secondary set with a drip factor of 15 gtt/mL; 100-mL bag D₅W; infusion pump.

a. *Drug calculation:* _____

b. *Infusion pump rate calculation (mL/hr):* _____

ANSWERS

I Direct IV Injection

1. a. 5 mL
   b. known drug : known minutes :: desired drug : desired minutes
   5 mg : 1 min :: 50 mg : X min
   5 X = 50
   X = 10 minutes

2. known drug : known minutes :: desired drug : desired minutes
   10 mL : 1 min :: 50 mL : X min
   10 X = 50
   X = 5 minutes

3. a. 10 mL
   b. known drug : known minutes :: desired drug : desired minutes
   2.7 mg : 1 min :: 40 mg : X min
   2.7 X = 40
   X = 14.8 or 15 minutes

4. a. 0.25 mL
   b. known drug : known minutes :: desired drug : desired minutes
   10 mcg : 1 min :: 12.5 mcg : X min
   10 X = 12.5
   X = 1.25 minutes

5. a. RP: H : V :: D : X
   10 mg : 1 mL :: 6 mg : X
   10 X = 6
   X = 0.6 mL

   or
   FE: $\dfrac{H}{V} = \dfrac{D}{X} = \dfrac{10\ mg}{1\ mL} = \dfrac{6\ mg}{X}$
   10 X = 6
   X = 0.6 mL

   b. known drug : known minutes :: desired drug : desired minutes
   10 mg : 4 min :: 6 mg : X min
   10 X = 24
   X = 2.4 minutes

6. a. 1 mL

   b. known drug : known minutes :: desired drug : desired minutes
   1 mL : 5 min :: X mL : 1 min
   5 X = 1
   X = 0.2 mL/minute

7. a. DA: mL $= \dfrac{1\ mL \times 2\ \cancel{mg}}{5\ \cancel{mg} \times 1} = \dfrac{2}{5} = 0.4\ mL$

   b. known drug : known minutes :: desired drug : desired minutes
   1 mg : 1 min :: 2 mg : X min
   X = 2 minutes

8. a. BF: $\dfrac{D}{H} \times V = \dfrac{6\ mg}{4\ mg} \times 1 = 1.5\ mL$
   b. known drug : known minutes :: desired drug : desired minutes
   2 mg : 1 min :: 6 mg : X min
   2 X = 6
   X = 3 minutes

9. a. RP: $\quad$ H $\;:\;$ V $\;::\;$ D $\;:\;$ V

$\qquad$ 25 mg : 5 mL :: 20 mg : X mL

$\qquad\qquad$ 25 X = 100

$\qquad\qquad\quad$ X = 4 mL

or
FE: $\dfrac{H}{V} = \dfrac{D}{X} = \dfrac{25\ mg}{5\ mL} = \dfrac{20\ mg}{X\ mL}$

(Cross multiply) 25 X = 100

$\qquad\qquad\qquad$ X = 4 mL

or
DA: $V = \dfrac{V \times D}{H \times 1}$

$mL = \dfrac{5\ mL \times \overset{4}{\cancel{20\ mg}}}{\underset{5}{\cancel{25\ mg}} \times 1} = \dfrac{20}{5} = 4\ mL$

b. $\dfrac{\text{Amount of drug}}{\text{Number of minutes}} = \dfrac{4\ mL}{2\ min} = 2\ mL/min$

Answer: Infuse 2 mL of cardizem per minute.

10. a. 140 lbs ÷ 2.2 = 64 kg

$\quad$ **b.** 10 mcg × 64 kg = 640 mcg

$\qquad$ Change micrograms (mcg) to milligrams by moving the decimal point three spaces to the *left:* 640 mcg = 0.640 mg or 0.6 mg.

$\quad$ **c.** Known drug : known seconds :: desired drug : desired seconds

$\qquad\quad$ 1 mg $\quad$: $\;$ 60 seconds $\;$ :: $\;$ 0.6 mg $\;$: $\quad$ X sec

$\qquad\qquad\qquad\qquad\qquad\qquad$ X = 36 seconds

$\qquad$ *Answer:* Infuse 0.6 mg of granisetron (Kytril) over 36 seconds.

II Continuous Intravenous Administration

1. a. Microdrip set because the patient is to receive 83 mL/hr

$\quad$ **b.** Three-step method: (a) $\dfrac{1000\ mL}{12\ hr} = 83\ mL/hr$

$\qquad\qquad\qquad\qquad\quad$ (b) $\dfrac{83\ mL/hr}{60\ min} = 1.38\ mL/min\ or\ 1.4\ mL$

$\qquad\qquad\qquad\qquad\quad$ (c) 1.4 mL/min × 60 gtt/mL = 84 gtt/min

$\qquad$ Using a microdrip set (60 gtt/mL), IV should run at 84 gtt/min.

2. a. 1 L = 1000 mL

$\quad$ **b.** Each liter should run for 8 hours.

$\quad$ **c.** Two-step method: 1000 ÷ 8 = 125 mL/hr

$\qquad \dfrac{125\ mL \times \overset{1}{\cancel{15}}\ gtt/min}{\underset{4}{\cancel{60}}\ min} = \dfrac{125}{4} = 31\text{–}32\ gtt/min$

$\qquad$ With a 15 gtt/mL drop set, IV should run at 31 to 32 gtt/min.

3. a. Microdrip set with drop factor of 60 gtt/mL is used because the hourly rate is low and would make drops easier to count.

$\quad$ **b.** One-step method: $\dfrac{250\ mL \times \overset{1}{\cancel{60}}\ gtt/min}{24\ hr \times \underset{1}{\cancel{60}}\ min/hr} = 10\ gtt/min$

$\qquad$ With a microdrip set, IV should run at 10 gtt/min.

4. a. 10 mL of KCl

$\quad$ **b.** Use a 10-mL syringe; withdraw 10 mL of KCl and inject into the rubber stopper part of the IV bag.

$\quad$ **c.** Microdrip set: 100 gtt/min

$\qquad$ Macrodrip set: drop factor of 20 gtt/mL; 33 gtt/min (33.3 gtt/min)

5. a. 700 mL of IV fluid is left and 4 hours are left.
  b. Recalculate using 700 mL and 4 hours to run.

Three-step method: (a) $\dfrac{700 \text{ mL}}{4 \text{ hr}} = 175 \text{ mL/hr}$

(b) $\dfrac{175 \text{ mL/hr}}{60 \text{ min}} = 2.9 \text{ mL/min}$

(c) $2.9 \text{ mL/min} \times 15 \text{ gtt/mL} = 43.5 \text{ gtt/min or } 44 \text{ gtt/min}$

6. 100 gtt/min

Two-step method: $\dfrac{100 \times \overset{1}{\cancel{60}} \text{ gtt/mL}}{\underset{1}{\cancel{60}} \text{ min}} = 100 \text{ gtt/min}$

7. a. KCl 40 mEq/20 mL
  b. 20 mL

  c. $\dfrac{1000 \text{ mL}}{125 \text{ mL/hr}} = 8 \text{ hours}$

8. a. KCl 20 mEq/10 mL
  b. 10 mL

  c. $\dfrac{1000 \text{ mL}}{100 \text{ mL/hr}} = 10 \text{ hours}$

  d. $\dfrac{100 \text{ mL} \times \overset{1}{\cancel{10}} \text{ gtt/mL}}{\underset{6}{\cancel{60}} \text{ min}} = \dfrac{100}{6} = 16.6 \text{ gtt/min or } 17 \text{ gtt/min}$

or

$\dfrac{1000 \text{ mL} \times \overset{1}{\cancel{10}} \text{ gtt/mL}}{\underset{1}{\cancel{10}} \text{ hr} \times 60 \text{ min}} = \dfrac{1000}{60} = 16.6 \text{ gtt/min or } 17 \text{ gtt/min}$

III Intermittent Intravenous Administration

1. a. 250 mg = 0.25 g
  b. *Drug calculation:*

BF: $\dfrac{D}{H} \times V = \dfrac{0.25 \text{ g}}{1 \text{ g}} \times 2.5 \text{ mL} = 0.6 \text{ mL}$

or

RP: H :   V   ::   D :   X
         1 g : 2.5 mL :: 0.25 g : X mL
            1 X = 2.5 × 0.25
               X = 0.6 mL

or

DA: $\text{mL} = \dfrac{2.5 \text{ mL} \times \quad 1 \text{ g} \quad \times 250 \text{ mg}}{1 \text{ g} \quad \times 1000 \text{ mg} \times \quad 1} = 0.6 \text{ mL}$

or

FE: $\dfrac{H}{V} = \dfrac{D}{X} = \dfrac{1 \text{ g}}{2.5 \text{ mL}} = \dfrac{0.25 \text{ g}}{X} = X = 0.6 \text{ mL}$

  c. *Flow rate calculation:* Amount of solution: 75 mL + 0.6 mL = 75.6 or 76 mL

$\dfrac{\text{Amount of solution} \times \text{gtt/mL}}{\text{Minutes to administer}} = \dfrac{76 \text{ mL} \times 60 \text{ gtt/mL}}{30 \text{ min}} = 152 \text{ gtt/min}$

Regulate flow rate for 152 gtt/min.

2. a. *Drug calculation:*

$$\text{BF:} \frac{D}{H} \times V = \frac{500 \text{ g}}{1000 \text{ mg}} \times 100 \text{ mL} = 50 \text{ mL}$$

or

$$\text{RP:} \quad H \ : \ V \ :: \ D \ : \ X$$
$$1000 \text{ g}:100 \text{ mL}::500 \text{ mg}:X \text{ mL}$$
$$1000 \text{ X} = 50{,}000$$
$$X = 50 \text{ mL}$$

or

$$\text{DA:} \text{ mL} = \frac{100 \text{ mL} \times 500 \text{ mg}}{1000 \text{ mg} \times 1} = 50 \text{ mL}$$

or

$$\text{FE:} \frac{H}{V} = \frac{D}{X} = \frac{1000 \text{ mg}}{100 \text{ mL}} = \frac{500 \text{ mg}}{X}$$
$$1000 \text{ X} = 50{,}000$$
$$(\text{Cross multiply}) \text{ X} = 50 \text{ mL}$$

b. *Flow rate calculation:*

$$\frac{\text{Amount of solution} \times \text{gtt/mL}}{\text{Minutes to administer}} = \frac{100 \text{ mL} \times 6 \text{ gtt/mL}}{15 \text{ minutes}} = 40 \text{ gtt/min}$$

Regulate flow rate of secondary tubing for 40 gtt/min.

3. a. *Drug calculation:*

$$\text{BF:} \frac{D}{H} \times V = \frac{500 \text{ mg}}{1000 \text{ mg}} \times 4 \text{ mL} = \frac{2000}{1000} = 2 \text{ mL is the dose for 500 mg of ticarcillin.}$$

b. *Flow rate calculation:* Amount of solution: 75 mL D_5W + 2 mL of drug solution = 77 mL
For Buretrol set:

$$\frac{77 \text{ mL} \times \overset{3}{\cancel{60}} \text{ gtt/mL (set)}}{\underset{2}{\cancel{40}} \text{ minutes}} = \frac{231}{2} = 115.5 \text{ or } 116 \text{ gtt/min}$$

c. *Infusion pump rate calculation:*

$$\text{Amount of solution} \div \frac{\text{Minutes to administer}}{60 \text{ min/hr}} = \text{mL/hr}$$

$$77 \text{ mL} \div \frac{\overset{2}{\cancel{40}} \text{ min to administer}}{\underset{3}{\cancel{60}} \text{ min/hr}} = 77 \times \frac{3}{2} = \frac{231}{2} = 116 \text{ mL/hr}$$

Set pump rate at 116 mL/hr to deliver Ticar 500 mg in 40 minutes.

4. a. *Drug calculation:*

$$\text{BF:} \frac{D}{H} \times V = \frac{2.5 \text{ g}}{\underset{2}{\cancel{4} \text{ g}}} \times \overset{5}{\cancel{10}} \text{ mL} = \frac{12.5}{2} = 6.25 \text{ mL}$$

or

$$\text{RP:} \ H : \ V \ :: \ D \ : \ X$$
$$4 \text{ g}:10 \text{ mL}::2.5 \text{ g}:X \text{ mL}$$
$$4 \text{ X} = 25$$
$$X = 6.25 \text{ mL}$$
piperacillin 2.5 g = 6.25 mL

or

$$\text{FE:} \frac{H}{V} = \frac{D}{X} = \frac{4 \text{ g}}{10 \text{ mL}} = \frac{2.5 \text{ g}}{X \text{ mL}}$$
$$(\text{Cross multiply}) \ 4 \text{ X} = 25$$
$$X = 6.25 \text{ mL}$$

or

$$\text{DA:} \text{ mL} = \frac{10 \text{ mL} \times 2.5 \text{ g}}{4 \text{ g} \times 1} = \frac{25}{4} = 6.25 \text{ mL}$$

b. *Flow rate calculation for Buretrol set:* amount of solution: 6.25 mL + 100 mL = 106.25 mL

$$\frac{106 \text{ mL} \times \overset{2}{\cancel{60}} \text{ gtt/mL}}{\underset{1}{\cancel{30}} \text{ min/hr}} = 212 \text{ gtt/min}$$

c. *Infusion pump rate calculation:* 100 mL + 6 mL medication = 106 mL

$$106 \text{ mL} \div \frac{\overset{1}{\cancel{30}} \text{ min to administer}}{\underset{2}{\cancel{60}} \text{ min/hr}} = 106 \times \frac{2}{1} = 212 \text{ mL/hr}$$

Set pump rate at 212 mL/hr to deliver piperacillin 2.5 g in 30 minutes.

5. a. *Drug calculation:* Staphcillin 4 g = 8 mL

$$\text{BF:} \frac{D}{H} \times V = \frac{1\,g}{4\,g} \times 8\,mL = \frac{8}{4} = 2\,mL \text{ dose of Staphcillin}$$

Amount of solution: 2 mL + 100 mL = 102 mL

b. *Flow rate calculation for secondary set:*

$$\frac{102\,mL \times 15\,gtt/mL\,(set)}{40\,minutes} = \frac{1530}{40} = 38.25 \text{ or } 38\,gtt/min$$

c. *Infusion pump rate calculation:* amount of solution: 100 mL + 2 mL = 102 mL

$$102\,mL \times \frac{\overset{2}{\cancel{40}}\,min\ to\ administer}{\underset{3}{\cancel{60}}\,min/hr} = 102 \times \frac{3}{2} = \frac{306}{2} = 153\,mL/hr$$

Set pump rate at 153 mL/hr to deliver Staphcillin 1 g in 40 minutes.

6. a. *Drug calculation:*

$$\text{BF:} \frac{D}{H} \times V = \frac{250\,mg}{\underset{10}{\cancel{400}}\,mg} \times \overset{1}{\cancel{40}}\,mL = \frac{250}{10} = 25\,mL$$

or

$$\text{RP:}\quad H\ :\ V\ ::\ D\ :\ X$$
$$400\,mg : 40\,mL :: 250\,mg : X\,mL$$
$$400\,X = 10{,}000$$
$$X = 25\,mL$$

or

$$\text{FE:} \frac{H}{V} = \frac{D}{X} = \frac{400}{40} = \frac{250}{X} =$$

(Cross multiply) 400 X = 10,000
X = **25 mL** of ciprofloxacin

or

$$\text{DA: mL} = \frac{\overset{1}{\cancel{40}}\,mL \times 250\,\cancel{mg}}{\underset{10}{\cancel{400}}\,\cancel{mg} \times 1} =$$

25 mL of ciprofloxacin

b. *Flow rate calculation (gtt/min):*
Amount of solution: 25 mL + 250 mL = 275 mL

$$\frac{275\,mL \times 15\,gtt/mL}{60\,min/hr} = \frac{4125}{60} = 68.75 \text{ or } 69\,gtt/min$$

7. a. *Flow rate calculation (gtt/min):*
Amount of solution: 10 mL + 100 mL = 110 mL

$$\frac{110\,mL \times \overset{3}{\cancel{15}}\,gtt/mL}{\underset{8}{\cancel{40}}\,min\ to\ admin} = \frac{330}{8} = 41.25 \text{ or } 41\,gtt/min$$

b. *Infusion pump rate calculation (mL/hr):*

$$110\,mL \div \frac{40\,min}{60\,min} = 110\,mL \times \frac{\overset{6}{\cancel{60}}}{\underset{4}{\cancel{40}}} = \frac{660}{4} = 165\,mL/hr$$

8. a. *Amount of solution:*

$$\frac{Min\ to\ administer}{60\,mL/hr} = 50\,mL \div \frac{15\,min}{60\,min} = 50\,mL \times \frac{\overset{4}{\cancel{60}}\,min}{\underset{1}{\cancel{15}}\,min} = 200\,mL/hr$$

Infusion pump rate calculation: 200 mL/hr

9. 1 g = 1000 mg (use conversion table as needed) of Maxipime
a. *Drug calculation:*

$$\text{BF:} \frac{D}{H} \times V = \frac{\overset{3}{\cancel{750}}\,mg}{\underset{4}{\cancel{1000}}\,mg} \times 10\,mL = \frac{30}{4} = 7.5\,mL \text{ drug solution}$$

Amount of solution: 7.5 mL + 100 mL = 107.5 mL

b. *Infusion pump rate calculation:*

$$107.5 \text{ mL} \div \frac{30 \text{ min to administer}}{60 \text{ min/hr}} = 107.5 \text{ mL} \times \frac{\overset{2}{\cancel{60}}}{\underset{1}{\cancel{30}}} = 215 \text{ mL/hr pump rate}$$

10. *Amount of solution:* 10 mL + 500 mL = 510 mL

a. *Infusion pump rate calculation:* $510 \text{ mL} \div \dfrac{180 \text{ min}}{60 \text{ min/hr}} = 510 \text{ mL} \times \dfrac{\overset{1}{\cancel{60}}}{\underset{3}{\cancel{180}}} = \dfrac{510}{3} = 170 \text{ mL/hr}$

11. **a.** Mix 2 g of cefoxitin (Mefoxin) using ADD-Vantage vial with ADD-Vantage 100 mL diluent bag. See p. 231 for mixing ADD-Vantage drugs.

   b. *Infusion pump rate calculation (mL/hr):*

   $$100 \text{ mL} \div \frac{30 \text{ min to administer}}{60 \text{ min/hr}} =$$

   $$100 \text{ mL} \times \frac{\overset{2}{\cancel{60}}}{\underset{1}{\cancel{30}}} = 200 \text{ mL/hr}$$

12. **a.** BSA· 1 74 m²; see Figure 7.1.

   b. *Drug calculation:*
   1.5 mg × 1.74 m² = 2.61 or 2.6 mg/m²/day

   $$\textbf{BF:}\ \frac{D}{H} \times V = \frac{2.6 \text{ mg}}{\underset{2}{\cancel{4}} \text{ mg}} \times \overset{3}{\cancel{6}} \text{ mL} = \frac{7.8}{2} = 3.9 \text{ mL or 4 mL}$$

   Amount of solution: 4 mL + 100 mL = 104 mL

   c. *Infusion pump rate calculation (mL/hr):*

   $$104 \text{ mL} \div \frac{30 \text{ min to administer}}{60 \text{ min/hr}} = 104 \times \frac{\overset{2}{\cancel{60}}}{\underset{1}{\cancel{30}}} = 208 \text{ mL/hr}$$

13. **a.** 2.05 m² (BSA)

   b. *Drug calculation:*
   3.7 mg × 2.05 m² = 7.58 or 7.6 mg/m²
   Velban 10 mg diluted in 10 mL
   Each mg = 1 mL; 7.6 mg = 7.6 mL
   Amount of solution: 7.6 mL + 250 mL = 257.6 mL

   c. *Infusion pump rate calculation (mL/hr):*

   $$257.6 \text{ mL} \div \frac{60}{60} = 257.6 \times \frac{\overset{1}{\cancel{60}}}{\underset{1}{\cancel{60}}} = 257.6 \text{ or 258 mL/hr}$$

14. **a.** *Drug calculation:*

   $$\textbf{BF:}\ \frac{D}{H} \times V = \frac{600 \, mg}{900 \, mg} \times 6 \text{ mL} = \frac{36}{9} = 4 \text{ mL} \qquad\qquad \textbf{DA:}\ \text{mL} = \frac{6 \, mL \times 600 \, mg}{900 \, mg \times 1} = \frac{36}{9} = 4 \text{ mL}$$

   $$\textbf{RP:}\quad \begin{array}{cccc} H & : & V & :: & D & : X \\ 900 \text{ mg} & : & 6 \text{ mL} & :: & 600 \text{ mg} : X \end{array}$$
   $$9 \text{ X} = 36$$
   $$\text{X} = 4 \text{ mL}$$

   $$\textbf{FE:}\ \frac{H}{V} = \frac{D}{X} = \frac{900 \text{ mg}}{6 \text{ mL}} = \frac{600 \text{ mg}}{X \text{ mL}}$$
   (cross multiply) $\quad 9 \text{ X} = 36$
   $$\text{X} = 4 \text{ mL}$$

Amount of solution: 50 mL + 4 mL = 54 mL

b. *Infusion pump rate calculation:*

$$54 \text{ mL} \div \frac{90 \text{ min } \textit{to administer}}{60 \textit{ min/hr}} = 54 \times \frac{6}{9} = 36 \text{ mL/hr}$$

Set pump rate at 36 mL/hr to deliver Cleocin 600 mg in 90 minutes.

15. *Drug calculation:*

a. 1 mL = 500 mg and 2 mL = 1 g

b. BF: $\dfrac{D}{H} \times V = \dfrac{5 \text{ g}}{1 \text{ g}} \times 2 = 10$ mL

or
RP: H : V :: D : X
     1 : 2 :: 5 : X
            X = 10
            X = 10 mL KCl magnesium sulfate

or
FE: $\dfrac{H}{V} = \dfrac{D}{X} = \dfrac{1 \text{ g}}{2 \text{ mL}} = \dfrac{5 \text{ g}}{X \text{ mL}}$

or
DA: mL $= \dfrac{1 \text{ mL} \times \overset{2}{\cancel{1000} \text{ mg}} \times 5 \text{ g}}{\underset{1}{\cancel{500} \text{ mg}} \times 1 \text{ g} \times 1} = 10$ mL

(Cross multiply) X = 10 mL of magnesium sulfate

Amount of solution: 10 mL + 100 mL = 110 mL

c. *Infusion pump rate calculation:*

$$110 \text{ mL} \div \frac{\overset{3}{\cancel{180}} \text{ min to administer}}{\underset{1}{\cancel{60}} \text{ min/hr}} = 110 \times \frac{1}{3} = 36.6 \text{ or } 37 \text{ mL/hr}$$

Set pump rate at 37 mL/hr to deliver magnesium sulfate 5 g in 3 hours.

16. a. *Drug calculation:*

BF: $\dfrac{D}{H} \times V = \dfrac{16 \text{ mEq}}{4.65 \text{ mEq}} \times 10 \text{ mL} = 34.4$ mL

or
RP: H : V ::   D : X
     4.65 mEq : 10 mL :: 16 mEq : X mL
            4.65 X = 160
                 X = 34.4 mL

or
FE: $\dfrac{H}{V} = \dfrac{D}{X} = \dfrac{4.65}{10} = \dfrac{16}{X}$
       4.65 X = 160
            X = 34.4 mL

or
DA: mL $= \dfrac{10 \text{ mL} \times 16 \text{ } \cancel{\text{mEq}}}{4.65 \text{ } \cancel{\text{mEq}} \times 1} = 34.4$ mL

Amount of solution: 34.4 mL + 100 mL = 134.4 mL

b. *Infusion pump rate calculation:*

$$134.4 \text{ mL} \div \frac{\overset{1}{\cancel{30}} \text{ min to administer}}{\underset{2}{\cancel{60}} \text{ min/hr}} = 134.4 \times \frac{2}{1} = 268.8 \text{ or } 269 \text{ mL/hr}$$

NEXT-GENERATION NCLEX® EXAMINATION-STYLE QUESTIONS

Choose the most likely option for the information missing from the statement provided by selecting from the lists of options provided.

A 75-year-old woman is admitted to a Rehabilitation facility after a right hip replacement surgery and develops acute heart failure (HF). The patient's healthcare provider orders furosemide (Lasix) 10mg IV now. Furosemide 20mg in 2ml is available to administer. The nurse would administer _A_ ml. The patient has a peripheral IV in her left hand which is capped. Prior to administering furosemide, the nurse's next action should be to _B_ . The nurse is unable to aspirate any blood from peripheral intravenous line (PIV) and when flushed, the surrounding skin is cool to the touch and is slightly edematous but the patient does not report any pain. The nurse suspects a grade I infiltration. The priority nursing action is to _C_ .

Option A	Option B	Option C
0.2	Flush PIV with 3ml of Heparin	Apply heat to PIV site
0.5	Take vital signs	Remove the PIV
1	Flush PIV with 3ml of Normal Saline	Start a new PIV
1.5	Assess for peripheral edema	Get an order for an oral dose of the medication
2	Assess bilateral radial pulses	Document the PIV assessment

ANSWERS NEXT-GENERATION NCLEX® EXAMINATION-STYLE QUESTIONS

Option A	Option B	Option C
0.2	Flush PIV with 3ml of Heparin	Apply heat to PIV site
0.5	Take vital signs	Remove the PIV
1	Flush PIV with 3ml of Normal Saline	Start a new PIV
1.5	Assess for peripheral edema	Get an order for an oral dose of the medication
2	Assess bilateral radial pulses	Document the PIV assessment

Rationale:

Option A:
D: V :: H : X20 mg : 2 ml :: 10mg : X
20 mg X = 20 mg/ml
X = 1 ml

Option B: Flush PIV with 3ml of Normal Saline

Option C: Start a new PIV

Furosemide (Lasix) is a loop diuretic which helps in the management and prevention of fluid overload seen in patients with heart failure (HF). The diuretic effect of furosemide helps to relieve fluid buildup which can produce: edema, shortness of breath and abdominal distention. Prior to administering furosemide, the patient's intravenous site should be assessed and flushed with normal saline to ensure it is patent. This is the most appropriate action this question is addressing. Additionally, the patient's vital signs should be taken prior to administering furosemide since the removal of fluid may cause the patient's blood pressure to decrease. Peripheral intravenous (PIV) infiltration occurs when fluid and or medication injected into that PIV leaks into the tissue around the IV site. On the infiltration scale, the clinical criteria for a grade I infiltration include: blanchable skin, cool to touch, edema (less than 1 inch) and the site may or may not be painful. It is important that this PIV is no longer used to prevent further tissue damage and thus should be removed. The most appropriate action for this nurse is to start a new PIV to administer the ordered medication. The nurse should also remove the infiltrated PIV and document an assessment of the infiltration site and the placement of the new PIV. Acute HF can progress rapidly, especially in the older adult. Furosemide was ordered to be given "now" and failure to administered this medication in a timely matter could result in a decline of the patient's condition. For this reason, starting a new PIV in order to administer the medication takes priority over discontinuing the infiltrated PIV.

For additional practice problems, refer to the Intravenous Flow Rates section of the Elsevier's Interactive Drug Calculation Application, Version 1 on Evolve.

PART IV

CALCULATIONS FOR SPECIALTY AREAS

CHAPTER 12

Anticoagulants

Objectives
- Identify the role of anticoagulants in clinical setting.
- Understand the importance of calculating and administering the correct heparin dose.
- Note differences between unfractionated heparin and low molecular weight heparin.
- Discuss differences between warfarin and new oral anticoagulants.
- Calculate heparin dosages when ordered in concentration and volume per hour.
- Use weight based heparin protocol to calculate correct heparin dosages.

Outline
HEPARIN
HEPARIN DOSING
UNFRACTIONATED HEPARIN
COAGULATION TESTS
WARFARIN
NEW ORAL ANTICOAGULANTS
REVERSAL AGENTS
INTRAVENOUS HEPARIN CALCULATIONS: CALCULATING CONCENTRATION AND VOLUME PER HOUR
WEIGHT-BASED HEPARIN PROTOCOL CALCULATIONS
CALCULATING HEPARIN DOSAGES BASED ON WEIGHT

Anticoagulants are a classification of medications that are prescribed to inhibit or prevent clot formation. Anticoagulants interfere with various processes of the clotting cascade by impeding the activation of certain clotting factors, thus prolonging the blood's clotting or coagulation time.

The use of anticoagulants is indicated in the management or prophylaxis treatment of thromboembolic events such as a deep vein thrombus (DVT) or pulmonary embolus (PE). If these conditions are left untreated or mismanaged, the thrombosis (blood clot) can dislodge resulting in a life-threatening myocardial infarction (MI) or stroke. Anticoagulation may also be prescribed for patients suffering from arrhythmias, prolonged immobility, cardiac events, or has a history of arterial or venous thromboembolic conditions. Additionally, anticoagulation may be ordered prophylactically in the perioperative setting for patients undergoing certain surgical procedures or needed to maintain patency of an indwelling venipuncture device.

All anticoagulants are considered high risk medications due to the significant harm it can cause patients if it is given in error. It is the nurse's responsibility to have a clear understanding of the medication to be delivered, identify the correct route of administration, and carefully read the drug's label for the concentration.

NOTE

Venous thromboembolism (VTE) — Conditions where a blood clot partially or completely blocks the circulation of blood. A term used to refer to both DVT and PE.

Deep vein thrombus (DVT) — A clot located in the deep vessels of the lower extremities, commonly found in the legs. Signs and symptoms include: pain, swelling, tenderness, and erythema at the site.

Pulmonary embolus (PE) — A blood clot that has become lodged in an artery located in the patient's lung. Related signs and symptoms include: dyspnea, hypotension, and chest pain.

HEPARIN

There are two types of heparin, unfractionated heparin (UFH) that is typically just referred to as heparin and Low Molecular Weight Heparin (LMWH). Both can be administered subcutaneously (subcut) or intravenously. Heparin is not active orally and intramuscular (IM) administration should be avoided due to the risk of hematoma formation at the injection site. Heparin therapy is often administered using a combination of intermittent IV boluses and continuous IV infusions to achieve and maintain a therapeutic level. Heparins play an important role in preventing and treating venous thromboembolism (VTE) and pulmonary embolism (PE). Heparins do lack fibrinolytic or clot busting activity and therefore cannot dissolve any existing thrombi.

HEPARIN DOSING

Heparin dosages are expressed and measured according to United States Pharmacopeia (USP) units. The United States Pharmacopeia (USP) is a recognized standard-setting organization for medications that is responsible for developing a standardized reference (USP units) to determine the potency activity of heparin.

Heparin is available in single-dose and multi-dose vials and is supplied in several different strengths (Figure 12.1). On heparin labels, the dose strength or concentration of the total volume is

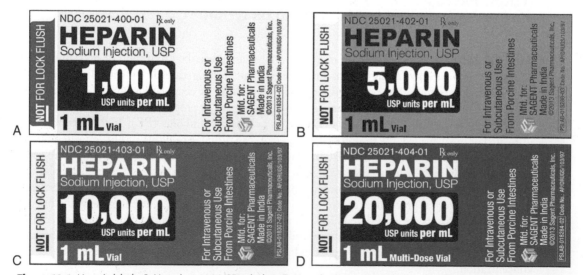

Figure 12.1 Heparin labels. **A,** Heparin 1,000 USP units/mL. **B,** Heparin 5,000 USP units/mL. **C,** Heparin 10,000 USP units/mL. **D,** Heparin 20,000 USP units/mL.

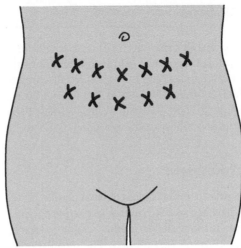

Figure 12.2 Abdominal subcutaneous injection sites for heparin administration.

emphasized in large bold print in an attempt to prevent the administration of the wrong dose. In a 1-mL vial, the heparin concentration can range from 1000 USP units to 20,000 USP units, where the latter is 20 times more concentrated. It is imperative that nurses examine each heparin label carefully to ensure that they are administering the correct concentration from the correct vial to prevent a lethal medication error. Fatal hemorrhages have occurred due to the administration of an incorrect dose of heparin.

Subcutaneous Heparin Administration

Heparin should be administered intravenously or subcutaneously using a syringe calibrated in milliliters. Insulin syringes are calibrated in 100 units per mL, these units are not equivalent to the USP units of heparin and should not be used in the dosing or administration of heparin. When administering heparin subcutaneously, a size 26- or 27-gauge, ½-inch needle is used, based on the patient's habitus to minimize tissue trauma. The injection uses a 90-degree angle to the skin to deposit the drug into the patient's subcutaneous tissue. Subcutaneous heparin injections are typically administered in the patient's abdomen due to its favorable absorption of the anticoagulant (Figure 12.2). Rotate injection sites on the abdomen, keeping approximately 2 inches away from the patient's umbilicus, and avoid massaging injection sites to reduce the risk of developing a hematoma. A standard dose of 5000 units of heparin subcut q8h or q12h is an order commonly prescribed by physicians in the hospital setting for DVT prevention in at risk patients. See Chapter 9 on Injectable Preparation for more information and calculations for subcutaneous injections.

NOTE

The maximum volume delivered for subcut injections should not exceed 1 mL. Therefore, the nurse should select the heparin concentration that will produce a volume that is equal to or less than 1 mL.

UNFRACTIONATED HEPARIN

Heparin or unfractionated heparin (UHF) is derived from the intestinal mucosa of porcine and standardized for its anticoagulant activity. UFH is indicated for short-term use, has a lower bioavailability (30%), shorter half-life (1 hour), and has a larger molecular weight when compared to Low Molecular Weight Heparin (LMWH) (Table 12.1). UFH dosing is adjusted based on a lab test called activated partial thromboplastin time (aPTT). This lab value is also used to monitor the effectiveness of heparin. Heparin is said to be therapeutic when a patient's aPTT is 1.5 to 2.5 times its normal lab value (30-40 seconds).

Low Molecular Weight Heparin

LMWH bind mostly to anticoagulant-related plasma proteins and thus have a more predictable pharmacology, a longer half-life which requires less redosing and an increased bioavailability which is why the subcutaneous route is the preferred method of administration. Since the anticoagulant response is predictable, laboratory monitoring isn't needed. The coagulation test Anti-factor Xa can be used to monitor the effect of LMWH such as Enoxaparin (Lovenox) and dalteparin (Fragmin). Enoxaparin is a LMWH that is administered once or twice (BID) a day subcutaneously for DVT prevention and it is supplied in a pre-filled syringe (Figure 12.3). Another LMWH used in the clinical setting is dalteparin (Fragmin) (Figure 12.4).

TABLE 12.1 Comparing UFH and LMWH

	Unfractionated Heparin (UFH)	Low Molecular Weight Heparin (LMWH)
Route	IV, subcut	subcut
Onset of action	3 min IV	4 hrs
Duration of action	1 hr IV	12 hrs
Lab test	aPTT, ACT	Anti-Xa
Reversal agent	Protamine	Protamine (partially)

ACT, activated clotting time; *aPTT,* activated partial thromboplastin time; *LMWH,* low molecular weight heparin; *subcut,* subcutaneously; *UFH,* Unfractionated heparin.

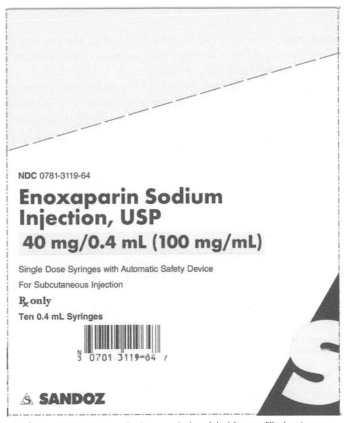

Figure 12.3. Enoxaparin (Lovenox) drug label for pre-filled syringes.

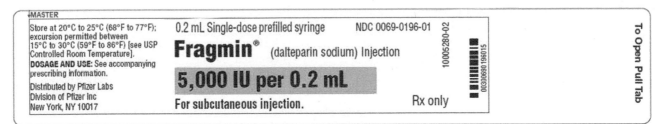

Figure 12.4. Dalteparin (Fragmin) drug label.

Heparin Flushes

A low dose concentration of heparin can be used to maintain the patency of venous access devices that have a greater risk of clotting off such as peripherally inserted central catheters (PICC), implanted venous access ports (e.g., Mediports), and dialysis catheters. It is important to understand that heparin lock flushes are not intended to anticoagulant the patient but to prevent the formation of clots in the patient's indwelling venipuncture device that could render it unusable. The physician will place a heparin flush order for certain indwelling venous access sites. Heparin lock flush solutions are labeled as such and are available in 10 USP units/mL and 100 USP units/mL (Figure 12.5). Heparin lock flush solutions and heparin sodium injections use different concentrations and should never be interchanged. Refer to your institution's policy on which venous access sites that heparin flushes are appropriate for, as well as the concentration of heparin lock flush solution to use and the flush's volume in milliliters that may vary depending on the lengthen of the indwelling venous access device.

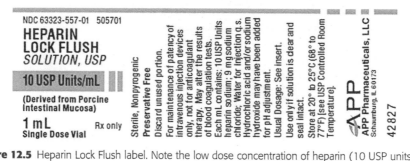

Figure 12.5 Heparin Lock Flush label. Note the low dose concentration of heparin (10 USP units/mL).

COAGULATION TESTS

Normal control values for specific tests are established by each facility's laboratory running the test. To ensure the accuracy of the test's measurement, coagulation tests are completed and evaluated daily. The goal coagulation range that will inhibit clot formation is known as the therapeutic range. This range is established by the control value that was previously determined by the laboratory's daily assessment. Table 12.2 outlines the most common coagulation tests used to guide patient anticoagulant therapy.

Therapeutic lab values are those that indicate the effectiveness of a drug in the blood. In the case of anticoagulants, when the lab values are considered therapeutic the patient should be adequately anticoagulated and no longer at risk for a thromboembolic event. By prolonging these bleeding times, it will prevent additional blood clots from forming. For example, the lab tests PT and INR both measure the time it takes for a clot to form. The longer it takes for blood to clot, the higher the PT and INR results, thus reducing the risk of a thromboembolic event.

TABLE 12.2 Coagulation Tests

Activated partial thromboplastin time (aPTT)	Primary tool used to monitor and guide dosing for unfractionated heparin (UFH) therapy. aPTT measures the time it takes for a clot to form and monitors the concentration of UFH in the blood and its therapeutic response. Therapeutic hepatization occurs when aPTT is 1.5-2.5 times normal. A normal control APTT is approximately 25-35 seconds; however, this reference range is established by each institution based on the test agents used.
Activated clotting time (ACT)	A rapidly performed test that measures the number of seconds it takes for blood to clot. Used to guide dosing and measure the anticoagulant effect of UFH. Typically used in cardiac surgical procedures, when higher doses of UFH are being administered. A normal ACT level is 90-120 seconds. A therapeutic level for anticoagulation can range from an ACT level of 150-660 seconds, depending on its indication.
Anti-factor Xa (Anti-Xa)	A newer lab test used to monitor the therapeutic levels of LMWH and UFH. It provides a better measure of the effects of heparin. Anti-Xa levels are considered therapeutic at 0.3-0.7 units/mL. The use of Anti-Xa is institution specific and may be utilized in patients who are elderly, obese, very young, pregnant, or have renal disease.
International normalized ratio (INR)	Uses a standardize formula to express the prothrombin time (PT) result. It monitors the therapeutic response to warfarin and offers guidance with dosing adjustments based on INR results. A normal value is 1.5-2.5 times the control. An INR ranging between 2.0-3.0 is considered a therapeutic target for anticoagulation.
Prothrombin time (PT)	A test used as an adjunct to INR to monitor warfarin dosing. Due to the sensitivity of the thromboplastin agents used in different laboratories, PT results were subject to variability. The therapeutic value of PT is 1.5 to 2.5 times (15.5 to 35 seconds) its normal value of 12-14 seconds.
Platelet count	Provides the quantity of platelets in the blood but does not provide any insight on the platelets' functionality. A normal platelet count is 150,000-300,000 mm^3. A platelet count less than 50,000 mm^3 poses an increased risk of bleeding during surgery.

WARFARIN

Warfarin (Coumadin) was first introduced in 1954 and for many years it was the only oral anticoagulant available. Warfarin's anticoagulant effect is the result of antagonizing vitamin K, an enzyme needed by the liver to produce important clotting factors. The effects of warfarin do not impact existing clotting factors that have already been synthesized. This explains why it takes 36 to 72 hours for a therapeutic range to be established. Regular anticoagulant monitoring with the International Normalized Ratio (INR) lab tests are necessary to evaluate and maintain adequate therapeutic levels of warfarin in the blood. Warfarin is dosed based on the patient's INR response and adjusted to maintain a target INR between 2.0-3.0. An INR level that falls below 2.0 is considered subtherapeutic and places the patient at risk for developing a VTE. An INR result greater than 3.0 is supratherapeutic and now the patient is at risk for bleeding. Warfarin has a narrow therapeutic range (index) that can be easily altered through interactions with various medications and foods. Therefore, it's important to closely monitor the patient's INR response when initiating warfarin therapy with daily INR lab draws and then every few weeks once INR results have stabilized in the therapeutic range. The duration of therapy is patient-dependent and is recommended to be discontinued once the threat of a VTE has subsided.

Coumadin dosing is highly individualized for each patient. Clinical factors such as age, gender, race, weight, diet, concomitant medication, and genetics account for the wide variance in warfarin dosing requirements. The cytochrome P450 (CYP) enzymes of the liver is responsible for the metabolism of warfarin. Exposure to certain environmental factors such as smoking, alcohol, and drugs can impact the individual's CYP enzyme activity. Interestingly, polymorphisms or variations in a patient's genetic makeup has an even greater influence on the activity of CYP enzymes. Thus, the CYP enzyme's ability to metabolize warfarin plays an important role in determining its therapeutic effect.

Warfarin is available in various doses, ranging from 1 to 10 mg. Each tablet is marked with a single-score and inscribed with the medication's name and dose strength. Additionally, manufacturers in the United States have developed a color scheme for warfarin tablets to help patients identify or remember their correct dosage. Each warfarin dose or strength is designated by a different color (Figure 12.6).

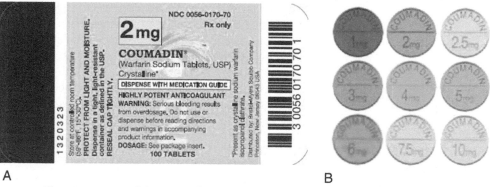

Figure 12.6 A, Warfarin (Coumadin) medication label. **B,** Color-coded Coumadin tablets.

NEW ORAL ANTICOAGULANTS

In recent years, a new class of oral anticoagulants known as target-specific oral anticoagulants (TSOACs) or novel oral anticoagulants (NOAC) have become much more prevalent in clinical practice and possess some notable advantages over older agents. Some common TSOACs include dabigatran (Pradaxa), apixaban (Eliquis), and rivaroxaban (Xarelto) (Figure 12.7). TSOACs have proven to be favorable due to their quick onset of action and stable pharmacokinetic profile which doesn't require routine lab tests to monitor its anticoagulant response. However, all TSOACs lack an antidote except dabigatran (Pradaxa). In 2015, the FDA approved the intravenous antidote idarucizumab (Praxbind), a reversal agent specifically for dabigatran (Pradaxa). The use of Idarucizumab is only indicated when the anticoagulant effects of dabigatran need to be reversed for an emergent surgical procedure or in the event of uncontrolled hemorrhaging. TSOACs are an alternative to warfarin and have demonstrated their effectiveness in treating and preventing thromboembolic events in high-risk patients (Table 12.3).

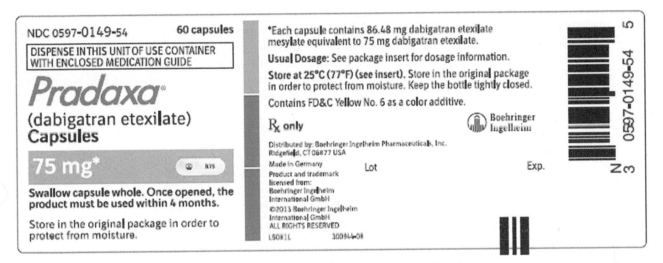

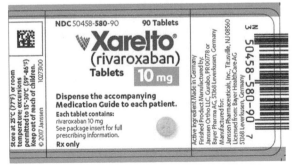

Figure 12.7 Target-specific oral anticoagulants (TSOACs) medication labels.

TABLE 12.3 Oral Anticoagulants

	Warfarin (Coumadin)	Dabigatran (Pradaxa)	Rivaroxaban (Xarelto)	Apixaban (Eliquis)
Route	PO	PO	PO	PO
Onset of action	36-72 hrs	1-2 hrs	2-4 hrs	3-4 hrs
Duration of action	36 hrs	14-17 hrs	7-11 hrs	8-14 hrs
Lab test	INR, PT	None	None	None
Reversal agent	Phytonadione (Vitamin K)	idarucizumab (Praxbind)	None	None

REVERSAL AGENTS

Protamine Sulfate

Protamine sulfate is the antidote for heparin (Figure 12.8). Protamine combines with heparin, neutralizing it, thus making it ineffective and reversing its anticoagulant effects. Protamine inhibits the anticoagulant effects of heparin causing the patient's Activated Clotting Time (ACT) to decrease, thus preventing bleeding. The onset of action of this medication is 1 minute and its duration of action is 2 hours. Protamine is given intravenously and should be administered slowly over 3 minutes to prevent adverse reactions such as: significant hypotension, hypertension, tachycardia, bradycardia, and even anaphylaxis. Protamine is dosed based on the route, duration, and dose of heparin administered. For every 1 mg of Protamine administered, 100 USP units of heparin is neutralized.

Phytonadione (Vitamin K)

Phytonadione (Vitamin K) is the antidote used to reverse the anticoagulant effects of warfarin, a vitamin K antagonist (Figure 12.9). Warfarin indirectly inhibits the production and activation of vitamin K dependent clotting factors. Therefore, the administration of Phytonadione reestablishes the normal clotting factor activity. Phytonadione requires 4-8 hours to restore the vitamin K dependent clotting factors and decrease bleeding. This medication's effect can be seen by a decrease in the patient's INR.

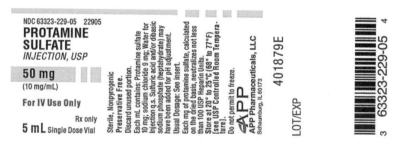

Figure 12.8 Protamine medication label.

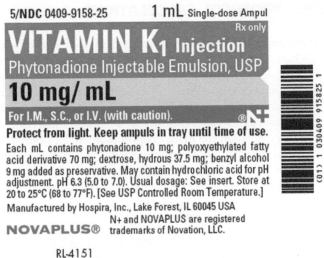

Figure 12.9 Phytonadione (Vitamin K) medication label.

INTRAVENOUS HEPARIN CALCULATIONS: CALCULATING CONCENTRATION AND VOLUME PER HOUR

It is crucial that nurses are able to demonstrate the ability to calculate the prescribed heparin infusion rates in units/hr and convert that dosage into mL/hr. Heparin is a high alert medication that will need to be infused using an electronic IV infusion pump, which is set to deliver in mL/hr.

Chapter 14 discusses calculating infusion rates of a medication for concentration and volume per unit time and for a specific body weight per unit time. Below is an example of calculating the rate in units/hr using the ratio and proportion formula.

EXAMPLE Order: Infuse heparin 5000 units in 250-mL D_5W at 30 mL/hr. Calculate the dose of heparin the patient is to receive per hour.

$$RP: \quad D \quad : \quad V \quad :: X : H$$
$$5000 \text{ units} : 250 \text{ mL} :: X : 30 \text{ mL}$$
$$250\,X = 150{,}000$$
$$X = 600 \text{ units/hr}$$

Answer: The concentration per hour of heparin that patient will receive is 600 units/hr.

EXAMPLE Order: Infuse heparin 950 units/hr. The provided concentration is heparin 20,000 units in 250 mL of D_5W. Calculate the rate in milliliters per hour that should be programmed into the IV infusion pump.

$$RP: \quad D \quad : \quad V \quad :: \quad H \quad : X$$
$$20{,}000 \text{ units} : 250 \text{ mL} :: 950 \text{ units} : X$$
$$20{,}000\,X = 237{,}500$$
$$X = 11.875 \text{ or } 12 \text{ mL/hr}$$

Answer: The volume per hour of heparin to be programmed into the IV pump is 12 mL/hr.

WEIGHT-BASED HEPARIN PROTOCOL CALCULATIONS

Weight-based heparin protocols have become the standard of care when it comes to managing heparin infusions. Hospitals have developed heparin protocols to aid in the administration and management of heparin infusions and to prevent heparin related medication errors. Heparin is dosed based on the patient's weight in kilograms. Heparin protocols use an IV heparin order set to administer IV bolus doses or titrate the infusion rate based on the patient's aPTT results. The aPTT blood test is used to guide the heparin therapy and should be drawn 6 hours after the infusion is initiated and 6 hours after any dose change. Once three consecutive aPTTs are within the therapeutic window, aPTTs can be drawn daily.

Providers will place an order for the heparin infusion protocol to be initiated. Heparin protocols will specify the loading or initial bolus dose and the initial continuous or maintenance dose. Table 12.4 offers an example of a heparin infusion protocol that can be used to guide the administration and management of a continuous IV heparin infusion.

 NOTE

Heparin is a high alert medication and must be administered by an infusion pump. As a safety measure, all boluses and rate changes must be double checked with another nurse.

TABLE 12.4 Heparin Infusion Protocol – Goal aPTT 50-70 Seconds

*Use standard premixed solution of heparin sodium 25,000 units in 250 mL D$_5$W for infusion (100 units/mL).
*Prior to initiation of heparin, obtain baseline Hgb, Hct, platelet count, aPTT, and INR.
*Round all bolus doses to the nearest 100 units and all infusion rates to nearest 50 units/hr.
*Adjust heparin infusion according to protocol and then repeat aPTT q6h.
*Collect aPTT daily after three consecutive aPTTs are within the target range (aPTT 50-70).

*Initial bolus dose: 70 units/kg
*Initial infusion rate: 20 units/kg/hr

aPTT (seconds)	IV Bolus	Hold Infusion (minutes)	Infusion Rate Change	Repeat aPTT
<30	60 units/kg	0 min	Increase by 4 units/kg/hr	6 hours
30-49	30 units/kg	0 min	Increase by 2 units/kg/hr	6 hours
50-70 **(goal)**	No bolus	0 min	No change	6 hours
71-95	No bolus	30 min and notify provider	Decrease by 2 units/kg/hr	6 hours
>95	No bolus	60 min and notify provider	Decrease by 3 units/kg/hr	6 hours

*Sample only. Not to be used in clinical setting.

CALCULATING HEPARIN DOSAGES BASED ON WEIGHT

Use the weight-based heparin protocol in Table 12.4 to answer the questions below.

EXAMPLE Calculate the initial loading (bolus) dose of IV heparin. Patient weighs 185 lbs. Per the heparin protocol, the initial bolus dose is 70 units/kg. How many units of heparin should be administered to this patient?

a. Convert pounds to kilograms:

Divide pounds by 2.2 $\dfrac{185\ lbs}{2.2} = 84.09$ or 84 kg

b. Calculate the heparin loading dose:

Multiply the patient's weight in kg by ordered bolus dose

70 units/kg × 84 kg = 5880 units

Answer: The patient should receive 5880 units of IV heparin as a loading dose.

NOTE

aPTT is the preferred laboratory test used to monitor and measure IV heparin therapy. APTT should be measured and evaluated every 6 hours and the continuous IV heparin drip should be adjusted based on the aPTT result per the facility's IV heparin infusion protocol. The IV heparin drip should prolong the aPTT lab result.

EXAMPLE Calculate the initial heparin loading dose and the initial infusion rate in units/hr and determine the rate in mL/hr to program into the infusion pump. Patient weighs 130 lbs. Per the heparin protocol, the initial loading dose is 70 units/kg and the initial infusion rate is 20 units/kg/hr.

a. Convert pounds to kilograms.

Divide pounds by 2.2 $\dfrac{130\ lbs}{2.2} = 59.09$ or 59kg

b. Calculate heparin loading dose.

Multiply the patient's weight in kg by ordered bolus dose: 70 units/kg × 59 kg = 4130 units.

The patient should receive 4130 units of IV heparin as a loading dose.

c. Calculate the infusion rate for heparin gtt.

Multiply patient's weight in kg by ordered initial infusion rate: 20 units/kg/hr × 59 kg = 1180 units/hr.

d. Determine the rate in mL/hr to program into infusion pump.

Note that the concentration of the heparin infusion is 100 units per mL. Set up a ratio and proportion (**RP**) or use dimensional analysis (**DA**).

RP: H : V ::   D   : X

100 units : 1 mL :: 1180 units/hr : X

$\quad\quad\quad$ 100 X = 1180 mL/hr

$\quad\quad\quad\quad$ X = 11.8 or 12 mL/hr

Or

$$\textbf{DA:}\ X = \frac{1\ mL \times 1180\ units}{100\ units \times 1\ hr} \quad\quad\quad X = \frac{1180}{100} \quad\quad\quad X = 11.8\ or\ 12\ mL/hr$$

Answer: The infusion pump would be set to deliver 1180 units/hr at 12 mL/hr.

EXAMPLE Using the patient and information collected from the example above, calculate the new infusion rate and determine the mL/hr to program into the infusion pump, based on the aPTT result.

Patient's weight is 59 kg. The heparin infusion is currently set 24 mL/hr to deliver 1180 units/hr. After 6 hours, the aPTT result is 35 seconds. According to the heparin protocol, re-bolus with 30 units/kg and increase infusion rate by 100 units/hr.

Calculate the new heparin continuous infusion dose (units/hr) based on the protocol.

a. Calculate the dosage in units of the heparin re-bolus.

30 units/kg × 59 kg = 1770 units

b. Determine the heparin re-bolus volume.

RP: H : V ::   D   : X

100 units : 1 mL = 1770 units : X mL

$\quad\quad\quad$ 100 X = 1770

$\quad\quad\quad\quad$ X = 17.7 or 18 mL bolus

c. Calculate new infusion rate (increase by 2 units/kg/hr).

2 units/kg/hr × 59 kg = 118 units/hr

The heparin infusion rate should be increased by 118 units/hr.

d. Calculate the increase made to the new rate in mL/hr.

RP: D : V :: H : X

100 units : 1 mL :: 118 units/hr : X mL

100 X = 118 mL/hr

X = 1.18 or 1.2 mL/hr

Add rate increase to current rate.

$$
\begin{array}{r}
12 \text{ mL/hr (current rate)} \\
+\ 1.2 \text{ mL/hr (rate increase)} \\
\hline
13.2 \text{ or } 13 \text{ mL/hr (new rate)}
\end{array}
$$

Increase the infusion pump to deliver 13 ml/hr.

NOTE

Weight-based heparin protocols differ at each facility. It is important for the nurse to be familiar with the heparin protocol dosing nomogram utilized at their speci c facility.

PRACTICE PROBLEMS

Answers can be found on pages 282 to 284.

For each practice problem, use the Heparin Infusion Protocol (Table 12.4).

1. Calculate the initial loading dose and infusion rate for a patient weighing 165 lbs.

   a. Bolus dose (units)_____   **c.** Infusion dose (units/hr)_____

   b. Bolus volume (mL)_____   **d.** Infusion rate (mL/hr)_____

2. A patient weighing 74 kg received an aPTT result of 27 seconds. The patient's heparin drip is currently infusing at 1000 units/hr. Based on the heparin infusion protocol, determine the following:

   a. Bolus dose (units)_____   **c.** Infusion dose (units/hr)_____

   b. Bolus volume (mL)_____   **d.** Infusion rate (mL/hr)_____

3. A patient weighing 95 kg received an aPTT result of 60 seconds. The patient's heparin drip is currently infusing at 26 units/kg/hr. Based on the heparin infusion protocol, determine the following:

   a. Bolus dose (units)_____   **c.** Infusion dose (units/hr)_____

   b. Bolus volume (mL)_____   **d.** Infusion rate (mL/hr)_____

4. A patient weighing 275 lbs received an aPTT result of 99 seconds. The patient's heparin drip is currently infusing at 1500 units/hr. Based on the heparin infusion protocol, determine the following:

   a. Bolus dose (units)_____   **c.** Infusion dose (units/hr)_____

   b. Bolus volume (mL)_____   **d.** Infusion rate (mL/hr)_____

5. A patient weighing 66 kg received an aPTT result of 41 seconds. The patient's heparin drip is currently infusing at 15 units/kg/hr. Based on the heparin infusion protocol, determine the following:

   a. Bolus dose (units)_____   **c.** Infusion dose (units/hr)_____

   b. Bolus volume (mL)_____   **d.** Infusion rate (mL/hr)_____

ANSWERS PRACTICE PROBLEMS

1. As stated in the heparin infusion protocol, initial bolus dose: 70 units/kg and initial infusion rate: 20 units/kg/hr.

   Convert pounds to kilograms: $\dfrac{165 \text{ lbs}}{2.2} = 75 \text{ kg}$

   a. 70 units/kg × 75 kg = 5250 units
   Bolus dose: 5250 units

   RP: D : V :: H : X

   b. 100 units : 1 mL :: 5250 units : X

   $$100\,X = 5250$$
   $$X = 52.5 \text{ or } 53 \text{ mL}$$

   Bolus volume: 53 mL

   c. 20 units/kg/hr × 75 kg = 1500 units/hr

   Infusion dose: 1500 units/hr

   RP: D : V :: H : X

   d. 100 units : 1 mL :: 1500 units/hr : X

   $$100\,X = 1500$$
   $$X = 15 \text{ mL/hr}$$

   Infusion rate: 15 mL/hr

2. A patient weighing 74 kg received an aPTT result of 27 seconds. The patient's heparin drip is currently infusing at 1000 units/hr. Based on the heparin infusion protocol, determine the following:

    a. 60 units/kg × 74 kg = 4440 units

       Bolus dose: 4440 units

    b. RP : D : V ::   H   : X

       100 units : 1 mL :: 4440 units : X

             100 X = 4440

                  X = 44.4 or 44 mL

       Bolus volume: 44 mL

    c. 1000 units/hr *(current infustion dose)*

       4 units/kg/hr × 74 kg = 296 units/hr

       Infusion dose increase: 296 units/hr

    d. RP: D : V ::   H   : X

       100 units : 1 mL :: 1000 units/hr : X

           100 X = 1000

               X = 10 mL/hr *(current infusion rate)*

      RP: D: V :: H   : X

       100 units : 1 mL :: 296 units/hr : X

           100 X = 296

              X = 2.96 or 3 mL/hr *(infusion rate increase)*

$$\begin{array}{r} 10 \text{ mL/hr } (\textit{current rate}) \\ + \ 3 \text{ mL hr } (\textit{rate increase}) \\ \hline 13 \text{ mL/hr } (\textit{new rate}) \end{array}$$

      New infusion rate: 13 mL/hr

3. A patient weighing 95 kg received an aPTT result of 60 seconds. The patient's heparin drip is currently infusing at 26 units/kg/hr. Based on the heparin infuoion protocol, determine the following:

    a. A bolus dose is not warranted. aPTT is at target range.

    b. A bolus dose is not warranted. aPTT is at target range.

    c. 26 units/kg/hr × 95 kg = 2470 units/hr

       Infusion dose: 2470 units/hr

    d. RP :   D :   V :: H   : X

       100 units : 1 mL :: 2470 units/hr : X

          100 X = 2470

             X = 24.7 or 25 mL/hr

      Infusion rate: 25 mL/hr

4. A patient weighing 275 lbs received an aPTT result of 99 seconds. The patient's heparin drip is currently infusing at 1500 units/hr. Based on the heparin infusion protocol, determine the following:

Convert pounds to kilograms:

$$\frac{275 \text{ lbs}}{2.2} = 125 \text{ kg}$$

    a. A bolus dose is not warranted. aPTT is above target range.

    b. A bolus dose is not warranted. aPTT is above target range.

   c. Place heparin infusion on hold for 60 minutes and notify provider.

      3 units/kg/hr × 125 kg = 375 units/hr

      When heparin infusion is restarted, decrease infusion rate by 375 units/hr

   d. **RP** :   D :   V ::   H : X

      100 units : 1 mL :: 1500 units/hr : X

               100 X = 1500

                      X = 15 mL/hr (*current infusion rate*)

      100 units : 1 mL:: 375 units/hr : X

               100 X = 375

                      X = 3.75 or 3.7 mL/hr (*infusion rate increase*)

     15 units/hr (*current rate*)
     − 3.7 mL/hr (*rate decrease*)
     ———————
     11.3 or 11 mL/hr (*new rate*)

   Infustion rate: 11 mL/hr

   The new infusion rate to be restarted after 60 minutes is 11 mL/hr.

5. A patient weighing 66 kg received an aPTT result of 41 seconds. The patient's heparin drip is currently infusing at 17 units/kg/hr. Based on the heparin infusion protocol, determine the following:

   a. 66 kg × 30 units/kg = 1980 units

      Bolus dose: 1980 units

   b. **RP** : D   : V   ::   H   : X

      100 units : 1 mL :: 1980 units : X

             100 X = 1980

                  X = 19.8 mL or 20 mL

      Bolus volume: 20 mL

   c. 17 units/kg/hr × 66 kg = 1122 units/hr

      Current Infusion dose: 1122 units/hr

      2 units/kg/hr × 66 kg = 132 units/hr

      Infusion dose increase: 132 units/hr

   d.   D :   V   ::   H   : X

      100 units : 1 mL   :: 1122 units/hr : X

              100 X = 1122

                 X = 11.2 or 11 mL/hr

                    (*current infusion rate*)

      100 units: 1 mL:: 132 units/hr: X

              100 X = 132

                 X = 1.32 or 1.3 mL/hr

     11 mL/hr (*current rate*)
     +1.3 mL/hr (*rate increase*)
     ———————
     12.3 or 12 mL/hr (*new rate*)

     Infusion rate 12 mL/hr

NEXT-GENERATION NCLEX® EXAMINATION-STYLE QUESTIONS

Part I

A 68-year-old male presented to the emergency room on Wednesday afternoon with pain and swelling of his left calf. The area is warm to the touch and erythema is noted. A nursing assessment and history find that the patient has stage 4 renal failure, receives dialysis Monday, Wednesday, and Friday via a right AV fistula, hypertension, and paroxysmal (intermittent) Atrial Fibrillation One week ago, he had carpal tunnel release surgery and hasn't felt like moving around much. The patient weighs 250 pounds. Vital signs: BP 92/50, HR 102, RR 22, Temp 37.5 C, O2 saturation 95% on room air. He rates his pain a 7/10 in his left calf on a 0 to 10 pain intensity scale. The patient states that he is a difficult stick when it comes to PIV placement.

TABLE 12.5 Weight-Based Nomogram for Intravenous Heparin Infusion — Guidelines for Adjusting Infusion Rates for DVT
aPTT therapeutic range: **72 - 116** seconds

aPTT (in seconds)	Dose
< 50	80 units/kg bolus once, then increase infusion rate by 4 units/kg/hour
50 – 71.9	40 units/kg bolus once, then increase infusion rate by 2 units/kg/hour
72 – 116	NO CHANGE
116.1 – 127	Decrease infusion rate by 1 unit/kg/hour
127.1 – 138	Hold infusion for 1 hour, then decrease infusion rate by 2 units/kg/hour
>138	Hold infusion for 2 hour, then decrease infusion rate by 3 units/kg/hour

Place an X (or drag and drop to indicate which client assessment findings require immediate follow up by the ED nurse.

Assessment Findings	Assessment Findings that require Immediate follow up
Left lower calf edema and erythema	
Dialysis Monday, Wednesday and Friday schedule	
Recent surgery and immobilization	
Blood pressure 90/50	
Heart rate 102 beats per minute	
Respirations 22 breaths per minute	
Temperature 37.5 C	
Oxygen saturation of 95% on room air	
7/10 left calf pain	
Difficult PIV placement	

Part II

IV access was established and the patient's d-dimer was found to be 650 nanograms/milliliter, an indicator of coagulation and a possible blood clot. Ultrasonography confirmed a diagnosis of a left lower extremity deep venous thrombosis (DVT). Because of the patient's renal impairment, the decision is made to initiate a heparin drip as a bridge for warfarin therapy. Baseline activated partial thromboplastin time (aPTT), partial thromboplastin time (PTT), prothrombin time (PT)/ INR, liver function tests (LFTs), serum creatinine (sCr) and complete blood count (CBC) were ordered and drawn.

Choose the most likely option for the information missing from the statement provided by selecting from the lists of options provided.

The patient's healthcare provider orders a bolus dose of heparin 80 units/kg intravenously (maximum dose of 10,000 units). The patient's bolus is A units. The emergency room stocks 5000 units/1 ml vials. The nurse should administer a volume of B mL for the heparin bolus. The physician orders an intravenous heparin drip with an initial rate of 18 units/kg/hr. If the hospital carries Heparin 25,000 units/ D5W 250 ml bags, the patient's heparin infusion will run at a rate of C ml/hr. Six hours after the heparin infusion is initiated, an aPTT is drawn and is 130 seconds. Based on the institutional specific nomogram below, the heparin infusion will be decreased by 2 ml/hr and the patient's new infusion rate will infuse at D ml/hr

Option A	Option B	Option C	Option D
8909	1.5	18.2	18.2
9040	1.8	20.5	18.8
9120	2.4	25.1	19.3
9410	3.1	30.4	19.8

ANSWERS NEXT-GENERATION NCLEX®
EXAMINATION-STYLE QUESTIONS

Part I

Assessment Findings	Assessment Findings that require Immediate follow up
Left lower calf edema and erythema	X
Dialysis Monday, Wednesday and Friday schedule	X
Recent surgery and immobilization	
Blood pressure 90/50	X
Heart rate 102 beats per minute	X
Respirations 22 breaths per minute	
Temperature 37.5 C	
Oxygen saturation of 95% on room air	
7/10 left calf pain	X
Difficult PIV placement	X

Rationale:

The patient's left lower extremity edema, erythema and pain need to be evaluated further since these are signs for a possible DVT. The patient has stage 4 renal failure, it is important to determine if the patient has received dialysis today or recently. Whether he received dialysis or not can help with the patient's care management such as fluid status and lab results. A blood pressure of 90/50 is low and the patient has a history of hypertension. It's important to determine what the patient's baseline normally is, if he took any blood pressure medication today, if this is a side effect of receiving dialysis or even another underlying disease process. A heart rate of 102 is high. The patient's heart rate might be high due to the pain he is experiencing but it is also critical that the nurse determine if his rhythm is regular due to his history of paroxysmal Afib. This patient will need labs and peripheral intravenous access. It is important that the nurse try to establish IV access on the patient's left arm since the patient has an AV fistula on his right arm. If possible, a proactive approach could be contacting the facility's IV team to help establish IV access with ultrasound guidance

Part II

Option A	Option B	Option C	Option D
8909	1.5	18.2	**18.2**
9040	**1.8**	**20.5**	18.8
9120	2.4	25.1	19.3
9410	3.1	30.4	19.8

Rationale:

Option A:

250 lbs ÷ 2.2 = 113.6 kg or 114 kg (round to the nearest whole number)

80 units/kg x 114 kg = 9,120 units

Option B:

RP: D: V :: H : X

5000 units : 1mL :: 9,120 units : X

5,000 units X = 9, 120 units/ml

X = 1.8 ml

Option C:

25,000 units ÷ 250 ml = 100 units/ml (concentration of heparin gtt carried by hospital)

18 units/kg/hr x 114 kg= 2052 units/hr

RP: D : V :: H : X

100 units : 1mL :: 2052 units/hr : X

100 units X = 2052 units/ml/hr

X = 20.5 ml/hr

Option D: According to the weight-based nomogram, an aPTT of 130 will require the infusion to be held for 1 hour and then the heparin infusion rate will be decreased by 2 units/kg/hr.

2 units/kg/hr x 114 kg = 228 units/hr

RP: D: V :: H : X

100 units : 1 ml :: 228 units/hr : X

100 units X = 228 units/ml/hr

X = 2.28 ml/hr or 2.3 ml/hr (round to the nearest whole number)

20.5 ml/hr (pervious infusion rate) − 2.3 ml/hr = 18.2 ml/hr

For additional practice problems, refer to the Dosages Measured in Units section of the Elsevier's Interactive Drug Calculation Application, Version 1 on evolve.

CHAPTER 13

Pediatrics

Objectives
- Use the two primary methods of determining pediatric drug dosages.
- State the reason for checking pediatric dosages before administration.
- Describe the dosage inaccuracies that can occur with pediatric drug formulas.
- Identify the steps in determining body surface area from a pediatric nomogram and with the square root method.

Outline
FACTORS INFLUENCING PEDIATRIC DRUG ADMINISTRATION
PEDIATRIC DRUG CALCULATIONS
PEDIATRIC DOSAGE FROM ADULT DOSAGE

FACTORS INFLUENCING PEDIATRIC DRUG ADMINISTRATION

Drug dosages for children differ greatly from those for adults because of the physiological differences between the two groups. Neonates and infants have immature kidney and liver function, which delays metabolism and elimination of many drugs. Drug absorption in neonates is different as a result of slow gastric emptying. Decreased gastric acid secretion in children younger than 3 years contributes to altered drug absorption. Neonates and infants have a lower concentration of plasma proteins, which can cause toxic effects with drugs that are highly bound to proteins. They have less total body fat and more total body water. Therefore lipid-soluble drugs require smaller doses because less than normal fat is present, and water-soluble drugs can require larger doses because of a greater percentage of body water. As children grow, changes in fat, muscle, body water, and organ maturity can alter the pharmacokinetic effects of drugs. Most drugs are dosed according to weight, and doses are specifically calculated for each child. For example, a dose of cefazolin for a 34-kg, 12-year-old child is larger than a dose for a 7-kg, 8-month-old infant. It is the nurse's responsibility to ensure that a safe drug dosage is given and to closely monitor for signs and symptoms of adverse reactions to drugs. The purpose of learning how to calculate pediatric drug doses is to ensure that each child receives the correct dose within its therapeutic range.

Oral

Oral pediatric drug delivery often requires the use of a metric dosing device because most drugs for small children are provided in liquid form. The metric measuring device can be a small plastic measuring cup, an oral dropper, a calibrated measuring spoon, an oral syringe, or a specially designed pediatric medication dispenser such as the medibottle (Figure 13.1). The medibottle is a specially designed pediatric medication dispenser that provides optimum drug delivery by allowing small volumes of medication to be swallowed with oral fluids. Some liquid medications come with their own calibrated droppers. The type of measuring device chosen depends on the developmental level of the child. For infants and toddlers, the oral syringe, dropper, and medibottle provide better drug delivery than is provided by a small cup. A young child who is cooperative is able to use a small cup or measuring spoon. All liquid medications can be drawn up with an oral syringe to ensure accuracy and then are transferred to a small cup or measuring spoon. It may be necessary to refill the cup or spoon with water or juice and to have the child drink that as well to ensure that all prescribed medication has been administered. Medicine should not be mixed in the infant's or toddler's bottle because the full dose will not be administered if the child doesn't finish the bottle. Any medication with a strong taste should not be mixed in formula because the infant could begin to refuse formula. Avoid giving oral medications to a crying child or infant, who could easily aspirate the medication. Some chewable medications are available for administration to the older child. Because many drugs are enteric-coated or are provided in timed-release form, the child must be told which medications are to be swallowed and not chewed.

Intramuscular

Intramuscular (IM) sites are chosen on the basis of the age and muscle development of the child (Table 13.1). All injections should be given in a manner that minimizes physical and psychosocial trauma. The child must be adequately restrained, if necessary, and provided with a momentary distraction. The procedure must be performed quickly, with comfort measures immediately following.

Common IM injection sites in the pediatric population include the quadriceps' vastus lateralis and the rectus femoris muscles of the thigh, the dorsal and ventrogluteal muscles of the buttocks, and the deltoid muscle of the upper arm. The vastus lateralis located on the lateral aspect of the thigh is considered the best IM injection site for both newborns and infants. See Figure 9.15 in Chapter 9 for IM injection sites. Nurses must be able to identify the anatomical landmarks specific to each of these IM injection sites in order to properly administer medications by this route and to this vulnerable patient population.

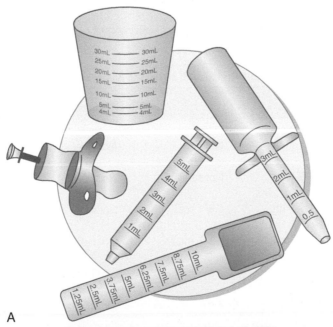

A

Figure 13.1 A, Calibrated measuring devices.

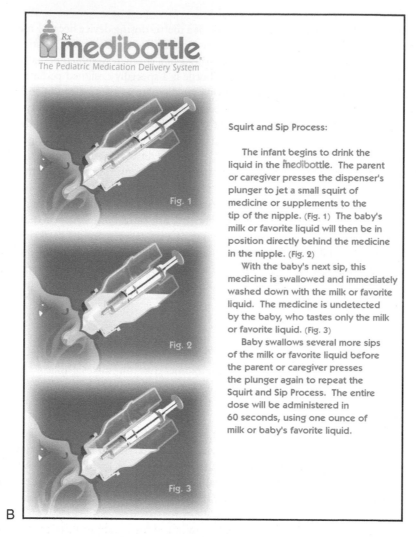

Squirt and Sip Process:

The infant begins to drink the liquid in the medibottle. The parent or caregiver presses the dispenser's plunger to jet a small squirt of medicine or supplements to the tip of the nipple. (Fig. 1) The baby's milk or favorite liquid will then be in position directly behind the medicine in the nipple. (Fig. 2)

With the baby's next sip, this medicine is swallowed and immediately washed down with the milk or favorite liquid. The medicine is undetected by the baby, who tastes only the milk or favorite liquid. (Fig. 3)

Baby swallows several more sips of the milk or favorite liquid before the parent or caregiver presses the plunger again to repeat the Squirt and Sip Process. The entire dose will be administered in 60 seconds, using one ounce of milk or baby's favorite liquid.

Figure 13.1, cont'd B, Medibottle. **(B,** From The Medicine Bottle Company, Inc.)

TABLE 13.1 Pediatric Guidelines for Intramuscular Injections According to Muscle Group*

	AMOUNT BY MUSCLE GROUP (mL)				
	Vastus Lateralis	**Rectus Femoris**	**Ventro-gluteal**	**Dorsal Gluteal**	**Deltoid**
Neonates	0.5 mL	Not safe	Not safe	Not safe	Not safe
Infants					
1-12 months	0.5-1 mL	Not safe	Not safe	Not safe	Not safe
Toddlers					
1-2 years	0.5-2 mL	0.5-1 mL	Not safe	Not safe	0.5-1 mL
Preschool					
3-5 years	0.5-2 mL	0.5-1 mL	0.5-1 mL	Not safe	0.5-1 mL
School age					
6-12 years	2 mL	2 mL	0.5-3 mL	0.5-2 mL	0.5-1 mL
Adolescent					
12-18 years	2 mL	2 mL	2-3 mL	2-3 mL	1-1.5 mL

*The safe use of all sites is based on normal muscle development and size of the child. Follow institutional policies and procedures.

NOTE

For IM injections, the usual needle length and gauge for pediatric clients are $^5/_8$ of an inch 1 inch long and 22 to 27 gauge. Another method of estimating needle length is to grasp the muscle for injection between the thumb and the forefinger; half the distance would be the needle length.

TABLE 13.2 Pediatric Guidelines for 24-Hour Intravenous Fluid Therapy

100 mL/kg for first 10 kg body weight
50 mL/kg for the next 10 kg body weight
20 mL/kg after 20 kg body weight

Example: Child's weight 25 kg

100 mL/kg × 10 kg = 1000 mL
50 mL/kg × 10 kg = 500 mL
20 mL/kg × 5 kg = 100 mL
1600 mL for 24 hours, or 66.6 mL/hr, or 67 mL/hr

Intravenous

For children, the maximum amount of intravenous (IV) fluid varies with age and body weight. Their 24-hour fluid status must be monitored closely to prevent overhydration and to ensure that fluid overload doesn't occur, volume control devices, such as IV pumps or volume control chambers are used (Figure 13.2). Volume control chambers used in the pediatric patient population are often designed with a safety feature, a floating valve or a membrane filter at the base of the calibrated cylinder. This safety mechanism prevents the free flow of fluid or air to the patient once the infusion is finished. In addition, the amount of fluid given with IV medications must be considered in planning their 24-hour intake (Table 13.2).

After the correct dosage of drug is obtained, it may need further dilution and to be given over a specified time, as mentioned in Chapter 11. Usually, the drug is diluted with 5 to 60 mL of IV fluid, depending on the drug or dosage, placed in a calibrated cylinder or syringe pump, and infused over 20 to 60 minutes, depending on the type of drug. After the drug has been infused, the cylinder is flushed with 3 to 20 mL of IV fluid to ensure that the child has received all of the medication and to prevent admixture. All fluid volume is considered intake. Refer to Chapter 11 for methods of calculating IV infusion rates.

The safety factors that must be considered when medications are administered to children are similar to those for adults. See Appendix A for more detailed information on safe nursing practice for drug administration.

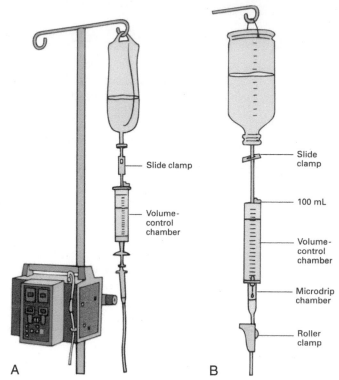

Figure 13.2 A, Electronic infusion pump with volume-control device. **B,** Gravity infusion with volume-control device and microdrip tubing.

PEDIATRIC DRUG CALCULATIONS

The two main methods of determining drug dosages for pediatric drug administration are body weight and body surface area (BSA). For both, a current weight is essential. The first method uses a specific number of milligrams, micrograms, or units for each kilogram of body weight (mg/kg, mcg/kg, unit/kg). Usually, drug data for pediatric dosage (mg/kg) are supplied by manufacturers in a drug information insert. BSA, measured in square meters (m^2), is considered a more accurate method than body weight. BSA takes into consideration the relation between basal metabolic rate and surface area, which correlates with blood volume, cardiac output, and organ growth and development. Although BSA has been used primarily to calculate the dosage of antineoplastic agents, BSA is used when there is a narrow margin between therapeutic and toxic doses. Pharmaceutical manufacturers are including BSA parameters (mg/m^2, mcg/m^2, units/m^2) in the drug information.

If the manufacturer does not supply data for pediatric dosing, the child's dosage can be determined from the adult dose. The BSA formula is used to calculate the pediatric dose. The BSA formula is considered more accurate than previously used formulas, such as Clark's, Young's, and Fried's rules. Drug calculations performed according to the BSA formula are safer than those done with formulas that rely solely on the child's age or weight. The West nomogram for infants and children (Figure 13.3) can also be used to determine BSA or to verify BSA results. It is important to follow institutional policies regarding the calculation of BSA (see Chapter 7). Although the BSA formula has improved the accuracy of drug dosing in infants and children, calculation of drug doses for neonates and preterm infants are weight based because BSA does not guarantee complete accuracy.

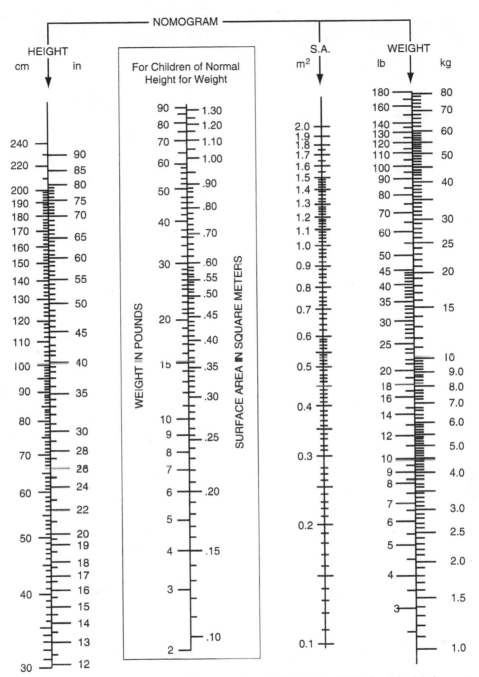

Figure 13.3 West nomogram for infants and children. *Directions: (1) Find height; (2) find weight; (3) draw a straight line connecting the height and weight. Where the line intersects on the S.A (surface area) column is the body surface area in square meters (m²).* (From Kliegman RM, St. Geme JW, Blum NJ, et al: *Nelson textbook of pediatrics,* ed. 21, Philadelphia, 2020, Saunders.)

NOTE

If the manufacturer states in the drug information insert that the medication is not for pediatric use, the alternative formulas should **NOT** be used for dosage calculation.

Dosage Per Kilogram Body Weight

The following information is needed to calculate the dosage:

a. Physician's order with the name of the drug, the dosage, and the frequency of administration.

b. The child's age and weight in kilograms:

$$1 \text{ kg} = 2.2 \text{ lbs}$$

c. The pediatric dosage as listed by the manufacturer or hospital formulary.

d. Information on how the drug is supplied.

EXAMPLES **PROBLEM 1:**

a. Order: amoxicillin (Amoxil) 60 mg, po, tid.
Child's age and weight: 4 months, 12.5 lbs.

b. Change pounds to kilograms.

$$\frac{12.5 \text{ lbs/kg}}{2.2 \text{ kg}} = 5.7 \text{ kg}$$

c. Pediatric dosage for children older than 3 months old: 20-40 mg/kg/day in three equal doses.

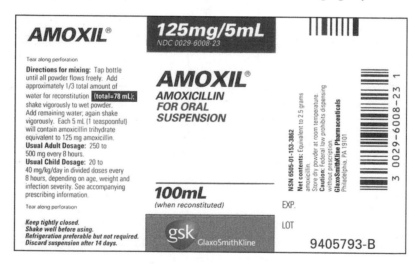

Step 1: Check dosing parameters by multiplying the child's weight by the minimum and maximum daily dose of the drug.

$$20 \text{ mg/kg/day} \times 5.7 \text{ kg} = 114 \text{ mg/day}$$

$$40 \text{ mg/kg/day} \times 5.7 \text{ kg} = 228 \text{ mg/day}$$

Step 2: Multiply the dosage by the frequency to determine the daily dose.
The order for amoxicillin 60 mg, po, tid means that three doses will be given per day.

$$60 \text{ mg} \times 3 = 180 \text{ mg}$$

Because the daily dose of amoxicillin 180 mg falls within the recommended range, it is considered a safe dose.

d. Drug preparation:

Use the basic formula **(BF)**, ratio and proportion **(RP)**, fractional equation **(FE)** method, or dimensional analysis **(DA)**.

Basic Formula

$$\text{BF:}\ \frac{D}{H} \times V = \frac{60\ \text{mg}}{125\ \text{mg}} \times 5\ \text{mL} = 2.4\ \text{mL}$$

or

RP: *Ratio and Proportion*

125 mg : 5 mL :: 60 mg : X mL

$$125\,X = 300$$
$$X = 2.4\ \text{mL}$$

or

$$\text{DA:}\ \text{mL} = \frac{5\ \text{mL} \times 60\ \text{mg}}{125\ \text{mg} \times 1} = \frac{300}{125} = 2.4\ \text{mL}$$

or

FE: *Fractional Equation*

$$\frac{H}{V} = \frac{D}{X} = \frac{125\ \text{mg}}{5\ \text{mL}} = \frac{60\ \text{mg}}{X}$$

(Cross multiply) 125 X = 300

$$X = 2.4\ \text{mL}$$

Answer: amoxicillin 60 mg, po = 2.4 mL

PROBLEM 2:

a. Order: ampicillin 350 mg, IV, q6h.

Child's weight and age: 61.5 lbs and 9 years old.

Dilution instructions: Mix with 20 mL of $D_5/1/4$ NS; infuse over 20 minutes.

Flush with 15 mL at same infusion rate.

b. Change pounds to kilograms.

$$\frac{61.5}{2.2} = 27.95\ \text{or}\ 28\ \text{kg}$$

c. Pediatric dose is 25 to 50 mg/kg/day in divided doses.

Step 1: Multiply weight by minimum and maximum daily dose:

$$25\ \text{mg} \times 28\ \text{kg} = 700\ \text{mg/day}$$

$$50\ \text{mg} \times 28\ \text{kg} = 1400\ \text{mg/day}$$

Step 2: Multiply the dose by the frequency:

$$350\ \text{mg} \times 4 = 1400\ \text{mg/day}$$

The dose is considered safe because it does not exceed the therapeutic range.

d. Drug available: When diluted, 500 mg = 2 mL. Use your selected formula to calculate the dosage.

NDC 0015-7403-20
NSN 6505-00-946-4700
EQUIVALENT TO
500 mg AMPICILLIN
STERILE AMPICILLIN
SODIUM, USP
For IM or IV Use
CAUTION: Federal law prohibits dispensing without prescription.

For IM use, add 1.8 mL diluent (read accompanying circular). Resulting solution contains 250 mg ampicillin per mL. Use solution within 1 hour. This vial contains ampicillin sodium equivalent to 500 mg ampicillin. Usual Dosage: Adults—250 to 500 mg IM q. 6h. READ ACCOMPANYING CIRCULAR for detailed indications, IM or IV dosage and precautions. APOTHECON® A Bristol-Myers Squibb Company Princeton, NJ 08540 USA   740320DRL-2

Cont:
Exp. Date:

$$\text{BF:}\ \frac{D}{H} \times V = \frac{350\ \text{mg}}{500\ \text{mg}} \times 2\ \text{mL} = 1.4\ \text{mL}$$

or
RP: 500 mg : 2 mL :: 350 mg : X mL
$$500 \, X = 700$$
$$X = 1.4 \text{ mL}$$

or
DA: no conversion factor

$$mL = \frac{2 \text{ mL} \times \overset{7}{\cancel{350}} \text{ mg}}{\underset{10}{\cancel{500}} \text{ mg} \times 1} = \frac{14}{10} = 1.4 \text{ mL}$$

or
$$FE: \frac{H}{V} = \frac{D}{X} = \frac{500 \text{ mg}}{2 \text{ mL}} = \frac{350 \text{ mg}}{X}$$
$$500 \, X = 700$$
$$X = 1.4 \text{ mL}$$

Answer: Each dose is 1.4 mL.
  e. Amount of fluid to infuse medication:

$$1.4 \text{ mL} + 20 \text{ mL (dilution)} = 21.4 \text{ mL}$$

  f. Flow rate calculation (60 gtt/mL set):

$$\frac{\text{Amount of solution} \times \text{gtt/mL (set)}}{\text{Minutes to administer}} = \text{gtt/min}$$

$$\frac{21.4 \text{ mL} \times \overset{3}{\cancel{60}} \text{ gtt/mL}}{\underset{1}{\cancel{20}} \text{ min}} = 64.2 \text{ gtt/min or } 64 \text{ gtt/min}$$

  g. Infusion pump setting

$$\text{Amount of solution} \div \frac{\text{Minutes to administer}}{60 \text{ min/hr}} = 21.4 \text{ mL} \div \frac{20 \text{ min}}{60 \text{ min}} =$$

$$21.4 \times \frac{60}{20} = 64.2 \text{ mL/hr or } 64 \text{ mL (round off to whole number)}$$

👆 YOU MUST REMEMBER

- The IV flush (3-20 mL) is part of the total IV fluids necessary for medication administration and must be included in patient intake. The flush is started after the IV medication infusion is completed, and it is infused at the same rate.
- For a 60-gtt/mL set, the drop per minute rate is the same as the milliliter per minute rate.

Dosage per Body Surface Area

The following information is needed to calculate the dosage:
  a. Physician's order with name of drug, dosage, and time frame or frequency.
  b. Child's height, weight in kilograms, and age.
  c. Information on how the drug is supplied.
  d. Pediatric dosage (in m²) as listed by manufacturer or hospital formulary.
  e. BSA with square root.
  f. BSA nomogram for children (see Figure 13.3).

EXAMPLE **PROBLEM**

   a. Order: methotrexate 50 mg, IV, × 1.
   b. Child's height, weight, age: 134 cm, 32.5 kg, 9 years.
   c. Pediatric dose: 25-75 mg/m^2 per week.
   d. Drug preparation: 25 mg/mL.
   e. BSA with square root (see BSA metric formula on p. 102)

$$\sqrt{\frac{134 \times 32.5}{3600}} = 1.09 \text{ m}^2$$

$$25 \text{ mg/m}^2 \times 1.09 \text{ m}^2 = 27.25 \text{ or } 27 \text{ mg}$$

$$75 \text{ mg/m}^2 \times 1.09 \text{ m}^2 = 81.75 \text{ or } 82 \text{ mg}$$

Compare answer with nomogram.

   f. BSA nomogram for children: The child's height (134 cm) and weight (32.5 kg) intersect at 1.11 m^2 BSA. Multiply the BSA, 1.11 m^2, by the minimum and maximum dose. (Substitute BSA for weight.)

$$25 \text{ mg/m}^2 \times 1.11 \text{ m}^2 = 28.0 \text{ mg}$$

$$75 \text{ mg/m}^2 \times 1.11 \text{ m}^2 = 83.0 \text{ mg}$$

This dose is considered safe because it is within the therapeutic range for the child's BSA.

   g. Calculate drug dose: For determination of the amount of drug to be administered, either formula can be used:

BF: $\dfrac{D}{H} \times V = \dfrac{50 \text{ mg}}{25 \text{ mg}} \times 1 \text{ mL} = 2 \text{ mL}$

or
FE: $\dfrac{H}{V} = \dfrac{D}{X} = \dfrac{25 \text{ mg}}{1 \text{ mL}} = \dfrac{50 \text{ mg}}{X \text{ mL}}$
(Cross multiply) 25 X = 50
X = 2 mL

or
RP: 25 mg : 1 mL :: 50 mg : X mL
25 X = 50
X = 2 mL

or
DA: mL $= \dfrac{1 \text{ mL} \times \overset{2}{\cancel{50 \text{ mg}}}}{\underset{1}{\cancel{25 \text{ mg}}} \times 1} = 2 \text{ mL}$

Answer: methotrexate 50 mg = 2 mL

SUMMARY PRACTICE PROBLEMS

In the following dosage problems for oral, IM, and IV administration, determine whether the ordered drug is a safe pediatric dose, and calculate the dose.

I Oral

Answers can be found on pages 310 to 312.

   1. Child with a streptococcal soft tissue infection.
   Order: clindamycin 90 mg, po, qid.
   Child's weight and age: 68 lbs, 6 years.
   Pediatric dose: 4-6 mg/lbs/day in 3 doses.

Drug available: clindamycin 75 mg/5 mL.

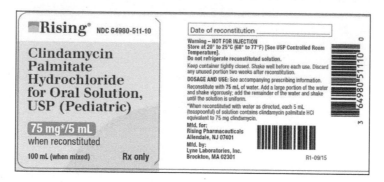

2. Child with seizures.
   Order: phenobarbital 25 mg, po, bid.
   Child's weight and age: 7.2 kg, 9 months.
   Pediatric dose: 5-7 mg/kg/day.
   Drug available: phenobarbital 20 mg/5 mL.

3. Child with lower respiratory tract infection.
   Order: cefprozil (Cefzil) 100 mg, po, q12h.
   Child's weight and age: 17 lbs, 6 months.
   Pediatric dose greater than 6 months: 15 mg/kg/q12h.
   Drug available:

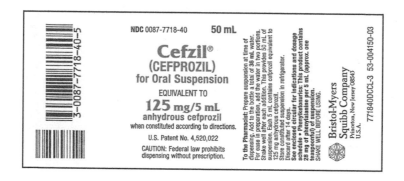

4. Child with pain.
   Order: codeine 7.5 mg, po, q4h, prn × 6 doses/day.
   Child's height, weight, and age: 43 inches, 50 lbs; 5 years.
   Pediatric dose: 100 mg/m²/day (see Figure 13.3), or solve by square root.
   Drug available: codeine 15-mg tablets.

5. Child with seizures.
   Order: Zarontin 125 mg, po, bid.
   Child's weight and age: 13 kg, 36 months.
   Pediatric dose: 15-40 mg/kg/day.

Drug available:

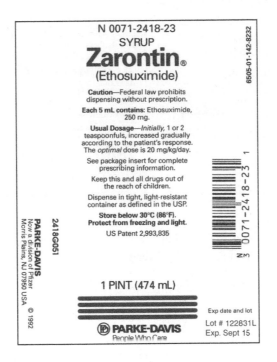

6. Child with seizures.
   Order: Dilantin 40 mg, po, bid.
   Child's weight and age: 6.7 kg, 3 months.
   Pediatric dose: 5-7 mg/kg/day.
   Drug available: Dilantin 125 mg/5 mL.

7. Child with acute urinary tract infection.
   Order: Bactrim 600 mg/120 mg, po, bid.
   Child's weight and age: 66 lbs, 9 years.
   Pediatric dose: Bactrim 6-10 mg/kg/day.
   Drug available: Bactrim 400 mg/80 mg.

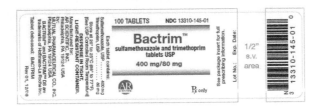

8. Infant with upper respiratory tract infection.
   Order: Augmentin oral suspension 75 mg, po, q8h.
   Child's weight and age: 8 kg, 7 months.
   Pediatric dose: 20-40 mg/kg/day.

Drug available:

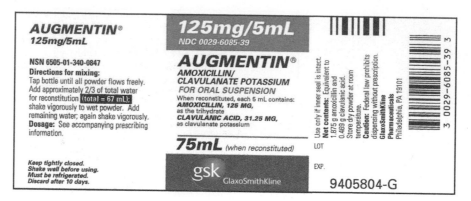

9. Child with poison ivy.
   Order: Benadryl 25 mg, po, q6h.
   Child's weight and age: 25 kg, 7 years.
   Pediatric dose: 5 mg/kg/day.
   Drug available: Benadryl 12.5 mg/5 mL.

10. Child with cystic fibrosis exposed to influenza A.
    Order: oseltamivir (Tamiflu) 45 mg, po, bid × 5 days.
    Child's weight and age: 16 kg, 4 years.
    Pediatric dose: 90 mg/day for 16-23 kg.
    Drug available: oseltamivir 12 mg/mL.

11. Order: cefaclor (Ceclor) 50 mg, qid.
    Child's weight and age: 15 lbs, age 4 months.
    Pediatric dose: 20-40 mg/kg/day in three or four divided doses.
    Drug available:

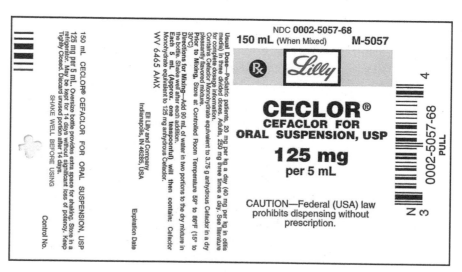

12. Child with nausea and vomiting from chemotherapy.
    Order: ondansetron (Zofran) 2 mg, po 30 minutes before administration, q8h, prn.
    Child's weight and age: 80 lbs, 10 years.
    Pediatric dose: 0.04-0.87 mg/kg/day.

Drug available:

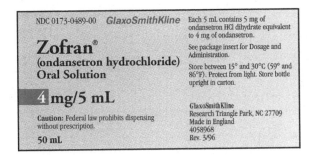

13. Child, 7 years old, with pinworms.
  Order: Pyrantel pamoate suspension 250 mg, daily.
  Child's weight: 50 lbs.
  Pediatric dose: 11 mg/kg.
  Drug available: Pyrantel pamoate 50 mg/mL.

II Intramuscular

Answers can be found on pages 313 to 314.

14. Child with pain after surgery.
  Order: Ketorolac 10 mg, IM × 1.
  Child's weight and age: 22 kg, 5 years.
  Pediatric dose: 0.5 mg/kg.
  Drug available: 30 mg/mL.

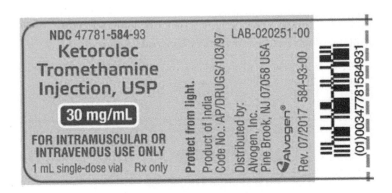

15. Child has strep throat (streptococcal pharyngitis).
  Order: Bicillin C-R, 1,000,000 units, IM × 1.
  Child's weight: 44 lbs.
  Pediatric dose: 30-60 lbs: 900,000-1,200,000 units daily.
  Drug available: Bicillin C-R, 1,200,000 units/2 mL.

16. Child receiving preoperative medication (may solve by nomogram or square root).
  Order: hydroxyzine (Vistaril) 25 mg, IM.
  Child's height and weight: 47 inches, 45 lbs.
  Pediatric dose: 30 mg/m^2.

Drug available:

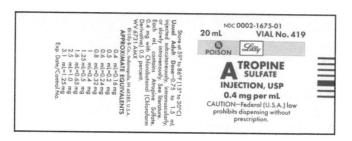

17. Child receiving preoperative medication.
    Order: atropine 0.2 mg, IM × 1.
    Child's weight and age: 12 kg, 7 months.
    Pediatric dose: 0.01-0.02 mg/kg/dose, not to exceed 0.4 mg/dose.
    Drug available:

18. Child with cancer.
    Order: methotrexate 40 mg, IM, weekly (may solve by nomogram or square root).
    Child's height and weight: 56 inches, 100 lbs.
    Pediatric dose: 7.5-30 mg/m²/wk.
    Drug available: methotrexate 2.5 mg/mL; 25 mg/mL; 100 mg/mL.

19. Order: A newborn is to receive AquaMEPHYTON (vitamin K) 0.5 mg IM immediately after delivery.
    Pediatric dose: 0.5-1 mg.
    Drug available:

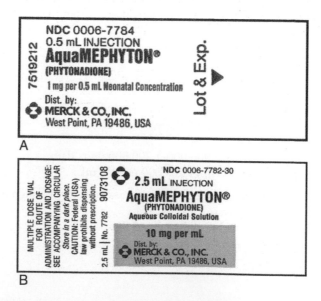

a. Which AquaMEPHYTON container would you select?_____
b. How many milliliters (mL) should the newborn receive?_____
c. Is drug dose within the safe range?_____

20. Child with severe croup.

Order: Dexamethasone 6 mg, IM × 1.

Child's height, weight, and age: 42 inches, 44 lbs, 4 years.

Pediatric dose: 0.6 mg/m^2 to 9 mg/m^2.

Drug available:

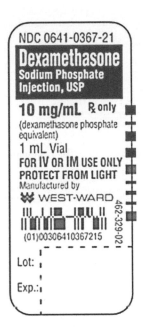

a. Determine if dosage is safe.

b. Calculate dose.

III Intravenous

Answers can be found on pages 314 to 317.

21. Adolescent with progressive hip pain secondary to rheumatoid arthritis.

Order: morphine sulfate 2.5 mg, one time dose, IV piggyback, in 10 mL NS over 5 minutes.

Flush with 5 mL.

Child's weight and age: 50 kg, 16 years.

Pediatric dose: 50-100 mcg/kg/dose for IV.

Drug available:

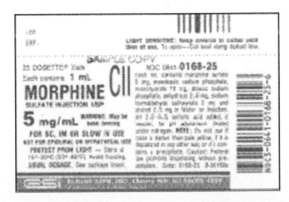

a. Determine if dosage is safe.

b. Calculate dose.

c. How many mL should infuse?

d. How many gtt/min should infuse?

e. What is the total amount of fluid given?

22. Treatment to reverse postoperative narcotic-induced respiratory depression.
    Order: Narcan (naloxone) 1.8 mg IV push, once. STAT.
    Child's weight and age: 18 kg, 3 years.
    Pediatric dose: 0.1 mg/kg.
    Drug available:

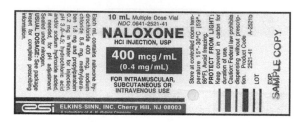

    a. Determine if dosage is safe.   **b.** Calculate dose.

23. Infant with sepsis.
    Order: Amikin 40 mg, IV, q12h, in D₅W 5 mL, over 20 minutes. Flush with 3 mL.
    Child's weight and age: 5.3 kg, 1 year.
    Pediatric dose: 15 mg/kg/day.
    Drug available:

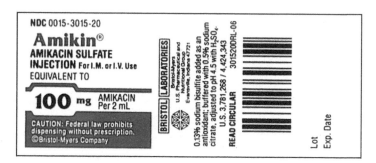

    a. Determine if dosage is safe.   **d.** How many gtt/min should infuse?
    b. Calculate dose.   **e.** What is the total amount of fluid given?
    c. How many mL should infuse?
    e. What is the total amount of fluid given?

24. Treatment for child with cerebral palsy having spasticity after spinal fusion.
    Order: lorazepam 3 mg IV q6h.
    Child's weight and age: 47 kg, 17 years.
    Pediatric dose: 0.05-0.1 mg/kg per dose.
    Drug available: lorazepam 4 mg/mL.

    a. Determine if dosage is safe.
    b. Calculate dose.

25. Child with pneumonia.
    Order: cefazolin (Ancef) 500 mg, IV, q6h, in D₅W 20 mL, over 30 minutes.
    Flush with 10 mL.
    Child's weight and age: 5.6 kg, 2 months.
    Pediatric dose: 25-100 mg/kg/day in four divided doses.
    Drug available:

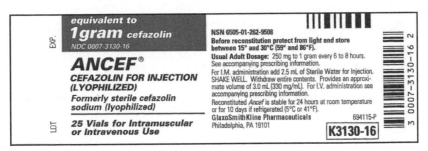

    a. Determine if dosage is safe.
    b. Calculate dose.
    c. How many mL should infuse?
    d. How many gtt/min should infuse?
    e. What is the total amount of fluid given?

26. Child with sepsis.
    Order: gentamicin 10 mg, IV, q8h, in D₅W, 4 mL, over 30 minutes. Flush with 3 mL.
    Child's height, weight, and age: 21 inches, 4 kg, 1 month.
    Pediatric dose: More than 7 days old: 5-7.5 mg/kg/day in three divided doses.
    Drug available: gentamicin 10 mg/mL.
        a. Determine if dosage is safe.
        b. Calculate dose.
        c. How many mL should infuse?
        d. How many gtt/min should infuse?
        e. What is the total amount of fluid given?

27. Child with postoperative wound infection.
    Order: cefazolin 185 mg, IV, q6h, in D₅W 20 mL, over 20 minutes. Flush with 15 mL.
    Child's weight: 15 kg.
    Pediatric dose: 25-50 mg/kg/day.
    Drug available:

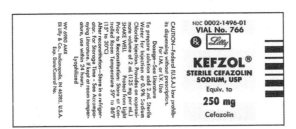

    a. Determine if dosage is safe.
    b. Calculate dose.
    c. How many mL should infuse?
    d. How many gtt/min should infuse?
    e. What is the total amount of fluid given?

28. Child with staphylococcus scalded skin syndrome.
    Order: clindamycin 50 mg IV q8h.
    Dilution instructions: Mix in 10 mL NS over 15 min via syringe pump.
    Child's weight and age: 7.5 kg, 5 months.
    Pediatric dose: 16-20 mg/kg/day.
    Drug available: clindamycin 150 mg/mL.
    a. Determine if dosage is safe.
    b. Calculate dose.

29. Child with congestive heart failure.
    Order: digoxin 40 mcg, IV, bid, in NS 2 mL, over 1 minute.
    Child's weight and age: 6 lbs, 1 month.
    Pediatric dose: 2 weeks to 2 years: 25-50 mcg/kg.
    Drug available: digoxin 0.1 mg/mL.
    a. Determine if dosage is safe.
    b. Calculate dose.

30. Child with lymphoma
    Order: Cytoxan 125 mg, IV, once, in D5½ NS, 300 mL, over 3 hours, no flush to follow.
    Child's weight and height: 16 kg, 75 cm (may solve by nomogram or square root).
    Pediatric dose: 60-250 mg/m²/day.
    Drug available:

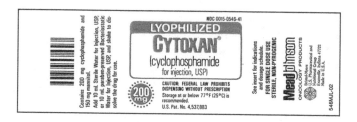

    a. Determine if dosage is safe.
    b. Calculate dose.

31. Child with pertussis.
    Order: azithromycin (Zithromax) 300 mg/day.
    Child's weight and age: 55 lbs, 8 years.
    Pediatric dose: 10 mg/kg/day × 5 days.
    Drug available: azithromycin 200 mg/5 mL.

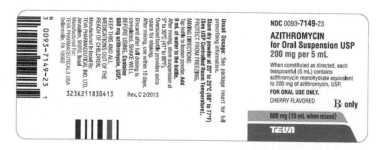

    a. Determine if dosage is safe.
    b. Calculate dose.

32. Child with severe systemic infection.
    Order: tobramycin (Nebcin) 15 mg, IV, q6h.
    Child's weight and age: 10 kg, 18 months.
    Pediatric dose parameters: 6-7.5 mg/kg/day in four divided doses.
    Drug available:

2 mL Multiple-dose   NDC 0409-3577-01
TOBRAMYCIN Injection, USP
Pediatric 20 mg/2 mL   ℞ only
WARNING: CONTAINS SULFITES
For I.V. or I.M. use. Must dilute for I.V. use.
RL-1992 (1/07)
Hospira, Inc., Lake Forest, IL 60045 USA

   a. Determine if dosage is safe.
   b. Calculate dose.

33. Child with acute lymphocytic leukemia.
    Order: daunorubicin HCl 40 mg, IV, daily.
    Pediatric dose parameters: More than 2 yr: 25-45 mg/m^2/day.
    Child's age, weight, and height: 10 years, 72 lbs, 60 inches.
    Drug available: daunorubicin 20 mg/4 mL.
    Instructions: Mix in 100 mL D$_5$W; infuse in 45 minutes via pump.

   a. The BSA is_____
   b. How many milliliters should be mixed in the D$_5$W?_____
   c. Is the drug dose within the safe range?_____
   d. How many milliliters per hour should infuse?_____

34. Child with a serious fungal infection.
    Order: fluconazole (Diflucan) 200 mg, IV, per day for 10 days.
    Child's weight and age: 55 lbs, 7 years.
    Pediatric dose: 6-12 mg/kg/day.
    Drug available: fluconazole 400 mg/200 mL.

   a. How many kilograms does the child weigh?_____
   b. Is the dose safe?_____
   c. How many milliliters should the child receive per dose?_____

IV Neonates

Answers can be found on pages 317 to 318.

35. Neonate with bradycardia, heart rate less than 60 beats/min.
    Order: epinephrine 0.25 mg IV × 1. STAT.
    Pediatric dose: 0.1 mg/kg.
    Neonate weight: 2.5 kg.

Drug available:

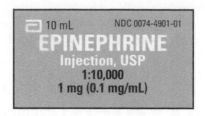

a. Determine if dosage is safe.

b. Calculate dose.

36. Neonate with respiratory depression after delivery; mother received Stadol during labor.
    Neonate weight: 8 lbs 12 oz.
    Order: naxolone 0.04 mg IM × 1. STAT.
    Pediatric dose: 0.01 mg/kg.
    Drug available: naxolone 0.4 mg/mL.

    a. Determine if dosage is safe.

    b. Calculate dose.

37. Neonate with bacterial meningitis.
    Neonate weight: 2.5 kg.
    Order: ampicillin 125 mg IV push, once, over 2 minutes.
    Pediatric dose parameters: 50-75 mg/kg/dose.
    Drug available:

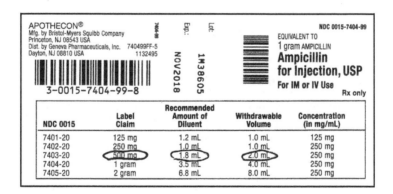

a. Determine if dosage is safe.

b. Calculate dose.

38. Neonate with IV fluids for sepsis.
    Neonate weight: 2.5 kg.
    Order: D₅W 80 mL/kg for 24 hours.

    a. How much D₅W should be given in 24 hours?

    b. How many milliliters per hour should be infused?

39. Neonate with meningitis.
    Neonate weight: 2.5 kg.
    Order: ampicillin 75 mg q4h.
    Pediatric dosing parameters: 400 mg/kg/day.
    Drug available: ampicillin 50 mg/mL.

    a. Determine if dosage is safe.

    b. Calculate dose.

PEDIATRIC DOSAGE FROM ADULT DOSAGE

Body Surface Area Formula

The following information is needed to calculate the pediatric dosage with the BSA formula:

a. Physician's order with the name of the drug, the dosage, and the time frame or frequency.

b. The child's height and weight.

c. A BSA nomogram for children (p. 293).

d. The adult drug dosage.

e. The BSA formula:

$$\frac{BSA(m^2)}{1.73\ m^2} \times \text{Adult dose} = \text{Child dose}$$

EXAMPLE **PROBLEM**

a. Erythromycin 80 mg, po, qid.

b. Child's height is 34 inches and weight is 28.5 lbs.

Note: *Height and weight do not have to be converted to the metric system.*

c. Height (34 inches) and weight (28.5 lbs) intersect the nomogram at 0.57 m². See BSA nomogram, Figure 13.3.

d. The adult drug dosage is 1000 mg/24 hr.

e. BSA formula:

$$\frac{BSA(m^2)}{1.73\ m^2} \times \text{Adult dose} = \frac{0.57\ m^2}{1.73\ m^2} \times 1000\ mg$$

$$= 0.33 \times 1000\ mg$$

$$= 330\ mg/24\ hr$$

Dose frequency: 330 mg ÷ 4 doses = 82.5 **or** 80 mg/dose

80 mg × 4 times per day = 320 mg/day

Dosage is safe.

Age Rules

Fried's rule and Young's rule are two methods for determining pediatric drug doses based on the child's age. Fried's rule is used primarily for children younger than 1 year of age, whereas Young's rule is used for children between 2 and 12 years of age. In current practice, these rules are infrequently used. Because the maturational development of infants and children is variable, age cannot be an accurate basis for drug dosing.

Fried's Rule:

$$\frac{\text{Age in months}}{150} \times \text{Adult dose} = \text{Infant dose}$$

Young's Rule:

$$\frac{\text{Child's age in years}}{\text{Age in years} + 12} \times \text{Adult dose} = \text{Child dose}$$

NOTE

The age rules should not be used if a pediatric dose is provided by the manufacturer.

ANSWERS SUMMARY PRACTICE PROBLEMS

I Oral

1. Dosage parameters: 4 mg × 68 lbs = 272 mg
   6 mg × 68 lbs = 408 mg
   Dosage frequency: 90 mg × 4 = 360 mg/day
   Dosage is safe.

   BF: $\dfrac{D}{H} \times V = \dfrac{90 \text{ mg}}{75 \text{ mg}} \times 5 \text{ mL} = 6 \text{ mL}$

   or

   DA: mL $= \dfrac{V \times D}{H \times X} = \dfrac{5 \text{ mL} \times 90 \text{ mL}}{75 \text{ mg} \times 1} = \dfrac{450}{75} = 6 \text{ mL}$

   or

   RP: H : V :: D : X
   75 mg : 5 mL :: 90 mg : X
   75 X = 450
   X = 6 mL

   or

   FE: $\dfrac{H}{V} = \dfrac{D}{X} = \dfrac{75 \text{ mg}}{5 \text{ mL}} = \dfrac{90 \text{ mg}}{X}$

   (Cross multiply) 75 X = 450
   X = 6 mL

2. Dosage parameters: 5 mg/kg/day × 7.2 kg = 36 mg/day
   7 mg/kg/day × 7.2 kg = 50.4 mg/day
   Dose frequency: 25 mg × 2 = 50 mg
   Dosage is safe.

   BF: $\dfrac{D}{H} \times V = \dfrac{25 \text{ mg}}{20 \text{ mg}} \times 5 \text{ mL} = 6.25 \text{ mL/dose}$

   or

   DA: mL $= \dfrac{5 \text{ mL} \times \overset{5}{25 \text{ mg}}}{\underset{4}{20 \text{ mg}} \times 1} = \dfrac{25}{4} = 6.25 \text{ mL}$

3. Dosage parameters: 15 mg/kg, q12h × 8 kg = 120 mg, q12h. 120 mg × 2 = 240mg total daily dose
   Dosage frequency: 100 mg, q12h
   Dosing is safe because a total daily dose of 200mg is less than the max daily dose of 240mg.

   BF: $\dfrac{D}{H} \times V = \dfrac{100 \text{ mg}}{125 \text{ mg}} \times 5 \text{ mL} = 4 \text{ mL/dose}$

   or

   FE: $\dfrac{H}{V} = \dfrac{D}{X} = \dfrac{125 \text{ mg}}{5 \text{ mL}} = \dfrac{100 \text{ mg}}{X}$

   (Cross multiply) 125 X = 500
   X = 4 mL

4. Height and weight intersect at 0.84 m² with nomogram.
   Dosage parameters: 100 mg/0.84 m²/day = 84 mg/day
   Dose frequency: 84 mg/day ÷ 6 = 14 mg/dose
   Dosage is safe.
   BSA with the Square Root: BSA Pounds and Inches Formula, see p. 99.

   $$\sqrt{\dfrac{43 \times 50}{3131}} = \sqrt{0.686} = 0.828 \text{ or } 0.83 \text{ m}^2$$

   Dosage parameters: 100 mg/0.83 m² = 83 mg/day (compare with nomogram)
   Dosage frequency: 83 mg/day/6 = 13.8 or 14 mg/dose
   Dosage is safe.

   BF: $\dfrac{D}{H} \times V = \dfrac{7.5 \text{ mg}}{15 \text{ mg}} \times 1 = 0.50 \text{ or } \frac{1}{2} \text{ tablet}$

   or

   RP: H : V :: D : X
   15 mg : 1 tab :: 7.5 mg : X
   15 X = 7.5
   X = ½ tablet

5. Dosage parameters: 15 mg/kg/day × 13 kg = 195 mg/day
   40 mg/day × 13 kg = 520 mg/day
   Dose frequency: 125 mg × 2 = 250 mg/day
   Dosage is safe.

   $$\textbf{BF:}\frac{D}{H} \times V = \frac{125 \text{ mg}}{250 \text{ mg}} \times 5 \text{ mL} = 2.5 \text{ mL}$$

6. Dosage parameters: 5 mg/kg/day × 6.7 kg = 33.5 mg/day
   7 mg/kg/day × 6.7 kg = 46.9 mg/day
   Dose frequency: 40 mg × 2 = 80 mg/day
   Dosage exceeds the therapeutic range. Dosage is *not safe.*

7. Pounds to kilograms

   $$\frac{66 \text{ lbs}}{2.2 \text{ lbs/kg}} = 30 \text{ kg}$$

   Dosage parameters: 6 mg/kg/day × 30 kg = 180 mg/day
   10 mg/kg/day × 30 kg = 300 mg/day
   Dosage frequency: 2 times a day × 120 mg = 240 mg/day
   Dosage is safe.

   $$\textbf{BF:}\frac{D}{H} \times \frac{120 \text{ mg}}{80 \text{ mg}} \times 1 = 1.5 \text{ tablets}$$

   or
   RP: H :V:: D :X
   80 mg: 1 ::120 mg:X
   80 X = 120
   X = 1.5 tablets

   or
   $$\textbf{DA: tab} = \frac{1 \text{ tab} \times 120 \text{ mg}}{80 \text{ mg} \times 1} = \frac{120}{80} = 1.5 \text{ tablets}$$

   or
   $$\textbf{FE:}\frac{H}{V} = \frac{D}{X} = \frac{80 \text{ mg}}{1 \text{ tab}} = \frac{120 \text{ mg}}{X}$$
   80 X = 120
   X = 1.5 tablets

8. Dosage parameters: 20 mg/kg/day × 8 kg = 160 mg/day
   40 mg/kg/day × 8 kg = 320 mg/day
   Dose frequency: 75 mg × 3 = 225 mg
   Dosage is safe.

   $$\textbf{BF:}\frac{D}{H} \times V = \frac{75 \text{ mg}}{125 \text{ mg}} \times 5 \text{ mL} = 3 \text{ mL}$$

   or
   RP: H : V :: D :X
   125 mg:5 mL::75 mg:X
   125 X = 375
   X = 3 mL

   or
   $$\textbf{FE:}\frac{H}{V} = \frac{D}{X} = \frac{125 \text{ mg}}{5 \text{ mL}} = \frac{75 \text{ mg}}{X} =$$
   125 X = 375
   X = 3 mL

9. Dosage parameters: 5 mg/kg/day × 25 kg = 125 mg/day
   Dose frequency: 25 mg × 4 = 100 mg/day
   Dosage is safe.

   $$\textbf{BF:}\frac{D}{H} \times V = \frac{25 \text{ mg}}{12.5 \text{ mg}} \times 5 \text{ mL} = 10 \text{ mL}$$

   or
   $$\textbf{DA: mL} = \frac{5 \text{ mL} \times \overset{2}{25} \text{ mg}}{\underset{1}{12.5} \text{ mg} \times 1} = 10 \text{ mL}$$

   or
   $$\textbf{FE:}\frac{H}{V} = \frac{D}{X} = \frac{12.5 \text{ mg}}{5 \text{ mL}} = \frac{25 \text{ mg}}{X \text{ mL}}$$
   12.5 X = 125
   X = 10 mL

10. Dosing parameters: 90 mg/day
    Dosing frequency: 45 mg $\times$ 2 = 90 mg
    Dosage is safe.

    BF: $\dfrac{D}{H} \times V = \dfrac{45 \text{ mg}}{12 \text{ mg}} \times 1 \text{ mL} = 3.75 \text{ mL}$

    or
    DA: $\text{mL} = \dfrac{1 \text{ mL} \times 45 \text{ mg}}{12 \text{ mg} \times 1} = 3.75 \text{ mL}$

11. 15 lbs $\div$ 2.2 = 6.8 kg
    Dosage parameters: 20 mg $\times$ 6.8 kg = 136 mg/day
     40 mg $\times$ 6.8 kg = 272 mg/day
    Dose frequency: 50 mg $\times$ 4 = 200 mg/day
    Dosage is safe.

    BF: $\dfrac{D}{H} \times V = \dfrac{50}{125} \times 5 = \dfrac{250}{125} = 2 \text{ mL}$

    or
    RP: $\quad$ H $\quad$: $\quad$ V $\quad$ :: $\quad$ D $\quad$: $\quad$ X
    $\qquad$ 125 mg : 5 mL :: 50 mg : X mL
    $\qquad\qquad$ 125 X = 250
    $\qquad\qquad\qquad$ X = 2 mL

    or
    FE: $\dfrac{H}{V} = \dfrac{D}{X} = \dfrac{125 \text{ mg}}{5 \text{ mL}} = \dfrac{50 \text{ mg}}{X}$

    (Cross multiply) 125 X = 250
    $\qquad\qquad\qquad$ X = 2 mL

    or
    DA: $\text{mL} = \dfrac{5 \text{ mL} \times \overset{2}{\cancel{50}} \text{ mg}}{\underset{5}{\cancel{125}} \text{ mg} \times 1} = \dfrac{10}{5} = 2 \text{ mL}$

12. Pounds to kilograms

    $\dfrac{80 \text{ lbs}}{2.2 \text{ lbs/kg}} = 36.4 \text{ kg}$

    Dosing parameters:
    $\quad$ 0.04 mg $\times$ 36.4 kg/day = 1.46 mg/kg/day
    $\quad$ 0.87 mg $\times$ 36.4 kg/day = 31.7 mg/kg/day
    Dosage frequency: 3 times a day $\times$ 2 mg = 6 mg
    Dosage is safe.

    BF: $\dfrac{D}{H} \times V = \dfrac{2 \text{ mg}}{4 \text{ mg}} \times 5 \text{ mL} = 2.5 \text{ mL}$

    or
    DA: $\text{mL} = \dfrac{5 \text{ mL} \times \overset{1}{\cancel{2}} \text{ mg}}{\underset{2}{\cancel{4}} \text{ mg} \times 1} = \dfrac{5}{2} = 2.5 \text{ mL}$

13. **a.** Pounds to kilograms

    $\dfrac{50 \text{ lbs}}{2.2 \text{ lbs/kg}} = 22.7 \text{ kg}$

    b. 22.7 kg $\times$ 11 mg/kg = 249.9 or 250 mg
     Dosage is safe.

    c. BF: $\dfrac{D}{H} \times V$

    $\qquad \dfrac{250 \text{ mg}}{50 \text{ mg}} \times 1 \text{ mL} = 5 \text{ mL}$

    or
    DA: $\text{mL} = \dfrac{1 \text{ mL} \times \overset{5}{\cancel{250}} \text{ mg}}{\underset{1}{\cancel{50}} \text{ mg} \times 1} = \dfrac{\overset{5}{\cancel{250}}}{\underset{1}{\cancel{50}}} = 5 \text{ mL}$

    or
    FE: $\dfrac{50 \text{ mg}}{1} = \dfrac{250 \text{ mg}}{X} =$
    $\qquad\qquad$ 50 X = 250
    $\qquad\qquad\qquad$ X = 5 mL

    or
    RP: $\quad$ H $\quad$: $\quad$ V $\quad$ :: $\quad$ D $\qquad$: X
    $\qquad$ 50 mg : 1 mL :: 250 mg : X
    $\qquad\qquad$ 50 X = 250 mg
    $\qquad\qquad\qquad$ X = 5 mL

II Intramuscular

14. Dosing parameters: 0.5 mg/kg × 22 kg = 11 mg
Dosing frequency: one time.
Dosing is safe.

$$\textbf{BF:}\ \frac{D}{H} \times V = \frac{10\ mg}{30\ mg} \times 1 = 0.33\ mL\ or\ 0.3\ mL$$

or

$$\textbf{DA:}\ mL = \frac{1\ mL \times 10\ mg}{30\ mg} = \frac{10}{30} = 0.33\ mL\ or\ 0.3\ mL$$

15. Dosage parameters: Child's weight is 44 lbs, which falls in the 30- to 60-lb pediatric dosage range.
Dose frequency: The one-time dose of 1,000,000 units falls within the pediatric dosage range.
Dosage is safe.

$$\textbf{BF:}\ \frac{D}{H} \times V = \frac{1,000,000\ Units}{1,200,000\ Units} \times 2\ mL = 1.666\ or\ 1.7\ mL\ (round\ off\ to\ tenths)$$

16. Height and weight intersect at 0.82 m² with the nomogram.
BSA with Square Root (Pounds and Inches Formula)

$$\sqrt{\frac{47\ inches \times 45\ pounds}{3131}} = \sqrt{0.675} = 0.82\ m^2\ (same\ as\ the\ nomogram)$$

Dosage parameters: 30 mg/m² × 0.82 m² = 24.6 mg or 25 mg
Dose frequency: 25 mg IM/dose
Dosage is safe.

$$\textbf{BF:}\ \frac{D}{H} \times V = \frac{25\ mg}{25\ mg} \times 1 = 1.0\ mL$$

or

$$\textbf{DA:}\ mL = \frac{1\ mL \times \overset{1}{\cancel{25}}\ \cancel{mg}}{\underset{1}{\cancel{25}}\ \cancel{mg} \times 1} = 1\ mL$$

17. Dosing parameters: 0.01 mg/kg/dose × 12 kg = 0.12 mg/dose
0.02 mg/kg/dose × 12 kg = 0.24 mg/dose

Dosage is safe.

$$\textbf{BF:}\ \frac{D}{H} \times V = \frac{0.2}{0.4} \times 1 = 0.5\ mL$$

18. Height and weight intersect at 1.38 m² with the nomogram.
Dosing parameters for nomogram: 7.5 mg × 1.38 m² = 10.35 mg/wk
30 mg × 1.38 m² = 41.4 mg/wk

BSA with Square Root (Pounds and Inches Formula)

$$\sqrt{\frac{56\ inches \times 100\ pounds}{3131}} = \sqrt{1.788} = 1.34\ m^2$$

Dosing parameter for BSA formula: 7.5 mg × 1.34 m² = 10.05 mg/wk
30 mg × 1.34 m² = 40.2 mg/wk

Dose frequency: 40 mg/wk IM
Dosage is safe.

$$\textbf{BF:}\ \frac{D}{H} \times V = \frac{40\ mg}{100\ mg} \times 1\ mL = 0.4\ mL$$

or

$$\textbf{DA:}\ mL = \frac{1\ mL \times 40\ \cancel{mg}}{100\ \cancel{mg} \times 1} = \frac{40}{100} = 0.4\ mL$$

19. a. Preferred selection is AquaMEPHYTON 1 mg = 0.5 mL. Drug container A.
b. *AquaMEPHYTON 1 mg = 0.5 mL:*

$$\textbf{BF:}\ \frac{D}{H} \times V = \frac{0.5\ mg}{1.0\ mg} \times 0.5\ mL = \frac{0.25}{1.0} = 0.25\ mL$$

or

RP: H : V :: D :X

$\quad$ 1 mg:0.5 mL::0.5 mg:X

$\qquad$ X = 0.25 mL

AquaMEPHYTON 10 mg = 1 mL:

BF: $\dfrac{D}{H} \times V = \dfrac{0.5 \text{ mg}}{10 \text{ mg}} \times 1.0 \text{ mL} = \dfrac{0.5}{10} = 0.05 \text{ mL}$

or

FE: $\dfrac{H}{V} = \dfrac{D}{X} = \dfrac{10 \text{ mg}}{1 \text{ mL}} = \dfrac{0.5 \text{ mg}}{X \text{ mL}}$

$\qquad 10\,X = 0.5$

$\qquad X = 0.05 \text{ mL}$

For AquaMEPHYTON 1 mg = 0.5 mL, give 0.25 mL (use a tuberculin syringe).

For AquaMEPHYTON 10 mg = 1 mL, give 0.05 mL (use a tuberculin syringe; however, it would be difficult to give this small amount).

c. Drug dose is within the safe range.

20. Height and weight intersect at 0.78 m² with the nomogram.

$\quad$ Dosage parameters: 0.6 mg/m² × 0.78 m² = 0.46 mg

$\qquad\qquad\qquad\quad$ 9 mg/m² × 0.78 m² = 7.02 mg

a. Dosage is safe.

b. BF: $\dfrac{D}{H} \times V = \dfrac{6 \text{ mg}}{10 \text{ mg}} \times 1 \text{ mL} = 0.6 \text{ mL}$

or

RP: H : V :: D :X

$\quad$ 10 mg:1 mL::6 mg:X

$\qquad$ 10 X = 6

$\qquad$ X = 0.6 mL

or

DA: mL $= \dfrac{1 \text{ mL}}{10 \text{ mg}} \times \dfrac{6 \text{ mg}}{1} = 0.6 \text{ mL}$

or

FE: $\dfrac{H}{V} = \dfrac{D}{H} = \dfrac{10 \text{ mg}}{1 \text{ mL}} = \dfrac{6 \text{ mg}}{X}$

(Cross multiply) 10 X = 6

$\qquad\qquad\qquad$ X = 0.6 mL

III Intravenous

21. Dosage parameters: 50 mcg/kg/dose × 50 kg = 2500 mcg/dose or 2.5 mg/dose

$\qquad\qquad\qquad\qquad$ 100 mcg/kg/dose × 50 kg = 5000 mcg/dose or 5 mg/dose

a. Dosage is safe.

b. BF: $\dfrac{D}{H} \times V = \dfrac{2.5}{5} \times 1 = 0.5 \text{ mL}$

or

DA: mL $= \dfrac{1 \text{ mL} \times \overset{1}{\cancel{2.5}} \text{ mg}}{\underset{2}{\cancel{5}} \text{ mg} \times 1} = \dfrac{1}{2}$ or 0.5 mL

c. Amount of fluid to be infused: 0.5 mL + 10 mL = 10.5 mL

d. $\dfrac{10.5 \text{ mL} \times \overset{12}{\cancel{60}} \text{ gtt/mL}}{\underset{1}{\cancel{5}} \text{ minutes}} = 126 \text{ gtt/min}$

e. Total fluid for medication infusion plus flush: 10.5 mL + 5 mL = 15.5 mL.

22. Dosing parameter: 0.1 mg/kg × 18 kg = 1.8 mg.

a. Dosage is safe.

b. BF: $\dfrac{D}{H} \times V = \dfrac{1.8 \text{ mg}}{0.4 \text{ mg}} \times 1 \text{ mL} = 4.5 \text{ mL by IV push}$

23. Dosage parameters: 15 mg/kg/day $\times$ 5.3 = 79.5 mg/day.

Dose frequency: 40 mg IV $\times$ 2 = 80 mg. 79.5 mg is rounded off to 80 mg.

a. Dosage is safe.

b. BF: $\dfrac{D}{H} \times V = \dfrac{40 \text{ mg}}{100 \text{ mg}} \times 2 = 0.8$ mL

or

RP: H : V :: D :X

100 mg:2 mL::40 mg:X

100 X = 80

X = 0.8 mL

or

FE: $\dfrac{H}{V} = \dfrac{D}{X} = \dfrac{100 \text{ mg}}{2 \text{ mL}} = \dfrac{40 \text{ mg}}{X}$

(Cross multiply) 100 X = 80

X = 0.8 mL

c. Amount of fluid to be infused: 0.8 mL + 5 mL = 5.8 mL

d. $\dfrac{5.8 \text{ mL} \times \overset{3}{\cancel{60}} \text{ gtt/mL}}{\underset{1}{\cancel{20}} \text{ minutes}}$ = 17.4 gtt/min or 17 gtt/min

e. Total fluid for medication infusion plus flush: 5.8 mL + 3 mL = 8.8 mL.

24. Dosing parameters: 0.05 mg/kg $\times$ 47 kg = 2.35 mg

0.1 mg/kg $\times$ 47 kg = 4.7 mg

a. Dosage is safe.

b. BF: $\dfrac{D}{H} \times V = \dfrac{3 \text{ mg}}{4 \text{ mg}} \times 1 \text{ mL} = 0.75$ mL

or

RP: H : V :: D :X

4 mg:1 mL::3 mg:X

4 X = 3

X = 0.75 mL

or

FE: $\dfrac{H}{V} = \dfrac{D}{X} = \dfrac{4 \text{ mg}}{1 \text{ mL}} = \dfrac{3 \text{ mg}}{X} =$

(Cross multiply) 4 X = 3

X = 0.75 mL

25. Dosage parameters: 25-100 mg/kg/day in four divided doses.

25 mg $\times$ 5.6 kg = 140 mg/day

100 mg $\times$ 5.6 kg = 560 mg/day

140 mg $\div$ 4 = 35 mg/dose

560 mg $\div$ 4 = 140 mg/dose

Dose frequency: 500 mg $\times$ 4 = 2000 mg/day

Dose exceeds therapeutic range of 560 mg/day. Dosage is *not safe*.

26. Dosage parameters: 5 mg/kg/day $\times$ 4 kg = 20 mg/day

7.5 mg/kg/day $\times$ 4 kg = 30 mg/day

Dose frequency: 10 mg $\times$ 3 times/day = 30 mg

a. Dosage is safe.

b. BF: $\dfrac{D}{H} \times V = \dfrac{10 \text{ mg}}{10 \text{ mg}} \times 1 \text{ mL} = 1$ mL

or

DA: mL = $\dfrac{1 \text{ mL} \times \overset{1}{\cancel{10 \text{ mg}}}}{\underset{1}{\cancel{10 \text{ mg}}} \times 1} = 1$ mL

or

RP: H : V :: D : X

10 mg:1 mL::10 mg:X mL

10 X = 10

X = 1 mL

or

FE: $\dfrac{H}{V} = \dfrac{D}{X} = \dfrac{10 \text{ mg}}{1 \text{ mL}} = \dfrac{10 \text{ mg}}{X \text{ mL}}$

(Cross multiply) 10 X = 10

X = 1 mL

c. Amount of fluid to be infused: 1 mL + 4 mL = 5 mL

d. $\dfrac{5 \text{ mL} \times \overset{2}{\cancel{60}} \text{ gtt/mL}}{\underset{1}{\cancel{30}} \text{ minutes}}$ = 10 gtt/min

e. Total fluid for medication infusion plus flush: 5 mL + 3 mL = 8 mL

27. Dosage parameters: 25 mg/kg/day $\times$ 15 kg = 375 mg/day
50 mg/kg/day $\times$ 15 kg = 750 mg/day
Dose frequency: 185 mg $\times$ 4 = 740 mg/day
a. Dosage is safe.

b. BF: $\dfrac{D}{H} \times V = \dfrac{185 \text{ mg}}{125 \text{ mg}} \times 1 \text{ mL} = 1.48$ or 1.5 mL

Reconstitution information: 125 mg = 1 mL

or

RP:$\quad$ H $\;:\;$ V $\;::\;$ D $\;:$ X
$\quad$125 mg : 1 mL :: 185 mg : X
$\qquad\qquad$125 X = 185
$\qquad\qquad\quad$X = 1.5 mL

c. Amount of fluid to be infused: 1.5 mL + 20 mL = 21.5 mL

d. $\dfrac{21.5 \text{ mL} \times \overset{3}{\cancel{60}} \text{ gtt/mL}}{\underset{1}{\cancel{20}} \text{ minutes}} = 64.5$ gtt/min

e. Total fluid for medication infusion plus flush: 21.5 mL + 15 mL = 36.5 mL

28. Dosing parameter: 16 mg/kg/day $\times$ 7.5 kg = 120 mg/day
20 mg/kg/day $\times$ 7.5 kg = 150 mg/day
Dosing frequency: 50 mg $\times$ 3 = 150 mg
a. Dosage is safe.

b. BF: $\dfrac{D}{H} \times V = \dfrac{50 \text{ mg}}{150 \text{ mg}} \times 1 \text{ mL} = 0.33 \text{ mL}$ or 0.3 mL

or

RP:$\quad$ H $\;:\;$ V $\;::\;$ D $\;:$ X
$\quad$150 mg : 1 mL :: 50 mg : X mL
$\qquad\qquad$150 X = 50
$\qquad\qquad\quad$X $= \dfrac{50}{150} = 0.3$ mL

or

DA: mL $= \dfrac{1 \text{ mL} \times \overset{1}{\cancel{50} \cancel{\text{mg}}}}{\underset{3}{\cancel{150} \cancel{\text{mg}}} \times 1} = 0.33$ mL or 0.3 mL

or

FE: $\dfrac{H}{V} = \dfrac{D}{X} = \dfrac{150 \text{ mg}}{1 \text{ mL}} = \dfrac{50 \text{ mg}}{X \text{ mL}} =$
(Cross multiply) 150 X = 50
$\qquad\qquad$X $= \dfrac{50}{150}$
$\qquad\qquad$X = 0.3 mL

29. Pounds to kilograms: 6 lbs $\div$ 2.2 lbs/kg = 2.72 kg
Dosage parameters: 25 mcg/kg/day $\times$ 2.72 kg = 68 mcg
50 mcg/kg/day $\times$ 2.72 kg = 136 mcg
Dose frequency: 40 mcg $\times$ 2 = 80 mcg
a. Dosage is safe.

b. BF: $\dfrac{D}{H} \times V = \dfrac{40 \text{ mcg}}{100 \text{ mcg}} \times 1 = 0.4$ mL

0.1 mg = 100 mcg

30. Height and weight intersect at 0.6 m^2 according to the nomogram.
Dosing parameters for nomogram: 60 mg/m^2/day $\times$ 0.6 m^2 = 36 mg/day.
250 mg/m^2/day $\times$ 0.6 m^2 = 150 mg/day.
BSA with the square root (metric formula)

$\dfrac{\sqrt{16 \text{ kg} \times 75 \text{ cm}}}{3600} = \sqrt{0.333} = 0.58 \text{ m}^2$

Dosage parameters for BSA formula: 60 mg/m^2/day $\times$ 0.58 m^2 = 34.8 mg/day
250 mg/m^2/day $\times$ 0.58 m^2 = 145 mg/day
a. Dosage is safe.

b. BF: $\dfrac{D}{H} \times V = \dfrac{125 \text{ mg}}{200 \text{ mg}} \times 10 \text{ mL} = 6.25$ mL

or

DA: mL $= \dfrac{10 \text{ mL} \times \overset{5}{\cancel{125} \cancel{\text{mg}}}}{\underset{8}{\cancel{200} \cancel{\text{mg}}} \times 1} = \dfrac{50}{8} = 6.25$ mL

31. Dosage parameters: 55 lbs ÷ 2.2 = 25 kg

$$25 \text{ kg} \times 10 \text{ mg/kg} = 250 \text{ mg}$$

a. Dosage is safe.

b. BF: $\dfrac{D}{H} \times V = \dfrac{300 \text{ mg}}{200 \text{ mg}} \times \dfrac{5 \text{ mL}}{1} = 7.5 \text{ mL}$

or

DA: mL $= \dfrac{300 \text{ mg} \times 5 \text{ mL}}{200 \text{ mg} \times \quad 1} = 7.5 \text{ mL}$

or

RP: H : V :: D : X

200 mg : 5 mL :: 300 mg : X mL

200 X = 1500

X = 7.5 mL

FE: $\dfrac{H}{V} = \dfrac{D}{X} = \dfrac{200 \text{ mg}}{5 \text{ mL}} = \dfrac{300 \text{ mg}}{X}$

(Cross multiply) 200 X = 1500

X = 7.5 mL

32. Pediatric dosage parameters: 6 mg × 10 kg/day = 60 mg/day

7.5 mg × 10 kg/day = 75 mg/day

15 mg × 4 (q6h) = 60 mg/day

a. Drug dosage per day is within the safe range.

b. BF: $\dfrac{15}{\cancel{20}_{10}} \times \overset{1}{\cancel{2}} \text{ mL} = \dfrac{15}{10} = 1.5 \text{ mL of Nebcin}$

or

RP: 20 mg : 2 mL :: 15 mg : X

20 X = 30

X = 1.5 of Nebcin

33. a. The BSA using inches and pound formula is 1.17.

b. 8 mL of daunorubicin HCl mixed in 100 mL D_5W.

c. Dosage parameters. 25 mg × 1.17 m² = 29.3 mg/day

45 mg × 1.17 m² = 52.7 mg/day or 53 mg/day

Child is to receive 40 mg of daunorubicin HCl per day.

Drug dose is within the safe range.

d. $108 \text{ mL} \div \dfrac{45 \text{ min}}{60 \text{ min}} = 108 \times \dfrac{\overset{4}{\cancel{60}}}{\underset{3}{\cancel{45}}} = 144 \text{ mL}$

Pump setting: 144 mL/hr

34. a. 55 lbs ÷ 2.2 lbs/kg = 25 kg

b. Yes. 6 mg/kg × 25 kg = 150 mg

12 mg/kg × 25 kg = 300 mg

Drug dosage is safe.

c. BF: $\dfrac{D}{H} \times V = \dfrac{200 \text{ mg}}{400 \text{ mg}} \times 200 \text{ mL} = 100 \text{ mL of Diflucan per dose}$

IV Neonates

35. a. 0.1 mg/kg × 2.5 kg = 0.25 mg

Drug dosage is safe.

b. BF: $\dfrac{0.25 \text{ mg}}{0.1 \text{ mg}} \times 1 \text{ mL} = 2.5 \text{ mL}$

or

FE: $\dfrac{H}{V} = \dfrac{D}{X} = \dfrac{0.1 \text{ mg}}{1 \text{ mL}} = \dfrac{0.25 \text{ mg}}{X} =$

(Cross multiply) 0.1 X = 0.25

X = 2.5 mL

or

DA: mL $= \dfrac{1 \text{ mL} \times 0.25 \text{ mg}}{0.1 \text{ mg} \times \quad 1} = \dfrac{0.25}{0.1} = 2.5 \text{ mL}$

36. a. $\dfrac{8.75}{2.2} = 3.97$ kg or 4 kg

0.01 mg/kg $\times$ 4 kg $= 0.04$ mg dose
Drug dosage is safe.

b. BF: $\dfrac{D}{H} \times V = \dfrac{0.04 \text{ mg}}{0.4 \text{ mg}} \times 1 \text{ mL} = 0.1 \text{ mL}$

or
RP: H : V :: D : X
0.4 mg : 1 mL :: 0.04 mg : X mL
0.4 X = 0.04
X = 0.1 mL

37. Dosage parameters: 50 mg/kg $\times$ 2.5 kg $= 125$ mg
75 mg/kg $\times$ 2.5 kg $= 187.5$ mg
a. Drug dosage is within safe range.

b. BF: $\dfrac{125 \text{ mg}}{500 \text{ mg}} \times 2 \text{ mL} = 0.5 \text{ mL}$

or
DA: mL $= \dfrac{2 \text{ mL} \times \overset{1}{\cancel{125 \text{ mg}}}}{\underset{4}{\cancel{500 \text{ mg}}} \times 1} = \dfrac{2}{4} = 0.5 \text{ mL}$

or
FE: $\dfrac{H}{V} = \dfrac{D}{X} = \dfrac{500 \text{ mg}}{2 \text{ mL}} = \dfrac{125 \text{ mg}}{X} =$
(Cross multiply) 500 X = 250
X = 0.5 mL

38. a. 80 mL/kg $\times$ 2.5 kg $= 200$ mL D_5W in 24 hours

b. $\dfrac{200 \text{ mL}}{24 \text{ hr}} = 8.3 \text{ mL/hr}$

39. Dosing parameters: 400 mg/kg/day $\times$ 2.5 kg $= 1{,}000$ mg/day
4 doses per day (q4h)
1,000 mg $\div$ 4 $= 300$ mg daily
a. Drug dosage is safe.

b. BF: $\dfrac{D}{H} \times V = \dfrac{75 \text{ mg}}{50 \text{ mg}} \times 1 \text{ mL} = 1.5 \text{ mL}$

or
RP: H : V :: D : X
50 mg : 1 mL :: 75 mg : X mL
50 X = 75
X = 1.5 mL

NEXT-GENERATION NCLEX® EXAMINATION-STYLE QUESTIONS

A 3-year-old child is brought to the Emergency Department by her mother. The child's mother states that since yesterday she has not been feeling well, has been coughing constantly, and not eating. The child appears agitated and tachypneic and has audible wheezing. Upon auscultation, breath sounds are found to be diminished throughout with expiratory wheezes. Vital signs: HR 125 beats per minute, respiratory rate of 35 per minute, BP 84/60 and oxygen saturation of 92% on room air. The child's past medical history includes eczema; she is otherwise healthy and fully immunized. She has an allergy to penicillin which gives her hives. According to the child's mother, her husband smokes cigarettes but never inside the house.

The health care provider has diagnosed the child with an acute asthma exacerbation and has ordered nebulized albuterol (Salbutamol) to be administered.

Use an X for the nursing action listed below that are **Indicated** (appropriate or necessary), **Contraindicated** (could be harmful), or **Non-essential** (makes no difference or not necessary) for the client's care at this time. Only one selection can be made for each nursing action.

Nursing Action	Indicated	Contraindicated	Non-essential
Ask mother to wait in the waiting room during IV access establishment			
Auscultate lungs			
Check temperature			
Prepare child for a chest x-ray			
Administer albuterol nebulizer when child is less agitated			
Perform neurological assessment			
Request antibiotics to treat potential upper respiratory infection			

ANSWERS-NEXT-GENERATION NCLEX® EXAMINATION-STYLE QUESTIONS

Nursing Action	Indicated	Contraindicated	Non-essential
Ask mother to wait in the waiting room during IV access establishment			X
Auscultate lungs	X		
Check temperature	X		
Prepare child for a chest x-ray			X
Administered albuterol nebulizer when child is less agitated		X	
Perform neurological assessment			X
Request antibiotics to treat potential upper respiratory infection		X	

Rationale:

This child has been diagnosed with an acute asthma exacerbation. Asthma is identified as a chronic inflammatory disease with periodic exacerbations caused by bronchial hyper-reactivity that can be reversed. Symptoms include wheezing, coughing, dyspnea and chest discomfort. The nurse will auscultate the child's lungs and check temperature for fever (in case of bacterial infection). The initial management is focused on symptomatic relief with bronchodilator therapy provided by an albuterol nebulizer. There is no indication that IV access is needed at this time; another consideration is that the patient is 3 years old and would likely benefit from the presence of a parent if IV access were needed. As the health care provider has already diagnosed the patient and ordered a nebulizer treatment, there is no indication for the need of a chest x-ray at this time. A neurological assessment is not needed, as no cognitive changes have been noted. Waiting to administer albuterol until the child is less agitated is contraindicated; the treatment is needed to address the symptoms associated with an asthma exacerbation. Holding the treatment allows the condition to worsen. Antibiotics are not indicated because there is no evidence of a bacterial infection.

For additional practice problems, refer to the Pediatric Dosages section of the Elsevier's Interactive Drug Calculation Application, Version 1 on evolve.

CHAPTER 14

Critical Care

Objectives
- Calculate the prescribed concentration of a drug in solution.
- Identify the units of measure designated for the amount of drug in solution.
- Describe the four determinants of infusion rates.
- Calculate the concentration of drug per unit of time for a specific body weight.
- Recognize the variables needed for the basic fractional formula.
- Describe how the titration factor is used when infusion rates are changed.
- Recognize the methods of determining the total amount of drug infused over time.

Outline
CALCULATING AMOUNT OF DRUG OR CONCENTRATION OF A SOLUTION
CALCULATING INFUSION RATE FOR CONCENTRATION AND VOLUME PER UNIT TIME
CALCULATING INFUSION RATES OF A DRUG FOR SPECIFIC BODY WEIGHT PER UNIT TIME
BASIC FRACTIONAL FORMULA
TITRATION OF INFUSION RATE
TOTAL AMOUNT OF DRUG INFUSED OVER TIME

In critical care areas, medication is primarily given intravenously and therefore has an immediate systemic effect on the patient. Drug dosages can be highly individualized, which necessitates close patient monitoring for improvement or stabilization in parameters such as vital signs, urine output, cardiac index, level of consciousness, or whatever is appropriate for the medication. Because intravenous (IV) medication can have immediate effects as well as a narrow therapeutic range, the patient can be at great risk if these medications are administered incorrectly. Therefore, it is essential that the nurse understand the drug's mechanism of action and the calculations necessary for safe drug administration.

Administration of potent drugs—drugs that cause major physiological changes—may be delivered in milligrams, micrograms, or units per body weight or unit time. The physician determines the drug dosage and rate of infusion either per body weight or unit time (per hour or per minute). Depending on the medication, the physician's order may specify the type of IV solution for the dilution. Most institutions have their own pharmacy guidelines or protocols for preparation of drugs for continuous IV infusion in critical care areas. Premixed, ready-to-use IV drugs in solution are also available from drug manufacturers with standardized dosages. The nurse is the last step in the administration process and must make sure that the dosage is accurate and the infusion rate is correct.

Medication errors can happen at any point during the medication delivery process, with a high incidence of IV drug errors committed by pharmacists, physicians, and nurses. Complete examination of medication processes is under way across the country in an effort to eliminate adverse drug errors. One step in the process has been to identify drugs with the highest potential to cause serious patient harm when used in error. Now these drugs are referred to as "high-alert" medications and identified in some facilities with special labeling (Table 14.1). Another effort under way is the increasing use of programmable infusion pump technology or "smart pumps." These pumps have drug menus called "libraries" entered into their software with safe dosing limits called guardrails. The pump will alarm if the limits are breached and prevent infusion of an unsafe dose. The smart pump's technology allows a facility to program the pump for specific areas, i.e., adult, pediatric, oncology, and anesthesia.

When the nurse uses the smart pump, she or he first selects the drug from the drug library. The library list of drugs is distinguished by capitalized letters that emphasize spelling differences for drugs with similar names. The nurse selects the amount of the drug and the amount of the prescribed soluton for infusion, and the pump calculates the *concentration of solution*. If the drug is dosed based on patient weight, the most current weight in kilograms is entered, allowing the smart pump to calculate the drug's dosage per kilogram of body weight per minute. Depending on the drug that is selected from the library, the smart pump will use volume per hour or volume per minute to calculate the dosage.

TABLE 14.1 High-Alert Drug Examples

Drug Class	Examples
Adrenergic agonists	Epinephrine, norepinephrine, dopamine, dobutamine, phenylephrine
Adrenergic antagonists	Esmolol
Anesthetics	Propofol, ketamine
Antiarrhythmics	Amiodarone, lidocaine
Anticoagulants	Heparin, bivalirudin, argatroban, lepirudin
Chemotherapeutic agents	
Dialysis solutions	
Dextrose, hypertonic, 20% or greater	
Electrolyte solutions	Potassium chloride, potassium phosphate, magnesium sulfate
Epidural or intrathecal medications	
Fibrinolytics	Streptokinase, anistreplase, alteplase
Glycoprotein llb/llla inhibitors	Eptifibatide
Hypoglycemic agents	
Inotropics	Milrinone, digoxin
Insulin	
Liposomal forms of drugs	Liposomal amphotericin
Moderate sedatives	Midazolam, lorazepam, diazepam, dexmedetomidine
Neuromuscular blockers	Rocuronium, vecuronium, succinylcholine
Opiates/Narcotics	
Radiocontrast agents	
Total parenteral nutrition solutions	
Vasodilators	Nitroglycerin, nitroprusside, nesiritide, epoprostenol

Adapted from: Institute for Safe Medication Practices. High-Alert Medications in Acute Care Settings. July 2014. Retrieved from: https://www.ismp.org/recommendations/high-alert-medications-acute-list.

The smart pump is an effective tool for drug administration, but the nurse must know all the drug calculation formulas used in the critical care setting and how they are applied to verify that the dose is correct before it is given to the patient. Nurses working in these areas need to be able to calculate for:

1. Concentration of the solution.
2. Concentration per hour or per minute.
3. Volume per hour or minute.
4. Dosage per kilogram body weight per minute.

For high-alert drugs it is recommended that two nurses independently do the drug calculations and verify the results. If any questions arise regarding dosing or infusion rates, the pharmacist and the physician should be consulted before the drug is administered to the patient.

CALCULATING AMOUNT OF DRUG OR CONCENTRATION OF A SOLUTION

The first step in administering a medication is to determine the concentration of the solution, which is the amount of drug in each milliliter (mL) of solution. This is written as units per milliliter, milligrams per milliliter, or micrograms per milliliter and must be calculated for individualized patient dosage. For all problems, remember to convert to like units before solving.

Calculating Units per Milliliter

EXAMPLE   Infuse heparin 5000 units in D_5W 250 mL at 30 mL/hr. What will be the concentration of heparin in each milliliter of D_5W?
Method: units/mL

<table>
<tr><td>Set up a ratio and proportion. Solve for X.</td><td>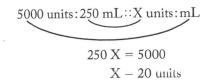</td></tr>
</table>

$$250\,X = 5000$$
$$X = 20\text{ units}$$

Answer: The D_5W with heparin will have a concentration of 20 units/mL of solution.

Calculating Milligrams per Milliliter

EXAMPLE   Infuse lidocaine 2 g in 500 mL D_5W at 2 mg/min. What will be the concentration of lidocaine in each milliliter of D_5W?
Method: mg/mL

<table>
<tr><td>Convert grams to milligrams. Set up a ratio and proportion and solve for X.</td><td>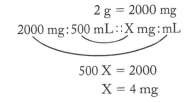</td></tr>
</table>

$$500\,X = 2000$$
$$X = 4\text{ mg}$$

Answer: The D_5W with lidocaine has a concentration of 4 mg/mL of solution.

> **NOTE**
>
> At the beginning of his or her shift, the nurse must check the infusion pump to verify the medication and concentration that are programmed in the device match the order on the MAR/eMAR. At some institutions, it is often required that two nurses check the infusion pump of high alert medications at change of shift.

Calculating Micrograms per Milliliter

EXAMPLE Infuse dobutamine 250 mg in 500 mL D₅W at 650 mcg/min. What is the concentration of dobutamine in each milliliter of D₅W?
Method: mcg/mL

Convert milligrams to micrograms. Set up a ratio and proportion and solve for X.

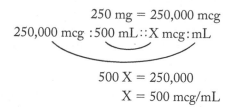

$$250 \text{ mg} = 250{,}000 \text{ mcg}$$
$$250{,}000 \text{ mcg} : 500 \text{ mL} :: X \text{ mcg} : \text{mL}$$

$$500 X = 250{,}000$$
$$X = 500 \text{ mcg/mL}$$

Answer: The D₅W with dobutamine will have a concentration of 500 mcg/mL of solution.

PRACTICE PROBLEMS: ▶ I CALCULATING CONCENTRATION OF A SOLUTION

Answers can be found on pages 337 to 338.

1. Order: ketamine 500 mg in 100 mL NS at 0.2 mg/kg/min.
2. Order: propofol 1000 mg in 100 mL at 30 mL/hr.
3. Order: regular insulin 100 units in 500 mL NS at 30 mL/hr.
4. Order: lidocaine 1 g in 1000 mL D₅W at 30 mL/hr.
5. Order: norepinephrine 4 mg in 500 mL D₅W at 15 mL/hr.
6. Order: dopamine 500 mg in 250 mL D₅W at 10 mL/hr.
7. Order: dobutamine 400 mg in 250 mL D₅W at 20 mL/hr.
8. Order: isuprel 2 mg in 250 mL D₅W at 10 mL/hr.
9. Order: streptokinase 750,000 units in 50 mL D₅W over 30 minutes.
10. Order: nitroprusside 50 mg in 500 mL D₅W at 50 mcg/min.
11. Order: aminophylline 1 g in 250 mL D₅W at 20 mL/hr.
12. Order: pronestyl 2 g in 250 mL D₅W at 16 mL/hr.
13. Order: heparin 25,000 units in 250 mL D₅W at 5 mL/hr.
14. Order: aminophylline 1 g in 500 mL D₅W at 40 mL/hr.
15. Order: nitroglycerin 50 mg in 250 mL D5W at 50 mcg/min.
16. Order: alteplase 100 mg in NS 100 mL over 2 hours.
17. Order: theophylline 800 mg in D₅W 500 mL at 0.5 mg/kg.
18. Order: milrinone 20 mg in D₅W 100 mL at 0.50 mcg/kg/min.
19. Order: esmolol 2500 mg in 250 mL NS at 50 mcg/kg/min.
20. Order: amiodarone 150 mg in D₅W 100 mL over 10 minutes.

CALCULATING INFUSION RATE FOR CONCENTRATION AND VOLUME PER UNIT TIME

The second step for administering medication is to calculate the *infusion rate* of the drug per *unit time*. Infusion rates can mean two things: the rate of volume (mL) given or the rate of concentration (units, mg, mcg) administered. *Unit time* means per hour or per minute. For drugs administered by continuous infusion, the four most important determinants are the concentration per hour and minute and the volume per hour and minute. Infusion rates are part of the physician's continuous infusion order, and they may be stated in concentration or volume per unit time.

Today's technology has produced smart pumps that are easily programmable, have built-in safety features, and can calculate and deliver appropriate drug dosages. The smart pump's conrol panel allows the user to select or enter (1) the name of the drug, (2) the concentration of the drug, (3) the volume of the solution, (4) the patient's weight in kilograms, and (5) the drug's dosage parameter per unit time (e.g., mg/min, units/hr, mcg/min) (Figure 14.1).

Not all facilities have infusion pumps with advanced technology; therefore the nurse must be able to calculate the infusion rates. For general-purpose infusion pumps that deliver mL/hr, the volume per hour of the drug must be known. *Remember:* If an infusion device is unavailable, a microdrip IV administration set is the appropriate set to use because the drops per minute rate (gtt/min) corresponds to the volume per hour rate (mL/hr).

Complete infusion rates for the volume and concentration are given in the examples and practice problems. In clinical practice, not all of the data is needed or pertinent for each drug to infuse. For example, when administering a heparin infusion, the concentration per minute is not as vital as the concentration per hour. However, vasoactive drugs such as dobutamine focus heavily on the concentration per minute and not the concentration per hour. Both of these drugs can use the same methods of calculation in order to obtain the same information. The nurse must have knowledge of pharmacology and clinical practice to determine the data that will be the most beneficial.

Concentration and Volume per Hour and Minute With a Drug in Units

EXAMPLES Infuse heparin 5000 units in D_5W 250 mL at 30 mL/hr. Concentration of solution is 20 units/mL. (Also note that volume/hour is given.) How many milliliters will be infused per minute?

Find volume per minute:
Method: mL/min

Set up a ratio and proportion. Use volume/hour, 30 mL/hr, or 30 mL/60 min as the known variable.	30 mL : 60 min :: X mL : min 60 X = 30 X = 0.5 mL

Answer: The infusion rate for volume per minute is 0.5 mL/min and the hourly rate is 30 mL/hr.

What is the concentration per minute and hour?
Find concentration per minute:
Method: units/min

Multiply the concentration of solution by the volume per minute.	20 units/mL × 0.5 mL/min = 10 units/min

Find concentration per hour:
Method: units/hr

Multiply the volume per minute by 60 min/hr.	10 units/min × 60 min/hr = 600 units/hr

Answer: The concentration per minute of heparin is 10 units/min and the concentration per hour is 600 units/hr.

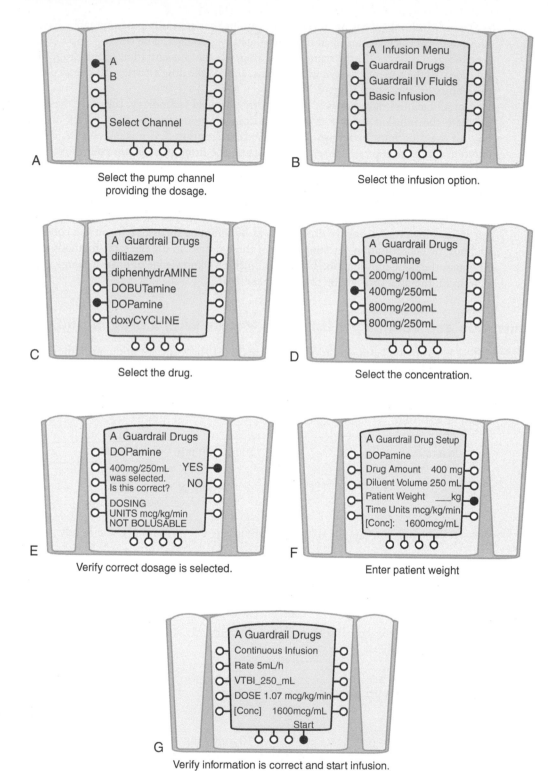

A Select the pump channel providing the dosage.

B Select the infusion option.

C Select the drug.

D Select the concentration.

E Verify correct dosage is selected.

F Enter patient weight

G Verify information is correct and start infusion.

Figure 14.1 Examples of display screens of a dose rate calculator on an advanced infusion pump. (Courtesy and © Becton, Dickinson and Company)

Concentration and Volume per Hour and Minute With a Drug in Milligrams

EXAMPLES   Infuse lidocaine 2 g in D$_5$W 500 mL at 2 mg/min. Concentration of solution is 4 mg/mL. (Also note that concentration/minute is given.) How many milligrams will be infused per hour?

Find concentration per hour:
Method: mg/hr

Find the concentration/minute. Multiply concentration/minute × 60 min/hr.	lidocaine 2 mg/min 2 mg/min × 60 min = 120 mg/hr

Answer: The amount of lidocaine infused per hour is 120 mg/hr.

How many milliliters of lidocaine will be infused in 1 hour?
Find volume per hour:
Method: mL/hr

Calculate concentration of solution. Divide the concentration/hour by the concentration of solution.	lidocaine 4 mg/mL $\dfrac{120 \text{ mg/hr}}{4 \text{ mg/mL}} = 30 \text{ mL/hr}$

Answer: The infusion rate in milliliters for lidocaine 2 mg/min is 30 mL/hr.

How many milliliters of lidocaine will be infused in 1 minute?

Divide the concentration/minute by the concentration of the solution.	$\dfrac{2 \text{ mg/min}}{4 \text{ mg/mL}} = 0.5 \text{ mL/min}$

Answer: The infusion rate for lidocaine 2 mg/min is 0.5 mL/min.

Concentration and Volume per Hour and Minute With a Drug in Micrograms

EXAMPLES   Infuse dobutamine 250 mg in D$_5$W 500 mL at 650 mcg/min. Concentration of solution is 500 mcg/mL. (Also note that concentration/minute is given in the order.) How many micrograms will be infused in 1 hour?

Find concentration per hour:
Method: mcg/hr

Find the concentration/minute. Multiply concentration/minute by 60 min/hr.	dobutamine 650 mcg/min 650 mcg/min × 60 min/hr = 39,000 mcg/hr

Answer: The concentration of dobutamine infused per hour is 39,000 mcg/hr.

How many milliliters of dobutamine will be infused in 1 hour?
Find volume per hour:
Method: mL/hr

Calculate concentration of solution. Divide the concentration/hour by the concentration of solution.	dobutamine 500 mcg/mL $$\frac{39{,}000 \text{ mcg/hr}}{500 \text{ mcg/mL}} = 78 \text{ mL/hr}$$

Answer: The infusion rate for dobutamine 650 mcg/min is 78 mL/hr.

How many milliliters of dobutamine should be infused in 1 minute?
Find volume per minute:
Method: mL/min

Divide concentration/minute by concentration of solution.	$$\frac{650 \text{ mcg/min}}{500 \text{ mcg/mL}} = 1.3 \text{ mL/min}$$

Answer: The infusion rate for dobutamine is 1.3 mL/min.

PRACTICE PROBLEMS: ▶ II CALCULATING INFUSION RATE

Answers can be found on pages 339 to 344.

Use the examples to find the following information:
• Concentration of the solution
• Infusion rates per unit time:
  a. Volume per minute
  b. Volume per hour
  c. Concentration per minute
  d. Concentration per hour

1. Order: heparin 1000 units in D_5W 500 mL at 50 mL/hr.
2. Order: nitroprusside 100 mg in D_5W 500 mL at 60 mL/hr.
3. Order: nitroprusside 25 mg in D_5W 250 mL at 50 mcg/min.
4. Order: dopamine 800 mg in D_5W 500 mL at 400 mcg/min.
5. Order: norepinephrine 2 mg in D_5W 250 mL at 45 mL/hr.
6. Order: dobutamine 1000 mg in D_5W 500 mL at 12 mL/hr.
7. Order: nicardipine 40 mg in D_5W 200 mL at 5 mg/hr.
8. Order: lidocaine 2 g in D_5W 500 mL at 4 mg/min.
9. Order: dopamine 400 mg in D_5W 250 mL at 60 mL/hr.
10. Order: isoproterenol 4 mg in D_5W 500 mL at 65 mL/hr.
11. Order: morphine sulfate 50 mg in 150 mL NS at 3 mg/hr.
12. Order: regular Humulin insulin 50 units in 250 mL NS at 4 units/hr.
13. Order: aminophylline 2 g in 250 mL D_5W at 20 mL/hr.
14. Order: nitroglycerin 50 mg in 250 mL D_5W at 24 mL/hr.
15. Order: vasopressin 20 units in 100 mL NS at 0.02 units/min.
16. Order: amiodarone 900 mg in D_5W 500 mL at 33.3 mL/hr.
17. Order: procainamide 1 g in D_5W 250 mL at 4 mg/min.
18. Order: diltiazem 100 mg in 100 mL NS at 10 mg/hr.
19. Order: streptokinase 750,000 units in 250 mL NS at 100,000 units/hr.
20. Order: bretylium 1 g in 250 mL D_5W at 1 mg/min.

CALCULATING INFUSION RATES OF A DRUG FOR SPECIFIC BODY WEIGHT PER UNIT TIME

The last method is calculating infusion rates for the amount of drug per unit time for a specific body weight. The weight parameter is an accurate means of dosing for a therapeutic effect. The metric system is used for all drug dosing, so pounds must be changed to kilograms. The physician orders the *desired dose per kilogram of body weight* and the *concentration of the solution*. From this information, infusion rates can be calculated for administering an individualized dose. Accurate daily weights are essential for the correct dosage.

The previous methods for calculating *concentration of solution* and *infusion rates* for concentration and volume are used, with one addition. The *concentration per minute* is obtained by multiplying the *body weight* by the *desired dose per kilogram per minute,* which must be done before the other infusion rates can be calculated. For many vasoactive drugs given as examples in this chapter, the most useful information clinically is the concentration per minute for the specific body weight, volume per minute, and volume per hour, because these parameters determine the infusion pump settings (see Figure 14.1).

New volumetric infusion pumps can now deliver fractional portions of a milliliter from tenths to hundredths in addition to calculating dosages for infusion rates. If the infusion pumps available do not have this feature and the volume per hour is a fractional amount, it must be rounded off to a whole number (1.8 mL/hr = 2 mL/hr). When calculating concentration per minute and hour and volume per minute, carry out the problem to three decimal places, if necessary, before rounding off. The volume per hour, if fractional, can then be rounded off, making the volume per hour as accurate as possible. There are two important factors to consider when rounding off fractional infusion rates:

1. If the patient's condition is labile, the difference between 1 or 2 mL could be significant.
2. The ordering physician should be consulted if rounding off would significantly change the drug dosage.

Micrograms per Kilogram Body Weight

EXAMPLES Infuse dobutamine 250 mg in 500 mL D₅W at 10 mcg/kg/min. Patient weighs 143 lb. Concentration of solution is 500 mcg/mL. How many micrograms of dobutamine would be infused per minute? Per hour?

Convert pounds to kilograms:

| Divide pounds by 2.2. | $\dfrac{143 \text{ lb}}{2.2 \text{ lb/kg}} = 65 \text{ kg}$ |

Find concentration per minute:
Method: mcg/min

| Multiply patient's weight by the desired dose of mcg/kg/min. | 65 kg × 10 mcg/kg/min = 650 mcg/min |

Find concentration per hour:
Method: mcg/hr

| Multiply concentration/min by 60 min/hr. | 650 mcg/min × 60 min/hr = 39,000 mcg/hr |

Answer: The concentration of dobutamine infused per minute and per hour is 650 mcg/min and 39,000 mcg/hr for the patient's body weight.

How many milliliters of dobutamine will be infused per minute? Per hour? Find volume per minute:
Method: mL/min

Divide the concentration/minute by the concentration of the solution.	$\dfrac{650 \text{ mcg/min}}{500 \text{ mcg/mL}} = 1.3 \text{ mL/min}$

Find volume per hour:
Method: mL/hr

Multiply volume/minute by 60 min/hr.	$1.3 \text{ mL/min} \times 60 \text{ min/hr} = 78 \text{ mL/hr}$

Answer: The volume of dobutamine infused per minute is 1.3 mL/min, and the infusion rate is 78 mL/hr.

BASIC FRACTIONAL FORMULA

A fractional equation can create a basic formula that can be used as another quick method to determine any one of the following quantities: concentration of solution, volume per hour, and desired concentration per minute ($\times$ kilogram of body weight, if required). The equation has one constant, the drop rate of the IV set, 60 gtt/mL. The unknown quantity can be represented by X. (See Chapter 6 for fractional equations.) The basic formula is not accurate to the nearest hundredth, as are the other methods in this section:

$$\frac{\text{Concentration of solution (units, mg, mcg/mL)}}{\text{Drop rate of set (60 gtt/mL)}} = \frac{\text{Desired concentration} \times \text{kg body weight}}{\text{Volume/hr (mL/hr or gtt/min)}}$$

Using Basic Formula to Find Volume per Hour or Drops per Minute

EXAMPLE Infuse fenoldopam 20 mg in 500 mL NS at 0.4 mcg/kg/min.

Patient weighs 70 kg. The concentration of solution is 40 mcg/mL.

Desired concentration/minute: 0.4 mcg/kg/min $\times$ 70 kg = 28 mcg/min

$$\frac{40 \text{ mcg/mL}}{60 \text{ gtt/mL}} = \frac{28 \text{ mcg/min}}{X(\text{mL/hr or gtt/min})}$$

$$40\,X = 1680$$

$$X = 42 \text{ mL/hr or 42 gtt/min}$$

Using Basic Formula to Find Desired Concentration per Minute

EXAMPLE Infuse lidocaine 2 g in 500 mL D_5W at 30 mL/hr. The concentration of the solution is 4 mg/mL.

$$\frac{4 \text{mg/mL}}{60 \text{ gtt/mL}} = \frac{X}{30 \text{ mL/hr}}$$

$$60\,X = 120$$

$$X = 2 \text{ mg/min}$$

Using Basic Formula to Find Concentration of Solution

EXAMPLE Infuse dobutamine 250 mg in D₅W 500 mL at 10 mcg/kg/min with rate of 78 mL/hr. Patient weighs 65 kg.

$$\text{Desired concentration per minute} = 10 \text{ mcg/kg/min} \times 65 \text{ kg}$$

$$= 650 \text{ mcg/min}$$

$$\frac{X}{60 \text{ gtt/mL}} = \frac{650 \text{ mcg/min}}{78 \text{ mL/hr}}$$

$$78 \, X = 39{,}000$$

$$X = 500 \text{ mcg/mL}$$

PRACTICE PROBLEMS: ▶ III CALCULATING INFUSION RATE FOR SPECIFIC BODY WEIGHT

Answers can be found on pages 344 to 347.

Determine the infusion rates for specific body weight by calculating the following:
- Concentration of the solution
- Weight in kilograms
- Infusion rates:
  a. Concentration per minute
  b. Concentration per hour (not always measured)
  c. Volume per minute
  d. Volume per hour
You can use the basic fractional formula and compare answers.

1. Infuse alteplase 100 mg in 100 mL NS at 0.8 mg/kg/hr. Patient weighs 192 lb.
2. Infuse amrinone 250 mg in 250 mL NS at 5 mcg/kg/min. Patient weighs 165 lb.
3. Infuse vecuronium 20 mg in 100 mL NS at 0.8 mcg/kg/min. Patient weighs 202 lb.
4. Infuse nitroprusside 100 mg in 500 mL D₅W at 3 mcg/kg/min. Patient weighs 55 kg.
5. Infuse Precedex 200 mcg in 50 mL NS at 0.3 mcg/kg/hr. Patient weighs 158 lb. Hourly rate only.
6. Infuse propofol (Diprivan) 500 mg/50 mL infusion bottle at 10 mcg/kg/min. Patient weighs 187 lb.
7. Infuse alfentanil (Alfenta) 10,000 mcg in D₅W 250 mL at 0.5 mcg/kg/min. Patient weighs 175 lb.
8. Infuse milrinone (Primacor) 20 mg in D₅W 100 mL at 0.375 mcg/kg/min. Patient weighs 160 lb.
9. Infuse theophylline 400 mg in D₅W 500 mL at 0.55 mg/kg/hr. Patient weighs 70 kg. Hourly rate only.
10. Infuse esmolol 2.5 g in NS 250 mL at 150 mcg/kg/min. Patient weighs 148 lb.

TITRATION OF INFUSION RATE

High-alert drugs are given to improve a physiological function that is causing a life-threatening condition for the patient. Every high-alert drug produces a physiological response that should be closely monitored and evaluated for effectiveness. For example, a patient receiving aminophylline should be monitored for improved respiratory rate and breath sounds. Another example is nitroprusside, where a patient's decrease in blood pressure is the goal of therapy. Monitoring parameters should be a part of the physician's order and followed closely by the nurse.

The purpose of titration in medication administration is to give the least amount of drug in the therapeutic range to elicit the appropriate targeted physiological response. With the smart pump, the therapeutic ranges are calculated. If a general-purpose infusion pump is used, the nurse should calculate the upper and lower limits of the therapeutic range.

Titration of drugs administered by infusion is based on (1) *concentration of solution*, (2) *infusion rates*, (3) *specific concentration per kilogram of body weight*, and (4) *titration factor*. The *titration factor* is the concentration of drug per drop in units (units/gtt), milligrams (mg/gtt), or micrograms (mcg/gtt). For the programmable volumetric infusion pump, the titration factor is the increment of increase or decrease in units, micrograms, or milligrams. If the only IV equipment available has the mL/hr feature, the titration factor of concentration per drop can be used. Smart pumps can infuse medication volume in increments of 0.01 mL/hr. Other pump features include a drug-specific dose calculator that allows the nurse to select a drug name and input the dosage, the concentration of the drug, and the weight of the patient (see Figure 14.1). These infusion pumps make drug delivery and titration easier for the nurse and safer for the patient. Any dose changes can be easily reprogrammed by the pump's drug-specific dose calculator. The smart pump's safety features help to decrease medication errors. Many drug manufacturers are recommending smart pumps for the delivery of all vasoactive medications used in the critical care setting.

Calculating the titration factor is necessary when the technology of the advanced infusion pump is unavailable. The titration factor can be added to or subtracted from the baseline infusion rate to determine the exact concentration of an infusion. Because the titration method of drug administration is primarily used when a patient's condition is labile, calculating the titration factor gives the nurse the means of determining the exact amount of drug to be infused.

Medication protocols of the institution or drug infusion charts (developed by the drug manufacturer or the hospital's pharmacy) can be used to adjust infusion rates at the appropriate increments when titrating medications via the physician's order. It is imperative that critical care nurses are knowledgeable on the expected effects of a given medication, its titration factor, and its minimum and maximum dosage when titrating. Often, the amount of drug being infused falls between calibrations on the charts. When this occurs, the titration factor can be used to determine the exact concentration of drug being administered. The titration factor can also be used to verify the correct selection from the chart.

EXAMPLE Infuse isuprel 2 mg in 250 mL D₅W. Titrate 1 to 3 mcg/min to maintain heart rate greater than 50 beats/min and less than 130 beats/min and blood pressure greater than 90 mm Hg systolic.

a. Find concentration of solution:

> Convert mg to mcg. Set up ratio and proportion.

$$2 \text{ mg} = 2000 \text{ mcg}$$
$$2000 \text{ mcg} : 250 \text{ mL} :: X \text{ mcg} : \text{mL}$$
$$250 X = 2000$$
$$X = 8 \text{ mcg}$$
$$8 \text{ mcg/mL}$$

b. Infusion rate by volume per unit time:
Desired infusion rate by concentration is stated in the problem.
Note that the upper dosage and lower dosage must be determined.

Find volume rate per minute: mL/min:

> Divide concentration/minute by concentration of solution.

Lower	*Upper*
$\dfrac{1 \text{ mcg/min}}{8 \text{ mcg/mL}}$	$\dfrac{3 \text{ mcg/min}}{8 \text{ mcg/mL}}$
$= 0.125 \text{ mL/min}$	$= 0.375 \text{ mL/min}$

Find volume rate per hour: mL/hr (equivalent to gtt/min):

Multiply volume rate/minute by 60 min.	*Lower* 0.125 mL/min × 60 min/hr = 7.5 mL/hr *Upper* 0.375 mL/hr × 60 min/hr = 22.5 mL/hr

Dosage range is 7.5 mL/hr at 1 mcg/min, the lowest dose ordered, to 22.5 mL/hr at 3 mcg/min, the highest dose ordered.

Determine Titration Factor Using Infusion Pump

When the amount of fluid being titrated is 1 mL or greater (0.1 mL/hr lowest increment of infusion), the concentration of the solution multiplied by the volume per hour will give the total concentration to be given in 1 hour. The total volume in 1 hour divided by 60 min/hr will yield the concentration per minute.

EXAMPLE   Increase isuprel from 7.5 mL/hr to 9 mL/hr.

Multiply concentration of solution by volume/hr. Then divide by 60 min/hr.	9 mL/hr × 8 mcg/mL = 72 mcg/hr $\dfrac{72 \text{ mcg/hr}}{60 \text{ min/hr}} = 1.2$ mcg/min

When increments of less than 1 mL are being titrated, multiply the concentration by the lowest increment of infusion.

Multiply concentration of solution by 0.1 mL/hr to get the concentration/hr.	8 mcg/mL × 0.1 mL/hr = 0.8 mcg/hr

Find rate in mcg/min by dividing concentration/hr by 60 min/hr.	$\dfrac{0.8 \text{ mcg/hr}}{60 \text{ min/hr}} = 0.013$ mcg/min

Titration factor is 0.8 mcg/hr or 0.013 mcg/min for the solution of isuprel 2 mg in 250 mL D_5W with 0.1 mL/hr as the lowest increment of infusion. If the baseline rate is 7.5 mL/hr and 1 mcg/min, increasing the rate by 0.1 mL/hr to 7.6 mL/hr will increase the per minute dose to 1.013 mcg/min. Since isuprel is ordered in mcg/min, using the titration factor in mcg/min would give a very accurate dose if increases or decreases are needed.

Increasing or Decreasing Infusion Rates Using Infusion Pump

When increasing infusion rate (0.1 mL/hr lowest increment of infusion) from baseline, multiply the titration factor by the number of increases and add to beginning rate.

EXAMPLE **Baseline Data**

Order	isuprel 2 mg in 250 mL
Concentration of solution	8 mcg/mL
Beginning rate	1 mcg/min
Volume per hour	7.5 mL/hr
Lowest increment of infusion	0.1 mL/hr (lowest pump setting)
Titration factors	0.8 mcg/hr or 0.013 mcg/min

Since the order is given in mcg/min, the titration factor of mcg/min should be used. To increase infusion rate from 7.5 mL/hr to 7.7 mL/hr, a 0.2-mL increase on the infusion pump, multiply titration factor by 2. Multiply 2×0.013 mcg/min = 0.026 mcg/min, then add to baseline of 1 mcg/min and now the concentration per minute is 1.026 mcg/min. Incremental increases can be easily calculated by multiplying the titration factor by the number of increases, then adding to baseline.

EXAMPLE

Hourly Rate (mL/hr)	Titration Factor	Concentration/min (ADD)
7.5 mL/hr	0.013 mcg/min	1 mcg/min
7.6 mL/hr	0.013 mcg/min × 1 = 0.013	1.013 mcg/min
7.7 mL/hr	0.013 mcg/min × 2 = 0.026	1.026 mcg/min
7.8 mL/hr	0.013 mcg/min × 3 = 0.039	1.039 mcg/min

To titrate downward, multiply titration factor by the number of decreases and subtract each decrease from current infusion rate.

EXAMPLE

Hourly rate (mL/hr)	Titration Factor	Concentration/min (SUBTRACT)
10 mL/hr	0.013 mcg/min	1.33 mcg/min
9.8 mL/hr	0.013 mcg/min × 2 = 0.026	1.299 mcg/min
9.4 mL/hr	0.013 mcg/min × 6 = 0.078	1.247 mcg/min

Determine Titration Factor Using a Microdrip IV Set

A microdrip IV set has a drop factor of 60 gtt/mL, so the number of drops per minute is the same as the hourly rate. In a situation where infusion pumps are not available, a microdrip IV set should be the only option to deliver small amounts of IV medication. Using the isuprel data, the mL/hr rate will be 7.5 gtt counted per minute from the drip chamber. The titration factor is the amount of isuprel in each drop.

Determine the titration factor:

Find rate in gtt/min. Divide concentration/minute by gtt/min.	7.5 gtt/min $$\frac{1 \text{ mcg/min}}{7.5 \text{ gtt/min}} = 0.133 \text{ mcg/gtt}$$

The *titration factor* is 0.133 mcg/gtt in a solution of isuprel 2 mg in 250 mL D$_5$W. In other words, changing drops per minute results in a corresponding change in milliliters per hour. If the baseline infusion rates are **1 mcg/min** for concentration and **7.5 mL/hr** for volume, increasing the infusion rate by **1 gt/min** changes the concentration/minute by **0.133 mcg** and increases the hourly volume by **1 mL** to give a rate of **8.5 mL/hr.**

Increasing or Decreasing Infusion Rates Using a Microdrip IV Set

To increase the infusion rate by 5 gtt/min from a baseline rate of 1 mcg/min, set up a ratio and proportion or multiply the titration factor (mcg/gt) by 5 to obtain the increment of increase.

EXAMPLES

Set up a ratio and proportion with rate in gtt/min as the known variable.	$7.5 \text{ gtt} : 1 \text{ mcg} :: 5 \text{ gtt} : X \text{ mcg}$ $7.5 X = 5$ $X = 0.666 \text{ mcg}$ $5 \text{ gtt}/0.66 \text{ mcg}$

or

Multiply titration factor in mcg/gt by 5.	$0.133 \text{ mcg/gt} \times 5 \text{ gtt} = 0.665 \text{ mcg}$

Adding 5 gtt/min increases the volume infusion rate by 5 mL/hr, from 7.5 to 12.5 mL/hr. The concentration of drug delivered is increased by 0.665 mcg/min to 1.665 mcg/min. For example,

$$\begin{array}{ll} 1.000 \text{ mcg/min} & \text{baseline rate} \\ \underline{+0.665 \text{ mcg/min}} & \text{increment of rate increased} \\ 1.665 \text{ mcg/min} & \text{adjusted infusion rate} \end{array}$$

Suppose the infusion rate was 3 mcg/min and a decrease was needed. To decrease the infusion rate by 10 gtt, set up another ratio and proportion or multiply the titration factor (mcg/gt) by 10.

EXAMPLES

Set up a ratio and proportion with rate in gtt/mcg as the known variable.	$7.5 \text{ gtt} : 1 \text{ mcg} :: 10 \text{ gtt} : X \text{ mcg}$ $7.5 X = 10$ $X = 1.33 \text{ mcg}$ $1.33 \text{ mcg}/10 \text{ gtt}$

or

Multiply titration factor in mcg/gt by 10.	$0.133 \text{ mcg/gt} \times 10 \text{ gtt} = 1.33 \text{ mcg}$

Subtracting 10 gtt/min decreases the infusion rate by 10 mL/hr, from 22.5 to 12.5 mL/hr. The amount of drug delivered is decreased by 1.33 mcg/min to 1.67 mcg/min. For example,

$$\begin{array}{ll} 3.00 \text{ mcg/min} & \text{baseline infusion rate} \\ \underline{-1.33 \text{ mcg/min}} & \text{increment of rate decreased} \\ 1.67 \text{ mcg/min} & \text{adjusted infusion rate} \end{array}$$

PRACTICE PROBLEMS: ▶ IV TITRATION OF INFUSION RATE

Answers can be found on pages 347 to 348.

1. What are the units of measure for the following terms?
   a. Concentration of solution per minute for specific body weight
   b. Concentration of solution
   c. Volume per hour
   d. Concentration per minute
   e. Volume per minute
   f. Concentration per minute
   g. Titration factor

2. Order: nitroprusside 50 mg in 250 mL D$_5$W. Titrate 0.5 to 1.5 mcg/kg/min to maintain mean systolic blood pressure at 100 mm Hg. Patient weighs 70 kg.

   Find the following:

   a. Concentration of solution
   b. Concentration per minute
   c. Volume per minute and hour
   d. Titration factor for infusion pump; for microdrop set
   e. Increase infusion rate of 10.5 mL/hr by 0.5 mL to 11 mL/hr with infusion pump. What is the concentration per minute?
   f. Increase infusion rate from 11 mL/hr to 20 mL/hr. What is the concentration per minute?
   g. Increase the infusion rate of 11 gtt/min by 5 gtt. What is the concentration per minute? What is the volume per hour?
   h. Increase the infusion rate of 16 gtt/mL by 13 gtt. What is the concentration per minute? What is the volume per hour?

3. Order: dopamine 400 mg in 250 mL D$_5$W. Titrate beginning at 4 mcg/kg/min to maintain a mean systolic blood pressure of 100 to 120 mm Hg. Patient weighs 75 kg.

   Find the following:

   a. Concentration of solution
   b. Concentration per minute
   c. Volume per minute and hour
   d. Titration factor for infusion pump; for microdrip set
   e. With the infusion pump, increase infusion rate from 11.4 mL/hr to 12 mL/hr. What is the concentration per minute?
   f. With the infusion pump, increase the infusion rate to 12.5 mL/hr. What is the concentration per minute?
   g. Using a microdrip set, increase the infusion rate of 13 gtt/min by 7 gtt. What is the concentration per minute? What is the volume per hour?
   h. Using a microdrip set, decrease the infusion rate of 20 mL/hr (20 gtt/min) by 5 gtt. What is the concentration per minute? What is the volume per hour?

TOTAL AMOUNT OF DRUG INFUSED OVER TIME

Determining the total amount of drug infused over time is useful when changes in drug therapy occur. If adverse effects, toxic levels, therapeutic failure, or discontinuance of a drug occurs, knowing the amount that was administered can be important for charting and for determining future therapies.

For this calculation, the concentration of the drug in its solution must be known, as well as the time that the drug therapy began to the nearest minute. Again, with 60-gtt sets, the hourly rate is the same as the drip rate per minute.

EXAMPLES Heparin 10,000 units in 250 mL D$_5$W at 30 mL/hr has been infusing for 3 hours. The drug is discontinued.

How much heparin did the patient receive?
Find concentration of solution:

Set up a ratio and proportion. Solve for X.	10,000 units : 250 mL :: X units : mL 250 X = 10,000 X = 40 units 40 units/mL

Find concentration per hour:

Multiply concentration of solution by volume/hour.	40 units/mL × 30 mL/hr = 1200 units/hr

Calculate total amount of drug infused.

Multiply concentration/hour by length of administration.	1200 units/hr × 3 hr = 3600 units/hr

Answer: The total amount of heparin infused over 3 hours was 3600 units.

PRACTICE PROBLEMS: ▶ V TOTAL AMOUNT OF DRUG INFUSED OVER TIME

Answers can be found on page 349.

Solve for the amount of drug infused over time.
1. In 1 hour, a patient received two boluses of lidocaine 100 mg and an IV infusion of 4 mg/mL at 40 mL/hr for 30 minutes. How many milligrams have been infused?

Note: Do not exceed 300 mg/hr of lidocaine.

2. Heparin 20,000 units in 500 mL D$_5$W at 50 mL/hr has been infused for 5½ hours. The drug is discontinued. How much heparin has been given?

ANSWERS

I Calculating Concentration of a Solution

1. 500 mg : 100 mL :: X mg : mL
   100 X = 500
   X = 5 mg
   The concentration of solution is 5 mg/mL.

2. 1000 mg : 100 mL :: X mg : mL
   100 X = 1000 mg
   X = 10 mg
   The concentration of solution is 10 mg/mL.

3. 100 units : 500 mL :: X units : mL
$$500 X = 100$$
$$X = 0.2 \text{ units}$$
The concentration of solution is 0.2 units/mL.

4.
$$1 \text{ g} = 1000 \text{ mg}$$
1000 mg : 1000 mL :: X mg : mL
$$1000 X = 1000$$
$$X = 1 \text{ mg}$$
The concentration of solution is 1 mg/mL.

5.
$$4 \text{ mg} = 4000 \text{ mcg}$$
4000 mcg : 500 mL :: X mcg : mL
$$500 X = 4000$$
$$X = 8 \text{ mcg}$$
The concentration of solution is 8 mcg/mL.

6. 500 mg : 250 mL :: X mcg : mL
$$250 X = 500$$
$$X = 2 \text{ mg}$$
The concentration of solution is 2 mg/mL.

7. 400 mg : 250 mL :: X mg : mL
$$250 X = 400$$
$$X = 1.6 \text{ mg}$$
The concentration of solution is 1.6 mg/mL.

8.
$$2 \text{ mg} = 2000 \text{ mcg}$$
2000 mcg : 250 mL :: X mcg : mL
$$250 X = 2000$$
$$X = 8 \text{ mcg}$$
The concentration of solution is 8 mcg/mL.

9. 750,000 units : 50 mL :: X units : mL
$$50 X = 750,000$$
$$X = 15,000 \text{ units}$$
The concentration of solution is 15,000 units/mL.

10.
$$50 \text{ mg} = 50,000 \text{ mcg}$$
50,000 mcg : 500 mL :: X mcg : mL
$$500 X = 50,000$$
$$X = 100 \text{ mcg}$$
The concentration of solution is 100 mcg/mL.

11.
$$1 \text{ g} = 1000 \text{ mg}$$
1000 mg : 250 mL :: X mg : mL
$$250 X = 1000$$
$$X = 4 \text{ mg}$$
The concentration of solution is 4 mg/mL.

12.
$$2 \text{ g} = 2000 \text{ mg}$$
2000 mg : 250 mL :: X mg : mL
$$250 X = 2000$$
$$X = 8 \text{ mg}$$
The concentration of solution is 8 mg/mL.

13. 25,000 units : 250 mL :: X mg : mL
$$250 X = 25,000$$
$$X = 100 \text{ units}$$
The concentration of solution is 100 units/mL.

14.
$$1 \text{ g} = 1000 \text{ mg}$$
1000 mg : 500 mL :: X mg : mL
$$500 X = 1000$$
$$X = 2 \text{ mg}$$
The concentration of solution is 2 mg/mL.

15.
$$50 \text{ mg} = 50,000 \text{ mcg}$$
50,000 mcg : 250 mL :: X mcg : mL
$$250 X = 50,000$$
$$X = 200 \text{ mcg}$$
The concentration of solution is 200 mcg/mL.

16. 100 mg : 100 mL :: X mg : mL
$$100 X = 100$$
$$X = 1 \text{ mg/mL}$$
The concentration of solution is 1 mg/mL.

17. 800 mg : 500 mL :: X mg : mL
$$500 X = 800$$
$$X = 1.6 \text{ mg/mL}$$
The concentration of solution is 1.6 mg/mL.

18. 20 mg : 100 mL :: X mg : mL
$$100 X = 20$$
$$X = 0.2 \text{ mg/mL}$$
The concentration of solution is 0.2 mg/mL.

19. 2500 mg : 250 mL :: X mg : mL
$$250 X = 2500$$
$$X = 10 \text{ mg}$$
The concentration of solution is 10 mg/mL.

20. 150 mg : 100 mL :: X mg : mL
$$100 X = 150$$
$$X = 1.5 \text{ mg/mL}$$
The concentration of solution is 1.5 mg/mL.

II Calculating Infusion Rate

1. *Concentration of solution:*
   1000 units : 500 mL = X units : mL
   $$500 X = 1000$$
   $$X = 2 \text{ units}$$
   The concentration of solution is 2 units/mL.
   Infusion rates:
   a. Volume/min:
   50 mL : 60 min :: X mL : min
   $$60 X = 50$$
   $$X = 0.833 \text{ mL or } 0.83 \text{ mL or } 0.8 \text{ mL}$$
   $$0.8 \text{ mL/min}$$
   b. Volume/hr:
   50 mL/hr

   c. Concentration/min:
   2 units/mL × 0.8 mL/min = 1.60 units/min

   d. Concentration/hr:
   1.60 units/min × 60 min/hr = 96 units/hr

2. *Concentration of solution:*
   100 mg : 500 mL :: X mg : mL
   $$500 X = 100$$
   $$X = 0.2 \text{ mg}$$
   The concentration of solution is 0.2 mg/mL.
   Infusion rates:
   a. Volume/min:
   60 mL : 60 min :: X mL : min
   $$60 X = 60$$
   $$X = 1 \text{ mL}$$
   $$1 \text{ mL/min}$$
   b. Volume/hr:
   60 mL/hr

   c. Concentration/min:
   0.2 mg/mL × 1 mL/min = 0.2 mg/min

   d. Concentration/hr:
   0.2 mg/min × 60 min/hr = 12 mg/hr

3. *Concentration of solution:*
   25 mg = 25,000 mcg
   25,000 mcg : 250 mL :: X mcg : mL
   $$250 X = 25,000$$
   $$X = 100 \text{ mcg}$$
   The concentration of solution is 100 mcg/mL.
   Infusion rates:
   a. Volume/min:
   $$\frac{50 \text{ mcg/min}}{100 \text{ mcg/mL}} = 0.5 \text{ mL/min}$$
   b. Volume/hr:
   0.5 mL/min × 60 min/hr = 30 mL/hr

   c. Concentration/min:
   50 mcg/min

   d. Concentration/hr:
   50 mcg/min × 60 min/hr = 3000 mcg/hr

4. *Concentration of solution:*

$$800 \text{ mg} = 800,000 \text{ mcg}$$
$$800,000 \text{ mcg} : 500 \text{ mL} :: X \text{ mcg} : \text{mL}$$
$$500 X = 800,000$$
$$X = 1600 \text{ mcg}$$

The concentration of solution is 1600 mcg/mL.

Infusion rates:

a. Volume/min:

$$\frac{400 \text{ mcg/min}}{1600 \text{ mcg/mL}} = 0.25 \text{ mL/min}$$

b. Volume/hr:

$$0.25 \text{ mL/min} \times 60 \text{ min/hr} = 15 \text{ mL/hr}$$

c. Concentration/min:

400 mcg/min

d. Concentration/hr:

$$400 \text{ mcg/min} \times 60 \text{ min/hr} = 24,000 \text{ mcg/hr}$$

5. *Concentration of solution:*

$$2 \text{ mg} = 2000 \text{ mcg}$$
$$2000 \text{ mcg} : 250 \text{ mL} :: X \text{ mcg} : \text{mL}$$
$$250 X = 2000$$
$$X = 8 \text{ mcg}$$

The concentration of solution is 8 mcg/mL.

Infusion rates:

a. Volume/min:

$$45 \text{ mL} : 60 \text{ min} :: X \text{ mL} : \text{min}$$
$$60 X = 45$$
$$X = 0.75 \text{ mL/min}$$

b. Volume/hr:

45 mL/hr

c. Concentration/min:

$$8 \text{ mcg/mL} \times 0.75 \text{ mL/min} = 6 \text{ mcg/min}$$

d. Concentration/hr:

$$6 \text{ mcg/min} \times 60 \text{ min/hr} = 360 \text{ mcg/hr}$$

6. *Concentration of solution:*

$$1000 \text{ mg} = 1,000,000 \text{ mcg}$$
$$1,000,000 \text{ mcg} : 500 \text{ mL} :: X \text{ mcg} : \text{mL}$$
$$500 X = 1,000,000$$
$$X = 2000 \text{ mcg}$$

The concentration of solution is 2000 mcg/mL.

Infusion rates:

a. Volume/min:

$$12 \text{ mL} : 60 \text{ min} :: X \text{ mL} : \text{min}$$
$$60 X = 12$$
$$X = 0.2 \text{ mL}$$
$$0.2 \text{ mL/min}$$

b. Volume/hr:

12 mL/hr

c. Concentration/min:

$$2000 \text{ mcg/mL} \times 0.2 \text{ mL/min} = 400 \text{ mcg/min}$$

d. Concentration/hr:

$$400 \text{ mcg/min} \times 60 \text{ min/hr} = 24,000 \text{ mcg/hr}$$

7. *Concentration of solution:*

$$40 \text{ mg} : 200 \text{ mL} :: X \text{ mg} : \text{mL}$$
$$200 X = 40$$
$$X = 0.2 \text{ mg/mL}$$

The concentration of solution is 0.2 mg/mL.

Infusion rates:

a. Volume/hr:

$$\frac{5 \text{ mg/hr}}{0.2 \text{ mg/mL}} = 25 \text{ mL/hr}$$

b. Volume/min:

$$\frac{25 \text{ mL/hr}}{60 \text{ min/hr}} = 0.416 \text{ mL/min}$$

c. Concentration/min:

$$0.2 \text{ mg/mL} \times 0.416 \text{ mL/min} = 0.083 \text{ mg/min}$$
or 0.08 mg/min

d. Concentration/hr:

5 mg/hr

8. *Concentration of solution:*

$$2\ g = 2000\ mg$$
$$2000\ mg : 500\ mL :: X\ mg : mL$$
$$500\ X = 2000$$
$$X = 4\ mg$$

The concentration of solution is 4 mg/mL.

Infusion rates:

a. Volume/min:

$$\frac{4\ mg/min}{4\ mg/mL} = 1\ mL/min$$

b. Volume/hr:

1 mL/min $\times$ 60 min/hr = 60 mL/hr

c. Concentration/min:

4 mg/min

d. Concentration/hr:

4 mg/min $\times$ 60 min/hr = 240 mg/hr

9. *Concentration of solution:*

$$400\ mg : 250\ mL :: X\ mg : mL$$
$$250\ X = 400$$
$$X = 1.6\ mg$$

The concentration of solution is 1.6 mg/mL.

Infusion rates:

a. Volume/min:

$$60\ mL : 60\ min :: X\ mL : min$$
$$60\ X = 60$$
$$X = 1\ mL$$
$$1\ mL/min$$

b. Volume/hr:

60 mL/hr

c. Concentration/min:

1.6 mg/mL $\times$ 1 mL/min = 1.6 mg/min

d. Concentration/hr:

1.6 mg/min $\times$ 60 min/hr = 96 mg/hr

10. *Concentration of solution:*

$$4\ mg = 4000\ mcg$$
$$4000\ mcg : 500\ mL :: X\ mcg : mL$$
$$500\ X = 4000$$
$$X = 8\ mcg$$

The concentration of solution is 8 mcg/mL.

Infusion rates:

a. Volume/min:

$$65\ mL : 60\ min :: X\ mL : min$$
$$60\ X = 65$$
$$X = 1.083\ mL\ or$$
$$1.08\ mL/min$$

b. Volume/hr:

65 mL/hr

c. Concentration/min:

8 mcg/mL $\times$ 1.08 mL/min = 8.64 mcg/min

d. Concentration/hr:

8.64 mcg/min $\times$ 60 min/hr = 518.4 mcg/hr or 518 mcg/hr

11. *Concentration of solution:*

$$50\ mg : 150\ mL :: X\ mg : mL$$
$$150\ X = 50$$
$$X = 0.33\ mg$$

The concentration of solution is 0.33 mg/mL.

Infusion rates:

a. Volume/min:

$$\frac{0.05\ mg/min}{0.33\ mg/mL} = 0.15\ mL/min$$

b. Volume/hr:

$$\frac{3\ mg/hr}{0.33\ mg/mL} = 9.09\ or\ 9\ mL/hr$$

c. Concentration/min:

$$3\ mg : 60\ min :: X\ mg : min$$
$$60\ X = 3$$
$$X = 0.05\ mg/min$$

d. Concentration/hr:

3 mg/hr

12. *Concentration of solution:*

    50 units : 250 mL :: X mg : mL

    $\qquad$ 250 X = 50

    $\qquad\qquad$ X = 0.2 units

    The concentration of solution is 0.2 units/mL.

    Infusion rates:

    a. Concentration/min:

    4 units : 60 min :: X units : min

    $\qquad$ 60 X = 4

    $\qquad\qquad$ X = 0.066 units/min or 0.07 units/min

    b. Concentration/hr:

    4 units/hr

    c. Volume/min:

    $$\frac{0.066 \text{ units/min}}{0.2 \text{ units/mL}} = 0.33 \text{ mL/min}$$

    d. Volume/hr:

    $$\frac{4 \text{ units/hr}}{0.2 \text{ units/mL}} = 20 \text{ mL/hr}$$

13. *Concentration of solution:*

    $\qquad$ 2 g = 2000 mg

    2000 mg : 250 mL :: X mg : mL

    $\qquad$ 250 X = 2000

    $\qquad\qquad$ X = 8 mg

    The concentration of solution is 8 mg/mL.

    Infusion rates:

    a. Volume/hr = 20 mL/hr

    b. Volume/min:

    20 mL : 60 min :: X mL : min

    $\qquad$ 60 X = 20

    $\qquad\qquad$ X = 0.3 mL/min

    c. Concentration/min:

    8 mg/mL × 0.3 mL/min = 2.4 mg/min

    d. Concentration/hr:

    2.4 mg/min × 60 min/hr = 144 mg/hr

14. *Concentration of solution:*

    $\qquad$ 50 mg = 50,000 mcg

    50,000 mcg : 250 mL :: X mg : mL

    $\qquad$ 250 X = 50,000

    $\qquad\qquad$ X = 200 mcg

    The concentration of solution is 200 mcg/mL.

    Infusion rates:

    a. Volume/hr = 24 mL/hr

    b. Volume/min:

    24 mL/hr : 60 min/hr :: X mL : min

    $\qquad$ 60 X = 24

    $\qquad\qquad$ X = 0.4 mL/min

    c. Concentration/min:

    200 mcg/mL × 0.4 mL/min = 80 mcg/min

    d. Concentration/hr:

    80 mcg/min × 60 min = 4800 mcg/hr

15. *Concentration of solution:*

    20 units : 100 mL :: X units : mL

    $\qquad$ 100 X = 20

    $\qquad\qquad$ X = 0.2 units

    The concentration of solution is 0.2 units/mL.

    Infusion rates:

    a. Volume/min:

    $$\frac{0.02 \text{ units/min}}{0.2 \text{ units/mL}} = 0.1 \text{ mL/min}$$

    b. Volume/hr:

    0.1 mL/min × 60 min/hr = 6 mL/hr

    c. Concentration/min:

    0.02 units/min

    d. Concentration/hr:

    0.02 units/min × 60 min/hr = 1.2 units/hr

16. *Concentration of solution:*
900 mg:500 mL::X mg:mL
500 X = 900
X = 1.8 mg/mL
The concentration of solution is 1.8 mg/mL.
Infusion rates:
a. Volume/hr:
33.3 mL/hr
b. Volume/min:
33.3 mL:60 min::X mL:min
60 X = 33.3
X = 0.55 mL/min

c. Concentration/hr:
1.8 mg/mL × 33.3 mL/hr = 59.9 mg/hr
d. Concentration/min:
1.8 mg/mL × 0.55 mL/min = 0.99 mg/mL or
1.0 mg/mL

17. *Concentration of solution:*
1 g = 1000 mg
1000 mg:250 mL::X mg:mL
250 X = 1000
X = 4 mg/mL
The concentration of solution is 4 mg/mL.
Infusion rates:
a. Volume/min:
$$\frac{4 \text{ mg/min}}{4 \text{ mg/mL}} = 1 \text{ mL/min}$$
b. Volume/hr:
1 mL/min × 60 min/hr = 60 mL/hr

c. Concentration/hr:
4 mg/min × 60 min/hr = 240 mg/hr
d. Concentration/min:
4 mg/min

18. *Concentration of solution:*
100 mg:100 mL::X mg:mL
100 X = 100
X = 1 mg/mL
The concentration of solution is 1 mg/mL.
Infusion rates:
a. Volume/hr:
$$\frac{10 \text{ mg/hr}}{1 \text{ mg/mL}} = 10 \text{ mL/hr}$$
b. Volume/min:
$$\frac{10 \text{ mL/hr}}{60 \text{ min/hr}} = 0.166 \text{ mL/min}$$

c. Concentration/hr:
10 mg/hr
d. Concentration/min:
1 mg/mL × 0.166 mL/min = 0.166 mg/min or
0.17 mg/min

19. *Concentration of solution:*
750,000 units:250 mL::X units:mL
250 X = 750,000
X = 3000 units/mL
The concentration of solution is 3000 units/mL.
Infusion rates:
a. Volume/hr:
$$\frac{100,000 \text{ units/hr}}{3000 \text{ units/mL}} = 33.3 \text{ mL/hr}$$
b. Volume/min:
$$\frac{33.3 \text{ mL/hr}}{60 \text{ min/hr}} = 0.55 \text{ mL/min}$$

c. Concentration/hr:
100,000 units/hr
d. Concentration/min:
$$\frac{100,000 \text{ units/hr}}{60 \text{ min/hr}} = 1666.6 \text{ units/min or } 1667 \text{ units/min}$$

20. *Concentration of solution:*

$$1 \text{ g} = 1000 \text{ mg}$$
$$1000 \text{ mg} : 250 \text{ mL} :: X \text{ mg} : mL$$
$$250 \text{ X} = 1000$$
$$X = 4 \text{ mg/mL}$$

The concentration of solution is 4 mg/mL.

Infusion rates:

a. Volume/min:

$$\frac{1 \text{ mg/min}}{4 \text{ mg/mL}} = 0.25 \text{ mL/min}$$

b. Volume/hr:

0.25 mL/min $\times$ 60 min/hr = 15 mL/hr

c. Concentration/hr:

4 mg/mL $\times$ 15 mL/hr = 60 mg/hr

d. Concentration/min:

1 mg/min

III Calculating Infusion Rate for Specific Body Weight

1. *Concentration of solution:*

$$100 \text{ mg} : 100 \text{ mL} :: X : mL$$
$$100 \text{ X} = 100$$
$$X = 1 \text{ mg/mL}$$

The concentration of solution is 1 mg/mL.

Infusion rates (hourly only, so no answers for a or c):

b. Concentration/hr:

Body weight $\times$ Desired dose/kg/hr

87.2 kg $\times$ 0.8 mg/kg/hr
= 69.76 mg/hr

2. *Concentration of solution:*

$$250 \text{ mg} = 250,000 \text{ mcg}$$
$$250,000 \text{ mcg} : 250 \text{ mL} :: X \text{ mcg} : mL$$
$$250 \text{ X} = 250,000$$
$$X = 1000 \text{ mcg}$$

The concentration of solution is 1000 mcg/mL.

Infusion rates:

a. Concentration/min:

Body weight $\times$ Desired dose/kg/min

75 kg $\times$ 5 mcg/kg/min = 375 mcg/min

b. Concentration/hr:

375 mcg/min $\times$ 60 min/hr = 22,500 mcg/hr

Patient weight:

lb to kg: $\dfrac{192}{2.2} = 87.2$ kg

d. Volume/hr:

$$\frac{69.76 \text{ mg/hr}}{1 \text{ mg/mL}} = 69.76 \text{ mL/hr or } 69.8 \text{ mL/hr}$$

Patient weight:

lb to kg: $\dfrac{165}{2.2} = 75$ kg

c. Volume/min:

$$\frac{375 \text{ mcg/min}}{1000 \text{ mcg/mL}} = 0.375 \text{ mL/min}$$

d. Volume/hr:

0.375 mL/min $\times$ 60 min/hr = 22.5 mL/hr

3. *Concentration of solution:*

$$20 \text{ mg} = 20,000 \text{ mcg}$$
$$20,000 \text{ mcg} : 100 \text{ mL} :: X \text{ mcg} : mL$$
$$100 \text{ X} = 20,000$$
$$X = 200 \text{ mcg}$$

The concentration of the solution is 200 mcg/mL.

Infusion rates:

a. Concentration/min:

Body weight × Desired dose/kg/min
$$92 \text{ kg} \times 0.8 \text{ mcg/kg/min}$$
$$= 73.6 \text{ mcg/min}$$

b. Concentration/hr:

73.6 mcg/min × 60 min/hr = 4416 mcg/hr

4. *Concentration of solution:*

$$100 \text{ mg} = 100,000 \text{ mcg}$$
$$100,000 \text{ mcg} : 500 \text{ mL} :: X \text{ mg} : mL$$
$$500 \text{ X} = 100,000$$
$$X = 200 \text{ mcg}$$

The concentration of solution is 200 mcg/mL.

Infusion rates:

a. Concentration/min:

3 mcg/kg/min × 55 kg = 165 mcg/min

b. Concentration/hr:

165 mcg/min × 60 min/hr = 9900 mcg/hr

5. *Concentration of solution:*

$$200 \text{ mcg} : 50 \text{ mL} :: X \text{ mcg} : mL$$
$$50 \text{ X} = 200$$
$$X = 4 \text{ mcg}$$

The concentration of solution is 4 mcg/mL.

Infusion rates (hourly only, so no answers for a or c):

b. Concentration/hr:

Body weight × Desired dose/kg/hr
$$72 \text{ kg} \times 0.3 \text{ mcg/kg/hr}$$
$$= 21.6 \text{ mcg/hr}$$

Patient weight:

lb to kg: $\dfrac{202}{2.2} = 92 \text{ kg}$

c. Volume/min:

$$\dfrac{73.6 \text{ mcg/min}}{200 \text{ mcg/mL}} = 0.368 \text{ mL/min}$$

d. Volume/hr:

0.368 mL/min × 60 min/hr = 22.08 or 22.1 mL/hr

Patient weight:

55 kg

c. Volume/min:

$$\dfrac{165 \text{ mcg/min}}{200 \text{ mcg/mL}} = 0.825 \text{ mL/min}$$

d. Volume/hr:

0.825 mL/min × 60 min/hr = 49.5 mL/hr

Patient weight:

lb to kg: $\dfrac{158 \text{ lb}}{2.2} = 72 \text{ kg}$

d. Volume/hr:

$$\dfrac{21.6 \text{ mcg/hr}}{4 \text{ mcg/mL}} = 5.4 \text{ mL/hr}$$

6. *Concentration of solution:*

$$500 \text{ mg} : 50 \text{ mL} :: X \text{ mg} : mL$$
$$50 X = 500$$
$$X = 10 \text{ mg/mL}$$

The concentration of solution is 10 mg/mL or 10,000 mcg/mL.

Infusion rates:

a. Concentration/min:
Body weight × Desired dose/kg/min
85 kg × 10 mcg/kg/min
= 850 mcg/min

b. Concentration/hr:
850 mcg/min × 60 min/hr = 51,000 mcg/hr
or 51 mg/hr

Patient weight:

lb to kg: $\dfrac{187}{2.2} = 85$ kg

c. Volume/min:

$$\dfrac{850 \text{ mcg/min}}{10,000 \text{ mcg/mL}} = 0.085 \text{ mL/min}$$

d. Volume/hr:
0.085 mL/min × 60 min/hr = 5.1 mL/hr

7. *Concentration of solution:*

$$10,000 \text{ mcg} : 250 \text{ mL} :: X \text{ mcg} : mL$$
$$250 X = 10,000$$
$$X = 40 \text{ mcg/mL}$$

Infusion rates:

a. Concentration/min:
Body weight × Desired dose/kg/min
79.5 kg × 0.5 mcg/kg/min
= 39.75 mcg/min

b. Concentration/hr:
39.75 mcg/min × 60 min/hr = 2385 mcg/hr
or 2.4 mg/hr

Patient weight:

lb to kg: $\dfrac{175}{2.2} = 79.5$ kg

c. Volume/min:

$$\dfrac{39.75 \text{ mcg/min}}{40 \text{ mcg/mL}} = 0.99 \text{ mL/min or 1 mL/min}$$

d. Volume/hr:
0.99 mL/min × 60 min/hr = 59.4 mL/hr

8. *Concentration of solution:*

$$20 \text{ mg} : 100 \text{ mL} :: X \text{ mg} : mL$$
$$100 X = 20$$
$$X = 0.2 \text{ mg/mL}$$
$$\text{or } 200 \text{ mcg/mL}$$

Infusion rates:

a. Concentration/min:
Body weight × Desired dose/kg/min
72.7 kg × 0.375 mcg/kg/min
= 27.2 mcg/min

b. Concentration/hr:
27.2 mcg/min × 60 min/hr = 1632 mcg/hr or
1.6 mg/hr

Patient weight:

lb to kg: $\dfrac{160}{2.2} = 72.7$ kg

c. Volume/min:

$$\dfrac{27.2 \text{ mcg/min}}{200 \text{ mcg/mL}} = 0.136 \text{ mL/min}$$

d. Volume/hr:
0.136 mL/min × 60 min/hr = 8.16 mL/hr or
8.2 mL/hr

Patient weight:
70 kg

9. *Concentration of solution:*

$$400 \text{ mg} : 500 \text{ mL} :: X \text{ mg} : mL$$
$$500 X = 400$$
$$X = 0.8 \text{ mg/mL}$$

Infusion rates (hourly only so no answers for a or c):

b. Concentration/hr:
Body weight × Desired dose/kg/min
70 kg × 0.55 mg/kg/min
= 38.5 mg/hr

d. Volume/hr:

$$\dfrac{38.5 \text{ mg/hr}}{0.8 \text{ mg/mL}} = 48.125 \text{ mL/hr or 48 mL/hr}$$

10. *Concentration of solution:*

$2500 \text{ mg} : 250 \text{ mL} :: X \text{ mg} : \text{mL}$

$$250 X = 2500$$
$$X = 10 \text{ mg/mL}$$

Infusion rates:

a. Concentration/min:

Body weight × Desired dose/kg/min

$67.3 × 150 \text{ mcg/kg/min}$
$= 10,095 \text{ mcg/min or } 10 \text{ mg/min}$

b. Concentration/hr:

$10 \text{ mg/min} × 60 \text{ min/hr} = 600 \text{ mg/hr}$

Weight:

lb to kg: $\dfrac{148}{2.2} = 67.27 \text{ or } 67.3 \text{ kg}$

c. Volume/min:

$\dfrac{10 \text{ mg/min}}{10 \text{ mg/mL}} = 1 \text{ mL/min}$

d. Volume/hr:

$1 \text{ mL/min} × 60 \text{ min/hr} = 60 \text{ mL/hr}$

IV Titration of Infusion Rate

1. a. (units, mg, mcg)/kg/min
　b. (units, mg, mcg)/mL
　c. mL/hr
　d. (units, mg, mcg)/min
e. mL/min
f. (units, mg, mcg)/min
g. (units, mg, mcg)/min with infusion pump
　(units, mg, mcg)/gtt with microdrip IV set

2. a. Concentration of solution:

$50 \text{ mg} = 50,000 \text{ mcg}$
$50,000 \text{ mcg} : 250 \text{ mL} :: X \text{ mcg} : 1 \text{ mL}$
$$250 X = 50,000$$
$$X = 200 \text{ mcg}$$

The concentration of solution is 200 mcg/mL.

b. Concentration/min:

Lower: $0.5 \text{ mcg/kg/min} × 70 \text{ kg} = 35 \text{ mcg/min}$
Upper: $1.5 \text{ mcg/kg/min} × 70 \text{ kg} = 105 \text{ mcg/min}$

c. Volume/min and volume/hr:

Lower

$\dfrac{35 \text{ mcg/min}}{200 \text{ mcg/mL}} = 0.175 \text{ mL/min} × 60 \text{ min/hr} = 10.5 \text{ or } 11 \text{ mL/hr}$

Upper

$\dfrac{105 \text{ mcg/min}}{200 \text{ mcg/mL}} = 0.525 \text{ mL/min} × 60 \text{ min/hr} = 31.5 \text{ or } 32 \text{ mL/hr}$

d. Titration factor for infusion pump:

$200 \text{ mcg/mL} × 0.1 \text{ mL/hr} = 20 \text{ mcg/hr}$

$\dfrac{20 \text{ mcg/hr}}{60 \text{ min/hr}} = 0.333 \text{ or } 0.3 \text{ mcg/min}$

Titration factor for microdrip

$11 \text{ mL/hr} = 11 \text{ gtt/min}$

$\dfrac{35 \text{ mcg}}{11 \text{ gtt/min}} = 3.18 \text{ or } 3 \text{ mcg/gt}$

e. Base rate 10.5 mL/hr or 35 mcg/min

$5 × 0.33/\text{min} = 1.65 \text{ mcg/min or } 1.7 \text{ mcg/min}$

Add to base rate　35　　mcg/min
　　　　　　+ 1.7 mcg/min
　　　　　　36.7 mcg/min

f. 200 mcg/hr $\times$ 20 mL/hr = 4000 mcg/hr

$$\frac{4000 \text{ mcg/hr}}{60 \text{ min/hr}} = 66.6 \text{ mcg/min}$$

g. Concentration/min and volume/hr using a microdrip set:
   5 gtt $\times$ 3 mcg/gt = 15 mcg
   15 mcg + 35 mcg/min = 50 mcg/min
   5 gtt + 11 gtt/min = 16 gtt/min or 16 mL/hr

h. Concentration/min and volume/hr using a microdrip set:
   13 gtt $\times$ 3 mcg/gt = 39 mcg
   39 mcg + 50 mcg = 89 mcg/min
   13 gtt + 16 gtt = 29 gtt/mL or 29 mL/hr

3. a. Concentration of solution:
   400 mg = 400,000 mcg
   400,000 mcg:250 mL::X mcg:1 mL
   250 X = 400,000 mcg
   X = 1600 mcg
   The concentration of solution is 1600 mcg/mL.

b. Concentration/min:
   4 mcg/kg/min $\times$ 75 kg = 300 mcg/min

c. Volume/min and volume/hr:
   $$\frac{300 \text{ mcg/min}}{1600 \text{ mcg/mL}} = 0.1875 \text{ mL/min} \times 60 \text{ min/hr} = 11.25 \text{ or } 11 \text{ mL/hr}$$

d. Titration factor for infusion pump:
   1600 mcg/mL $\times$ 0.1 mL/hr = 160 mcg/hr
   $$\frac{160 \text{ mcg/hr}}{60 \text{ min/hr}} = 2.66 \text{ or } 2.7 \text{ mcg/min}$$
   Titration factor for microdrip:

   11 mL/hr = 11 gtt/min

e. Base rate 11 mL/hr or 300 mcg/min
   6 $\times$ 2.7 mcg/min = 16.2 mcg/min

$$\frac{300 \text{ mcg/min}}{11 \text{ gtt/min}} = 27.2 \text{ or } 27 \text{ mcg/gtt}$$

$$\begin{array}{r} 300 \quad \text{mcg/min} \\ +16.25 \text{ mcg/min} \\ \hline 316.2 \quad \text{mcg/min} \end{array}$$

f. 12.5 mL/hr $\times$ 1600 mcg/mL = 333 mcg/min
   = 20,000 mcg/hr
   $$\frac{20,000 \text{ mcg/hr}}{60 \text{ min/hr}} = 333 \text{ mcg/min}$$

g. Concentration/min and volume/hr using a microdrip set:
   20 gtt/min $\times$ 27 mcg/gt = 540 mcg/min
   7 gtt + 13 gtt/min = 20 gtt/min or 20 mL/hr

h. Concentration/min and volume/hr using a microdrip set:
   15 gtt/min $\times$ 27 mcg/gt = 405 mcg/min
   20 gtt/min − 5 gtt = 15 gtt/min or 15 mL/hr

V Total Amount of Drug Infused Over Time

1. Lidocaine bolus:

   $100\ mg$
   $\underline{+100\ mg}$
   $200\ mg$

   Lidocaine IV infusion:

   a. Concentration of solution: given as 4 mg/mL in problem.

   b. Concentration/hr:

   4 mg/mL × 40 mL/hr = 160 mg/hr

   c. Concentration over ½ hour:

   $160\ \text{mg/hr} \times \dfrac{30\ \text{min}}{60\ \text{min/hr}} = 80\ \text{mg over 30 min}$

   d. Amount of IV drug infused:

   Lidocaine per two boluses: 200 mg
   Lidocaine per IV infusion: $\underline{+80\ \text{mg}}$

   280 mg total amount infused over 1 hr

   Note: The infusion rate is close to exceeding the maximum therapeutic range, which is 200 to 300 mg/hr.

2. Concentration of solution:

   20,000 units : 500 mL :: X units : 1 mL
   $500\ X = 20,000$
   $X = 40\ \text{units}$

   a. The concentration of solution is 40 units/mL.

   b. Concentration/hr:

   40 units/mL × 50 mL/hr = 2000 units/hr

   c. Amount of IV drug infused over 5½ hours:

   $2000\ \text{units} \times \dfrac{\overset{1}{\cancel{30}}\ \text{min}}{\underset{2}{\cancel{60}}\ \text{min/hr}} = 1000\ \text{units over ½ hr}$

   2000 units × 5 hr = 10,000 units/5 hr

   $10,000\ \text{units}$
   $\underline{+1,000\ \text{units}}$
   $11,000\ \text{units over 5½ hr}$

NEXT-GENERATION NCLEX® EXAMINATION-STYLE QUESTIONS

Question 1

At change of shift the nurse is taking over the care of a 72-year-old male in the Surgical Intensive care unit. The patient was admitted with new onset atrial fibrillation (Afib) and for glucose control after an open reduction and internal fixation (ORIF) of the femur after a fall. The patient's past medical history includes: uncontrolled diabetes type 2, hypertension, obesity (BMI 50), sleep apnea, smoker (1 pack per day), peripheral neuropathy, arthritis, and chronic alcoholism. The patient is currently on an amiodarone gtt @ 1 mg/min and insulin gtt @ 5 units/hour. The patient's last fasting blood sugar was 101 at 0600. In report, the nurse was told that the patient's vital signs have been normal and stable overnight. Current vital signs: HR 110, BP 82/49, Resp 20, SpO2 89% on room air. Upon entering the room at 0700 to begin an assessment, the patient reports feeling light headed. The nurse notes that he appears sweaty and restless.

Use an X to indicate which actions listed in the left column should be implemented by the nurse.

Potential Steps	Appropriate Steps
Place patient in a Reverse Trendelenburg position in bed	
Recheck blood pressure	
Document the need for rest and reassess vital signs in an hour	
Increase the maintenance intravenous fluid (MIVF) infusion	
Notify health care provider of current vital signs	
Place O2 at 2L/min via nasal cannula	
Initiate norepinephrine infusion	
Check blood glucose with glucometer	
Assess neurologic status to determine orientation	
Discontinue insulin infusion	

Question 2

A 72-year old male was admitted to the Surgical Intensive Care Unit (SICU) after undergoing a Whipple procedure for pancreatic cancer. The patient's past medical history includes: pancreatic cancer, hypertension, obesity (297lbs), sleep apnea and smoker (1 pack per day). Current vital signs: HR 105, BP 72/49, Resp 20, Sp02 95% on 4L nasal cannula and temp 38.3. The patient remains hypotensive despite 2-liter Normal Saline (NS) fluid boluses.

Choose the most likely option for the information missing from the statements below by selecting from the lists of options provided.

Due to the patient's hypotension, the health care provider orders a norepinephrine (levophed) infusion to be initiated at 0.02 mcg/kg/min. If the hospital's pharmacy provides norepinephrine 4 mg in 250 mL NS, the concentration of the solution will be _A_ mcg/mL. The nurse can expect to administer an initial volume of _B_ mL/min on the infusion pump for the norepinephrine infusion. Additionally, the health care provider's order states to titrate the norepinephrine infusion 0.05 mcg/kg/min every 5 min to keep the systolic blood pressure (SBP) > 100 with a max of 2 mcg/kg/min. The patient is able to maintain a SBP >100 with the norepinephrine infusion @ 0.12 mcg/kg/min. At this rate, the patient is now receiving _C_ mL/hr.

Option A	Option B	Option C
4	0.10	59.8
8	0.15	60.2
12	0.17	60.6
16	0.20	61.1
20	0.24	61.4

ANSWERS NEXT-GENERATION NCLEX® EXAMINATION-STYLE QUESTIONS

Question 1

Potential Steps	Appropriate Steps
Place patient in a Reverse Trendelenburg position in bed	
Recheck blood pressure	X
Document the need for rest and reassess vital signs in an hour	
Increase the maintenance intravenous fluid (MIVF)infusion	
Notify health care provider of current vital signs	X
Place O2 at 2L/min via nasal cannula	X
Initiate norepinephrine infusion	
Check blood glucose with glucometer	X
Assess neurologic status to determine orientation	X
Discontinue insulin infusion	

Rationale:

Vital signs are no longer within normal limits; the patient is hypotensive and has a low oxygen saturation. Recheck blood pressure to verify hypotension. Notify the health care provider of change in current vital signs. Place oxygen at 2L/min via nasal cannula since oxygen saturation has dropped below 90%. Patients on insulin infusions require blood glucose checks every hour. The nurse should check the patient's blood glucose with a glucometer now (and at the top of every hour) and assess neurologic status to determine orientation. The nurse will also assess for signs and symptoms of hypoglycemia which include sweating, dizziness, tachycardia, confusion, irritability and hunger.

Placing the patient's head of bed down and feet up (Trendelenburg) can help increase the patient's blood pressure temporarily. Placing the head of bed up and feet down (reverse Trendelenburg) is contra-indicated because blood will be pulled distally away from the patient's heart and brain thus decreasing their blood pressure even more. Documenting the need for rest and delaying reassessment for an hour would be detrimental because the patient already exhibits signs of hypoglycemia. Also, an order by the healthcare provider is needed to increase MIVF or initiate an infusion of a vasopressor (norepinephrine). The insulin infusion should not be discontinued by the nurse; this could be detrimental to the management of the patient's glucose. The hospital's insulin infusion protocol should be followed based on the patient's next blood glucose result.

Question 2

Option A	Option B	Option C
4	0.10	59.8
8	0.15	60.2
12	**0.17**	**60.6**
16	0.20	61.1
20	0.24	61.4

Option A:

4mg = 4000mcg

4000 mcg : 250 mL :: X : mL

250 mL X = 4000 mcg/mL

X = 16 mcg/mL

Option B:

297 lbs ÷ 2.2 = 135 kg

0.02 mcg/kg/min x 135 kg = 2.7 mcg/min (desired concentration per min)

2.7 mcg/min ÷ 16mcg/mL = 0.168 or 0.17 mL/min

Option C:

0.12 mcg/kg/min x 135kg = 16.2 mcg/min.

16.2 mcg/min ÷ 16 mcg/mL = 1.01 ml/min

1.01 mL/min x 60 min/hr = 60.6 mL/hr.

Rationale:

Norepinephrine (levophed) is the vasopressor selected by the healthcare provider to correct the patient's hypotension since the patient's blood pressure did not respond to the fluid boluses.

For additional practice problems, refer to the critical care Dosages section of the Elsevier's Interactive Drug calculation application, Version 1 on evolve.

CHAPTER 15

Pediatric Critical Care

Objectives
- Recognize factors that contribute to errors in drug and fluid administration.
- Identify the steps in calculating dilution parameters.
- Determine the accuracy of the dilution parameters in a drug order.

Outline
FACTORS INFLUENCING INTRAVENOUS ADMINISTRATION
CALCULATING ACCURACY OF DILUTION PARAMETERS

In delivery of emergency drugs with complex dilution calculations, it is important for the nurse to evaluate the accuracy of the prescriber's order and to ensure the child doesn't receive the incorrect dose of medication or fluid. Many health care institutions are attempting to standardize the concentration of pediatric intravenous (IV) dosages to decrease the occurrence of miscalculations.

As noted in Chapter 14, the same concepts of solution concentration, infusion rates and volume, and drug concentration based on body weight or body surface area are also utilized in pediatric critical care.

FACTORS INFLUENCING INTRAVENOUS ADMINISTRATION

Volume needs for pediatric patients vary based on the weight and age of the child. Excess fluid can be given when the volume of the drug is not considered in the 24-hour fluid intake. To ensure that fluid overload doesn't occur, volume-control devices are often used. An IV pump or a buretrol (gravity infusion) may be used to control the rate of the infusion (Figure 15.1).

CALCULATING ACCURACY OF DILUTION PARAMETERS

The nurse may find it necessary to calculate the dilution parameters of a drug order that specifies the concentration per kilogram per minute and the volume per hour infusion rate. The physician should determine all drug dose parameters, including concentration per kilogram per minute, volume per hour, and dilution parameters. The nurse should check the accuracy of the dilution parameters to ensure that the correct drug dosage is given. These methods are also used to prepare the pediatric dose. In many pediatric critical care areas, IV fluids for drug administration are limited to prevent fluid overload. If the physician changes the drug dosage, rather than increasing the volume (mL), the concentration of the solution will be changed. It is important that all health care providers follow the policies and procedures of their institution regarding medication administration.

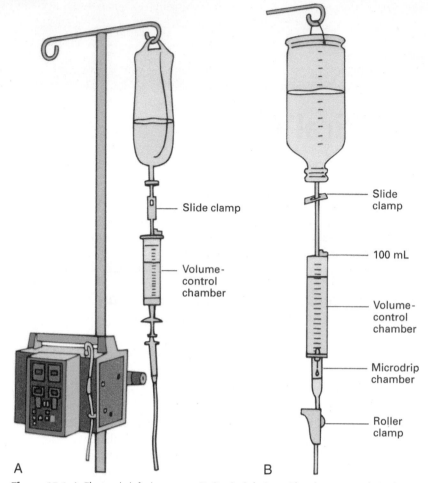

Slide clamp

Volume-
control
chamber

Slide
clamp

100 mL

Volume-
control
chamber

Microdrip
chamber

Roller
clamp

A

B

Figure 15.1 A. Electronic infusion pump. B. Gravity infusion with volume control trip device.

EXAMPLES **PROBLEM 1:** A 5-year-old child, weight 14 kg, with septic shock.

Order: dobutamine 10 mcg/kg/min at 2.1 mL/hr; titrate to keep SBP >90.

Dilute as follows: dobutamine 200 mg in D₅W to make a total volume of 50 mL for a
    syringe pump.

Pediatric dosage: 2-20 mcg/kg/min.

Drug available: dobutamine 250 mg/20 mL.

Here are the following checks that can determine whether the infusion rate and the dilution
orders will result in the correct concentration delivered according to weight.

Step 1: Calculate infusion concentration rates per minute and hour.

    a. Concentration per minute.

$$\text{Child's weight} \times \text{concentration/kg/min} =$$
$$14 \text{ kg} \times 10 \text{ mcg/kg/min} = 140 \text{ mcg/min}$$

    b. Concentration per hour.

$$140 \text{ mcg/min} \times 60 \text{ min/hr} = 8400 \text{ mcg/hr}$$

Step 2: Calculate the concentration of the solution. Check order by dividing concentration per hour by the ordered mL per hour. Results should match.

$$200 \text{ mg} = 200{,}000 \text{ mcg}$$

$$200{,}000 \text{ mcg} : 50 \text{ mL} :: X \text{ mcg} : 1 \text{ mL} \quad \textbf{and} \quad \frac{8400 \text{ mcg/hr}}{2.1 \text{ mL/hr}} = 4000 \text{ mcg/mL}$$

$$50 X = 200{,}000$$

$$X = 4000 \text{ mcg/mL}$$

The concentration solution matches.

Step 3: Calculate the infusion rate, volume per hour. Divide concentration per hour by concentration of solution. Results should confirm the infusion rate in order.

$$\frac{8400 \text{ mcg/hr}}{4000 \text{ mcg/mL}} = 2.1 \text{ mL/hr}$$

Infusion rate is correct.

Step 4: Calculate drug order.

$$\textbf{BF: } \frac{D}{H} \times V = \frac{200}{250} \times \frac{20}{1} = \frac{4000}{250} = 16 \text{ mL} \quad \textbf{or}$$

$$\textbf{RP: } H : V :: D : V$$

$$250 \text{ mg} : 20 \text{ mL} :: 200 \text{ mg} : X \text{ mL}$$

$$250 X = 4000$$

$$X = 16 \text{ mL}$$

Dobutamine 200 mg is 16 mL. Find the amount of D_5W by subtracting 16 mL of dobutamine drug volume from 50 mL; 34 mL of D_5W is needed to fill the 50-mL syringe.

PROBLEM 2: A 3-week-old premature infant, weight 1.6 kg, in shock.
Order: dopamine 2.5 mcg/kg/min at 0.6 mL/hr.
Dilute as follows: dopamine 20 mg in D_5W to make a total of 50 mL for syringe pump.
Dosage range: 2-20 mg/kg/min.
Drug available: dopamine 200 mg/5 mL.

Check to determine whether the infusion rate and the dilution orders will result in the correct concentration delivered according to weight.

Step 1: Calculate the concentration per minute and per hour, based on weight.
   a. Concentration rate per minute

$$\text{Infant's weight } 1.6 \text{ kg} \times 2.5 \text{ mcg/kg/min} = 4 \text{ mcg/min}$$

   b. Concentration rate per hour

$$4 \text{ mcg/min} \times 60 \text{ min/hr} = 240 \text{ mcg/hr}$$

Step 2: Calculate the concentration of the solution. Check order by dividing concentration per hour by the ordered mL per hour. Results should match.

$$20 \text{ mg} = 20{,}000 \text{ mcg}$$

$$20{,}000 \text{ mcg} : 50 \text{ mL} :: X \text{ mcg} : \text{mL} \quad \textbf{and} \quad \frac{240 \text{ mcg/hr}}{0.6 \text{ mL/hr}} = 400 \text{ mcg/mL}$$

$$50 X = 20{,}000$$

$$X = 400 \text{ mcg/mL}$$

The concentration of solution matches.

Step 3: Calculate the infusion rate, volume per hour. Divide concentration per hour by concentration solution. Results should confirm the infusion rate in order.

$$\frac{240 \text{ mcg/hr}}{400 \text{ mcg/mL}} = 0.6 \text{ mL/hr}$$

Infusion rate is correct.

Step 4: Calculate dilution orders.

$$\textbf{BF:}\ \frac{D}{H} \times V = \frac{20 \text{ mg}}{200 \text{ mg}} \times 5 \text{ mL} = 0.5 \text{ mL} \quad \textbf{or}$$

$$\textbf{RP:} H :\ V\ ::\ D\ :\ V$$
$$200 \text{ mg} : 5 \text{ mL} :: 20 \text{ mg} : X \text{ mL}$$
$$200\,X = 100$$
$$X = 0.5 \text{ mL}$$

Dopamine 20 mg is 0.5 mL. Find the amount of D$_5$W needed by subtracting 0.5 mL of dopamine drug volume from 50 mL; 49.5 mL of D$_5$W is needed to fill the 50-mL syringe.

PROBLEM 3: For the same infant, the physician increases the dose of dopamine.
Order: dopamine 15 mcg/kg/min at 1.8 mL/hr.
Dilution: Same, dopamine 20 mg in 50 mL with a syringe pump.
Pediatric dosage range: 2-20 mcg/kg/min.
Drug available: dopamine 200 mg/5 mL.

Check to determine whether the infusion rate and the dilution orders will result in the correct concentration delivered according to weight.

Step 1: Calculate the concentration per minute and per hour based on weight.
    a. Concentration rate per minute

$$\text{Infant's weight } 1.6 \text{ kg} \times 15 \text{ mcg/kg/min} = 24 \text{ mcg/min}$$

    b. Concentration rate per hour

$$24 \text{ mcg/min} \times 60 \text{ min/hr} = 1440 \text{ mcg/hr}$$

Step 2: Calculate the concentration of the solution. Check order by dividing concentration per hour by the ordered mL per hour.

$$400 \text{ mcg/mL (same as previous problem)} \quad \textbf{and} \quad \frac{1440 \text{ mcg/hr}}{1.8 \text{ mL/hr}} = 800 \text{ mcg/mL}$$

Concentrations do not match. Physician must be consulted.

Step 3: Calculate the correct infusion rate per hour. Divide concentration per hour by concentration of solution.

$$\frac{1440 \text{ mcg/hr}}{400 \text{ mcg/mL}} = 3.6 \text{ mL/hr}$$

SUMMARY PRACTICE PROBLEMS

Answers can be found on pages 358 to 361.

Determine whether dilution orders will yield the correct concentration of solution.

1. A 5-year-old child with acute status asthmaticus.
   Child weighs 21 kg.
   Order: terbutaline 0.1 mcg/kg/min. Dilute 25-mg terbutaline in D₅W to make a total volume of
   50 mL. Infuse at 0.25 mL/hr with syringe pump.
   Pediatric dosage range: 0.02-0.25 mcg/kg/min.
   Drug available: terbutaline 1 mg/mL.

2. A 9-year-old child who is intubated postoperatively.
   Child weighs 30 kg.
   Order: fentanyl 0.03 mcg/kg/min. Dilute 2.5-mg fentanyl in 0.9% saline to make a total volume
   of 50 mL. Infuse at 1 mL/hr with syringe pump.
   Pediatric dosage range: 0.01-0.05 mcg/kg/min.
   Drug available: fentanyl 2.5 mg/20 mL.

3. A 1-year-old child with septic shock.
   Child weighs 9 kg.
   Order: dopamine 5 mcg/kg/min. Dilute 40-mg dopamine in D₅W to make a total volume of
   50 mL. Infuse at 3.4 mL/hr with syringe pump.
   Pediatric dosage range: 2-20 mcg/kg/min.
   Drug available: dopamine 400 mg/5 mL.

4. A 3-year-old child with hypertension related to a tumor.
   Child weighs 16 kg.
   Order: sodium nitroprusside 2 mcg/kg/min. Dilute 50-mg nitroprusside in D₅W to make a
   total volume of 50 mL. Infuse at 3 mL/hr with syringe pump.
   Pediatric dosage range: 200-500 mcg/kg/hr.
   Drug available: sodium nitroprusside 50 mg/5 mL.

5. A 10-year-old child with diabetic ketoacidosis.
   Child weighs 32 kg.
   Order: regular insulin 0.1 units/kg/hr.
   Dilute: regular insulin 50 units in 0.9% saline, total volume 50 mL at 6.4 mL/hr with syringe pump.
   Pediatric dosage: 0.1 units/kg/hr.
   Drug available: regular insulin 100 units/mL.

6. A 2-day-old child with patent ductus arteriosus.
   Child weighs 3.4 kg.
   Order: alprostadil 0.1 mcg/kg/min.
   Dilute 0.1 mg of alprostadil in 50-mL D₅W to run at 2 mL/hr with syringe pump.
   Pediatric dosage range: 0.05-0.1 mcg/kg/min.
   Drug available: alprostadil 500 mcg/mL.

7. A 7-year-old child with pulmonary embolism.
   Child weighs 20 kg.
   Order: heparin 25 units/kg/hr using a premixed bag with a standard concentration of 200 units/mL.
   Run at 2.5 mL/hr with IV pump.
   Pediatric dosage range: 15-25 units/kg/hr.
   Drug available: heparin 50,000 units/250 mL.

ANSWERS   SUMMARY PRACTICE PROBLEMS

1. *Step 1:* Calculate the concentration per minute and hour based on weight.
   a. Concentration per minute.

$$21 \text{ kg} \times 0.1 \text{ mcg/kg/min} = 2.1 \text{ mcg/min}$$

   b. Concentration per hour.

$$2.1 \text{ mcg/min} \times 60 \text{ min/hr} = 126 \text{ mcg/hr} = 0.126 \text{ mg/hr}$$

   Step 2: Calculate the concentration of solution. Check order by dividing concentration per hour by the order mL per hour.

$$25 \text{ mg}:50 \text{ mL}::X \text{ mg}:1 \text{ mL} \quad \textbf{and} \quad \frac{126 \text{ mcg/hr}}{0.25 \text{ mL/hr}} = 504 \text{ mcg/mL} = 0.5 \text{ mg/mL}$$
$$50 \, X = 25$$
$$X = 0.5 \text{ mg/1 mL}$$

   The concentration of solution matches.

   Step 3: Calculate the infusion rate, volume per hour. Divide concentration per hour by concentration of solution.

$$\frac{0.126 \text{ mg/hr}}{0.5 \text{ mg/mL}} = 0.25 \text{ mL/hr}$$

   Step 4: Calculate the drug order.

$$\textbf{BF:} \frac{D}{H} \times V = \frac{25 \text{ mg}}{1 \text{ mg}} \times 1 \text{ mL} = \frac{25}{1} = 25 \text{ mL} \quad \textbf{or} \quad \textbf{RP:} 1 \text{ mg}:1 \text{ mL}::25 \text{ mg}:X \text{ mL}$$
$$X = 25 \text{ mL}$$

   Drug order is correct.

2. *Step 1:* Calculate the concentration per minute and hour based on weight.
   a. Concentration per minute.

$$30 \text{ kg} \times 0.03 \text{ mcg/kg/min} = 0.9 \text{ mcg/min}$$

   b. Concentration per hour.

$$0.9 \text{ mcg/min} \times 60 \text{ min/hr} = 54 \text{ mcg/hr} = 0.054 \text{ mg/hr}$$

   Step 2: Calculate the concentration of solution. Check order by dividing concentration per hour by the order mL per hour.

$$2.5 \text{ mg}:50 \text{ mL}::X \text{ mg}:1 \text{ mL} \quad \textbf{and} \quad \frac{54 \text{ mcg/hr}}{1 \text{ mL/hr}} = 54 \text{ mcg/mL} = 0.05 \text{ mg/mL}$$
$$50 \, X = 2.5$$
$$X = 0.05 \text{ mg/mL}$$

   The concentration of solution matches.

   Step 3: Calculate the infusion rate, volume per hour. Divide concentration per hour by concentration of solution.

$$\frac{0.054 \text{ mg/hr}}{0.05 \text{ mg/mL}} = 1 \text{ mL/hr}$$

   Step 4: Calculate the drug order.

$$\textbf{BF:} \frac{D}{H} \times V = \frac{2.5 \text{ mg}}{2.5 \text{ mg}} \times 20 \text{ mL} = \frac{1}{1} \times 20 \text{ mL} = 20 \text{ mL} \quad \textbf{or} \quad \textbf{RP:} 2.5 \text{ mg}:20 \text{ mL}::2.5 \text{ mg}:X \text{ mL}$$
$$2.5 \, X = 50$$
$$X = 20 \text{ mL}$$

   Drug order is correct.

3. *Step 1:* Calculate the concentration per minute and hour based on weight.
   a. Concentration per minute.

$$9 \text{ kg} \times 5 \text{ mcg/kg/min} = 45 \text{ mcg/min}$$

   b. Concentration per hour.

$$45 \text{ mcg/min} \times 60 \text{ min/hr} = 2700 \text{ mcg/hr} = 2.7 \text{ mg/hr}$$

Step 2: Calculate the concentration of solution. Check order by dividing concentration per hour by the order mL per hour.

$$40 \text{ mg} : 50 \text{ mL} :: X \text{ mg} : 1 \text{ mL} \qquad \textbf{and} \qquad \frac{2700 \text{ mcg/hr}}{3.4 \text{ mL/hr}} = 794 \text{ mcg/mL} \qquad \textbf{or} \qquad 0.8 \text{ mg/mL}$$

$$50 \, X = 40$$

$$X = 0.8 \text{ mg/mL or } 800 \text{ mcg/mL}$$

The concentration of solution matches.

Step 3: Calculate the infusion rate, volume per hour. Divide concentration per hour by concentration of solution.

$$\frac{2.7 \text{ mg/hr}}{0.8 \text{ mg/mL}} = 3.4 \text{ mL/hr } (3.375 \text{ mL/hr before rounding})$$

Step 4: Calculate the drug order.

$$\textbf{BF:} \ \frac{D}{H} \times V = \frac{40 \text{ mg}}{400 \text{ mg}} \times 5 \text{ mL} = \frac{200}{400} = 0.5 \text{ mL} \qquad \textbf{or} \qquad \textbf{RP:} \ 400 \text{ mg} : 5 \text{ mL} :: 40 \text{ mg} : X \text{ mL}$$

$$400 \, X = 200 \text{ mL}$$

$$X = 0.5 \text{ mL}$$

Drug order is correct.

4. *Step 1:* Calculate the concentration per minute and hour based on weight.
   a. Concentration per minute.

$$16 \text{ kg} \times 2 \text{ mcg/kg/min} = 32 \text{ mcg/min}$$

   b. Concentration per hour.

$$32 \text{ mcg/min} \times 60 \text{ min/hr} = 1920 \text{ mcg/hr} = 1.92 \text{ mg/hr}$$

Step 2: Calculate the concentration of solution. Check order by dividing concentration per hour by the order mL per hour.

$$50 \text{ mg} : 50 \text{ mL} :: X \text{ mg} : 1 \text{ mL} \qquad \textbf{and} \qquad \frac{1920 \text{ mcg/hr}}{3 \text{ mL/hr}} = 640 \text{ mcg/mL}$$

$$50 \, X = 50$$

$$X = 1 \text{ mg/mL or } 1000 \text{ mcg/mL}$$

The concentration of solution does not match and the order is incorrect. The physician must be consulted.

Step 3: Calculate the correct infusion rate, volume per hour. Divide concentration per hour by concentration of solution.

$$\frac{1920 \text{ mcg/hr}}{1000 \text{ mcg/mL}} = 1.9 \text{ mL/hr}$$

The concentration of solution is incorrect, and infusion rate cannot be confirmed until concentration of solution is clarified.

Step 4: Calculate the drug order.

$$\text{BF: } \frac{D}{H} \times V = \frac{50 \text{ mg}}{50 \text{ mg}} \times 5 \text{ mL} = \frac{250}{50} = 5 \text{ mL} \quad \textbf{or} \quad \text{RP: } 50 \text{ mg} : 5 \text{ mL} :: 50 \text{ mg} : X \text{ mL}$$
$$50 \text{ X} = 250$$
$$X = 5 \text{ mL}$$

Drug order is correct.

5. *Step 1:* Calculate the concentration per hour based on weight.

$$32 \text{ kg} \times 0.1 \text{ units/kg/hr} = 3.2 \text{ units/hr}$$

Step 2: Calculate the concentration of the solution. Check order by dividing the concentration per hour by the order per mL per hour.

$$50 \text{ units} : 50 \text{ mL} :: X \text{ units} : 1 \text{ mL} \quad \textbf{and} \quad \frac{3.2 \text{ units/hr}}{6.4 \text{ mL/hr}} = 0.5 \text{ units/mL}$$
$$50 \text{ X} = 50$$
$$X = 1 \text{ unit/mL}$$

The concentration of solution does not match. The physician must be consulted.

Step 3: Calculate the correct infusion rate, volume per hour. Divide concentration per hour by concentration of solution.

$$\frac{3.2 \text{ units/hr}}{1 \text{ unit/mL}} = 3.2 \text{ mL/hr}$$

The concentration of solution is incorrect and infusion rate cannot be confirmed.

Step 4: Calculate the drug order.

$$\text{BF: } \frac{D}{H} = \frac{50 \text{ units}}{100 \text{ units}} \times 1 \text{ mL} = 0.5 \text{ mL} \quad \textbf{or} \quad \text{RP: } 100 \text{ units} : 1 \text{ mL} :: 50 \text{ units} : X \text{ mL}$$
$$100 \text{ X} = 50$$
$$X = 0.5 \text{ mL}$$

Drug order is correct.

6. *Step 1:* Calculate the concentration per minute and hour based on weight.

    a. Concentration per minute.

$$3.4 \text{ kg} \times 0.1 \text{ mcg/kg/min} = 0.34 \text{ mcg/min}$$

    b. Concentration per hour.

$$0.34 \text{ mcg/min} \times 60 \text{ min} = 20.4 \text{ mcg/hr}$$

Step 2: Calculate the concentration of solution. Check order by dividing concentration per hour by the order mL per hour.

$$0.1 \text{ mg} = 100 \text{ mcg}$$
$$100 \text{ mcg} : 50 \text{ mL} :: X \text{ mcg} : \text{mL} \quad \textbf{and} \quad \frac{20.4 \text{ mcg/hr}}{2 \text{ mL/hr}} = 10.2 \text{ mcg/mL}$$
$$50 \text{ X} = 100$$
$$X = 2 \text{ mcg/mL}$$

The concentration of solution does not match. The physician must be consulted.

Step 3: Calculate the correct infusion rate, volume per hour. Divide the concentration per hour by the concentration of solution.

$$\frac{20.4 \text{ mcg/hr}}{2 \text{ mcg/mL}} = 10.2 \text{ mL/hr}$$

The concentration of solution is incorrect and infusion rate cannot be confirmed.

Step 4: Calculate the drug order.

BF: $\dfrac{D}{H} = \dfrac{0.1 \text{ mg}}{0.5 \text{ mg}} \times 1 \text{ mL} = 0.2 \text{ mL}$ **or**   **RP:** $0.5 \text{ mg} : 1 \text{ mL} :: 0.1 \text{ mg} : X \text{ mL}$

$$0.5 \text{ X} = 0.1$$
$$\text{X} = 0.2 \text{ mL}$$

Drug order is correct.

7. *Step 1:* Calculate the concentration per hour based on weight.
   Concentration per hour.

$$20 \text{ kg} \times 25 \text{ units/kg/hr} = 500 \text{ units/hr}$$

Step 2: Calculate the concentration of solution. Check order by dividing concentration per hour by the order mL per hour.

$50,000 \text{ units} : 250 \text{ mL} :: X \text{ units} : mL$ **and** $\dfrac{500 \text{ units/hr}}{2.5 \text{ mL/hr}} = 200 \text{ units/mL}$

$$250 \text{ X} = 50,000$$
$$\text{X} = 200 \text{ units/mL}$$

The concentration of solution matches.

Step 3: Calculate infusion rate, volume per hour. Divide concentration per hour by concentration of solution.

$$\frac{500 \text{ units/hr}}{200 \text{ units/mL}} = 2.5 \text{ mL/hr}$$

Step 4: Calculate the drug order.

Premixed bag of heparin 50,000 units/250 mL.

CHAPTER 16

Labor and Delivery

Objectives
- Describe the complications related to intravenous fluid administration in the obstetric patient population.
- Recognize the different types of fluid administration used in obstetric nursing.
- Identify medications commonly administered to patients in this specialty area.
- Determine the infusion rates of a drug in solution when the drug is prescribed by concentration or volume.

Outline
FACTORS INFLUENCING INTRAVENOUS FLUID AND DRUG MANAGEMENT
TITRATION OF MEDICATIONS WITH MAINTENANCE INTRAVENOUS FLUIDS
INTRAVENOUS LOADING DOSE
INTRAVENOUS FLUID BOLUS

Drug calculations for labor and delivery are the same as those used in the critical care setting. Determining the concentration of the solution, infusion rates and titration factors are the primary calculation skills used in this specialty area. Accurate calculations are essential in obstetric nursing, as is the measurement and monitoring of intravenous (IV) fluid intake for medications and anesthetic procedures.

Pregnancy causes the woman's body to undergo various changes in order to adapt and support the growing demands of the fetus. The physiologic changes brought on by pregnancy can impact each system of the body. For example, parturients acquire a notable increase in the intravascular fluid volume circulating around their body, which is why fluid status has major effects on labor and maternal outcomes. It is key to avoid dehydration to prevent episodes of maternal hypotension as well as fluid overload. Maternal hypotension must be avoided because the well-being of the fetus depends on adequate blood flow supplied by the mother. Fluid overload can result in peripheral edema which can make peripheral IV placement and regional anesthesia more challenging, but more importantly, it can compromise the parturient's respiratory status and facilitate the development of acute pulmonary edema, especially in women at high risk for complications.

Physicians' orders and hospital protocols give specific guidelines for administering IV drugs. Careful labeling of all IV fluids, IV medications, and IV lines is essential in preventing drug errors. The nurse is responsible for managing the IV drug therapy, monitoring the patient's fluid balance, and assessing the patient's response to drug therapy.

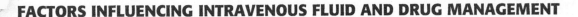

FACTORS INFLUENCING INTRAVENOUS FLUID AND DRUG MANAGEMENT

The most important concept in labor and delivery is that the drugs given to the mother also affect the unborn baby. Therefore the responses of both the mother and the unborn baby must be closely monitored. Vital signs and laboratory results, such as platelet counts, liver function studies, renal function, magnesium levels, reflexes, and contraction patterns, are the main indicators of the mother's status. For the fetus, the fetal heart rate and variability is the primary guide.

TITRATION OF MEDICATIONS WITH MAINTENANCE INTRAVENOUS FLUIDS

During the parturient's admission process, it's important to establish adequate peripheral IV access that will be used to administer IV fluids and IV medications. Typically, 500 to 1000 mL of crystalloid IV fluids may be given to initially hydrate the mother, especially in preterm labor or before the implementation of regional anesthesia to prevent hypotension. Obstetric patients should have a primary IV line and a secondary IV line for the administration of IV medications. All IV medications should be delivered by a volumetric infusion pump to ensure that the specific volume and correct dosage are provided to the patient. The titration of any IV medication should be recorded as part of the hourly IV rate.

The administration and titration of IV medications in the obstetric patient population is usually to stimulate labor, inhibit preterm labor, or treat pregnancy-induced complications such as preeclampsia. Tocolytic agents are used to stop or slow the progression of preterm labor by causing uterine relaxation. Some common tocolytic agents used in this specialty area are: magnesium sulfate and terbutaline. Uterotonic agents such as oxytocin (Pitocin) are frequently used to augment or induce labor and prevent or reduce bleeding after delivery.

In the following example, oxytocin (Pitocin) and the primary IV rate is adjusted with the secondary IV drug line to achieve a therapeutic effect and maintain adequate maternal hydration. Note that the drug is ordered to be given by concentration and that the infusion rates for volume per minute and hour must be determined.

NOTE

Important concepts to understand:

Preterm labor — Regular uterine contractions before 37 weeks of gestation.

Preeclampsia — A hypertensive disorder of pregnancy that typically presents with new onset high blood pressure and protein in the urine (proteinuria). If mismanaged or left untreated it can result in maternal and fetal morbidity and mortality.

Tocolytic Drugs — A class of medications used to stop or slow preterm labor by preventing contractions through uterine relaxation.

Uterotonic Agents — A class of medications that stimulate and enhance uterine contractions.

Administration by Concentration

EXAMPLES
1. Give IV fluids at 100 mL/hr with lactated ringer's solution (LR).
2. Mix 10 units of oxytocin in 1000 mL normal saline solution (NS). Start at 1 milliunit/min, increase by 1 or 2 milliunits/min, every 15-30 min, until uterine contractions are 2-3 minutes apart. Do not exceed 40 milliunits/min.

   Note: 1 unit = 1000 milliunits

Available: Secondary set:
        oxytocin 10 units/mL
        1000 mL NS
        IV set drop factor 20 gtt/mL
        infusion pump
    Primary set:
        1000 mL LR
        IV set drop factor 20 gtt/mL
        infusion pump

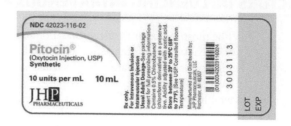

For the *secondary* IV set, the following calculations must be made:
1. Concentration of solution.
2. Infusion rates: Volume per minute and volume per hour.
3. Titration factor in concentration per minute (milliunits/min).

For the *primary* IV set, the following calculations must be made:
1. Pump is used; set the rate at mL/hr.
2. Balance primary IV flow with secondary IV rate to achieve 100 mL/hr.

Secondary IV (see Chapter 8 for formulas)

1. Concentration of solution:

$$10 \text{ units} : 1000 \text{ mL} :: X : 1 \text{ mL}$$
$$1000\,X = 10$$
$$X = 0.01 \text{ unit or } 10 \text{ millliunits}$$

The concentration of solution is 10 milliunits/mL.
2. Infusion rates for volume:

$$\frac{\text{Concentration/minute}}{\text{Concentration of solution}} = \text{Volume/min} \times 60 \text{ min} = \text{Volume/hr}$$

Volume per minute	**Volume per hour**
$\dfrac{1 \text{ milliunit/min}}{10 \text{ milliunits/mL}} = 0.1 \text{ mL/min}$	$\times\; 60 \text{ min} = 6 \text{ mL/hr}$
$\dfrac{2 \text{ milliunits/min}}{10 \text{ milliunits/mL}} = 0.2 \text{ mL/min}$	$\times\; 60 \text{ min} = 12 \text{ mL/hr}$
$\dfrac{4 \text{ milliunits/min}}{10 \text{ milliunits/mL}} = 0.4 \text{ mL/min}$	$\times\; 60 \text{ min} = 24 \text{ mL/hr}$

3. Titration factor (see Chapter 14): To increase the concentration by increments of 1 milliunit/min, the hourly rate on the pump must be increased by 6 mL/hr. The titration factor for this problem is 6 mL/hr. To increase the concentration to a higher rate, multiply the rate of increase times 6 mL/hr. (Example: To increase infusion to 4 milliunits/min, multiply 4 by 6 mL = 24 mL/hr.)
    For the secondary IV line, the concentration of the solution is 10 milliunits/mL of oxytocin, with the infusion rate of 6 mL/hr to be increased in increments of 1 to 2 milliunits every 15 to 30 minutes until contractions are 2 to 3 minutes apart.

Primary IV

The secondary IV rate will start at 6 mL/hr; therefore the primary rate will be 94 mL/hr. (A balance is needed to achieve 100 mL/hr.)

For every increase in rate from the secondary line, a corresponding decrease must be made with the primary IV line. If the rate of the secondary line exceeds the ordered hourly rate, the primary IV line may be shut off completely. The concentration of the solution may be changed by the physician if the parturient is receiving too much fluid.

Administration by Volume

In the previous example, oxytocin (Pitocin) was ordered to be infused by concentration (milliunits/min), which is the safety method of administration for this medicaion. Sometimes in clinical practice, the infusion rate may be ordered by volume (mL/hr).

EXAMPLES   Mix 30 units of oxytocin (Pitocin) in 500 mL NS. Start infusion at 1 mL/hr and increase by 1-2 mL every 15-30 min until uterine contractions are 2-3 apart. Notify physician before exceeding 40 milliunits/min.

To determine the concentration per hour of infusion, multiply concentration of the solution by volume/hr.

$$60 \text{ milliunits/mL} \times 1 \text{ mL/hr} = 60 \text{ milliunits/hr}$$

To determine the concentration of the infusion per minute, divide:

$$\frac{\text{Concentration/hr}}{60 \text{ min/hr}} = \text{Concentration/min}$$

$$\frac{60 \text{ milliunits/hr}}{60 \text{ min/hr}} = 1 \text{ milliunit/min}$$

Therefore, an oxytocin solution with a concentration of 60 milliunits/mL infused at 1 mL/hr will administer 1 milliunit of the drug per minute.

INTRAVENOUS LOADING DOSE

Some situations require a larger initial dose of an IV medication be infused over a short period of time to quickly establish an adequate serum concentration to achieve its intended therapeutic effect. This type of IV drug administration is called a *loading dose*.

In the following example, a patient with preeclampsia is receiving magnesium sulfate to prevent seizures. This parturient will receive a loading dose of magnesium sulfate, followed by a maintenance dose via the secondary IV line. A primary IV line is also maintained after the loading dose is given. At the end of this example, the total IV intake is determined for an 8-hour period.

EXAMPLES   1. Mix magnesium sulfate 40 g in 1000 mL of sterile NS.
2. Infuse 4 g over 20 minutes, then maintain at 2 g/hr.
3. Start LR at 75 mL/hr after magnesium sulfate loading dose.

Available: Secondary set:
    magnesium sulfate 50%
    (5 g in 10-mL ampules)
    1000 mL IV fluid
    IV set 20 gtt/mL
    infusion pump
  Primary set:
    1000 mL LR
    IV set drop factor 20 gtt/mL
    infusion pump

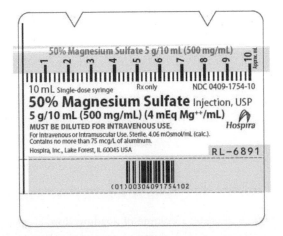

For the *secondary* IV line, the following calculations must be made:
1. Dose of magnesium sulfate in IV.
2. Concentration of solution.
3. Volume of loading dose and flow rate for infusion pump (see Chapter 11).
4. Infusion rate: Volume per hour of magnesium sulfate infusion.

For the *primary* IV line, the following calculation must be made:
1. Drop rate per minute.

For the total IV intake, the following solutions must be added:
1. Volume of loading dose.
2. Volume of secondary IV for 8 hours.
3. Volume of primary IV for 8 hours.

Secondary IV

1. $\dfrac{D}{H} \times V = \dfrac{40\,g}{5\,g} \times 10\ mL = 80\ mL$ of magnesium sulfate or 8 ampules

2. Concentration of solution:

$$40\,g = 40,000\ mg$$
$$40,000\ mg : 1000\ mL :: X : 1\ mL$$
$$1000\,X = 40,000$$
$$X = 40\ mg$$

The concentration of solution is 40 mg/mL.

3. Volume of loading dose:

$$4\,g = 4000\ mg$$
$$40\ mg : 1\ mL :: 4000\ mg : X\ mL$$
$$40\,X = 4000$$
$$X = 100\ mL$$

Flow rate for the pump:

$$100\ mL \div \dfrac{20\ min}{60\ min/hr} = 100 \times \dfrac{\overset{3}{\cancel{60}}}{\underset{1}{\cancel{20}}} = 300\ mL/hr$$

The rate on the infusion pump for the 4 g infusion of magnesium sulfate over 20 minutes is 300 mL/hr. When the infusion rate is this high, it must be monitored closely, and the patient must be observed for response to drug therapy.

4. Infusion rate: volume per hour:

$$2\,g = 2000\ mg$$

$$\dfrac{\text{Concentration/hr}}{\text{Concentration of solution}} = \text{Volume/hr} \qquad \dfrac{2000\ mg/hr}{40\ mg/mL} = 50\ mL/hr$$

The rate on the pump for the 2 g/hr infusion is 50 mL/hr.

Primary IV

After the loading dose of magnesium sulfate, the primary IV will run at 75 mL/hr.

Total IV Intake Over 8 Hours

Volume of loading dose		100 mL
Volume of secondary IV	50 mL × 8 =	400 mL
Volume of primary IV	75 mL × 8 =	+600 mL
		1100 mL

Since the development of fluid overload is a potential problem for Labor and Delivery patients, especially those with preeclampsia, all IV fluids must be calculated accurately and administered with an infusion pump.

INTRAVENOUS FLUID BOLUS

An IV fluid *bolus* is a large volume, 500 to 1000 mL, of IV fluid infused over a short time (1 hour or less). A bolus may be given before administration of regional anesthesia or to a patient experiencing preterm labor.

In the next example, calculate the flow rate of an IV bolus from the primary IV followed by an infusion of a tocolytic drug given by titration. At the end of this example, calculate the patient's fluid intake for 8 hours.

EXAMPLES

1. Start 1000 mL LR at 300 mL/10 min, then reduce to 125 mL/hr.
2. Mix terbutaline 7.5 mg in 500 mL of NS; start at 2.5 mcg/min; increase 2.5 mcg/min every 20 min until contractions subside.

Available: Primary set:
  1000 mL LR
  IV set drop factor 20 gtt/mL
  infusion pump
 Secondary set:
  terbutaline 1 mg/mL
  500 mL NS
  IV set 20 gtt/mL
  infusion pump

For the *secondary* IV line, the following calculations must be made:
1. The dose of terbutaline in IV.
2. Concentration of solution.
3. Infusion rates: Volume per minute and hour.
4. Titration factor for 2.5 mcg/mL.

For the *primary* IV line, determine the following:
1. Set pump to infuse 300 mL over 10 minutes and then 125 mL/hr.
2. Balance the primary IV with the secondary IV to achieve a rate of 125 mL/hr.
Total the IV fluids for 8 hours.

Secondary IV

1. **BF:** $\dfrac{D}{H} \times V = \dfrac{7.5 \text{ mg}}{1 \text{ mg}} \times 1 \text{ mL} = 7.5 \text{ mL of terbutaline}$

2. Concentration of solution:
$$7.5 \text{ mg} = 7500 \text{ mcg}$$
$$7500 \text{ mcg}: 500 \text{ mL}:: X \text{ mcg}: 1 \text{ mL}$$
$$500 \text{ X} = 7500$$
$$X = 15 \text{ mcg}$$

The concentration of solution is 15 mcg/mL.

3. Infusion rates: Volume per minute and volume per hour.

$$\frac{2.5 \text{ mcg/min}}{15 \text{ mcg/mL}} = 0.166 \text{ mL/min} \times 60 \text{ min/hr} = 9.96 \text{ mL/hr or } 10 \text{ mL/hr}$$

4. Titration factor: To increase the concentration by increments of 2.5 mcg/min, the volume of the increment of change must be calculated per minute and per hour:

$$\frac{\text{Concentration/minute}}{\text{Concentration of solution}} = \text{mL/min} \qquad \frac{2.5 \text{ mcg/min}}{15 \text{ mcg/mL}} = 0.166 \text{ mL/min}$$

$$\text{Volume/min} \times 60 \text{ min/hr} = \text{Volume/hr}$$
$$0.166 \text{ mL/min} \times 60 \text{ min/hr} = 9.96 \text{ mL/hr or } 10 \text{ mL}$$

The titration factor is 0.166 mL/min or 10 mL/hr. Increasing or decreasing the infusion rate by 2.5 mcg/min will correspond to an increase or decrease in volume by 0.166 mL/min or 10 mL/hr.

Primary IV

1. Set infusion pump at 300 mL over 10 minutes, then reduce rate to 125 mL/hr.

Total IV Intake Over 8 Hours

Volume of loading dose		300 mL
Volume of primary set	115 mL × 8 =	920 mL
Volume of secondary set	10 mL × 8 =	+ 80 mL
		1300 mL

Assume that an average of 10 mL/hr of terbutaline was given.

SUMMARY PRACTICE PROBLEMS

Answers can be found on pages 370 to 372.

1. Preeclamptic labor.

   a. Mix magnesium sulfate 20 g in 500 mL NS.

   b. Infuse 4 g over 30 minutes, then maintain at 2 g/hr.

   c. Start LR 1000 mL at 75 mL/hr after loading dose of magnesium sulfate.

   Available: Secondary set:
            magnesium sulfate 50% (5 g in 10 mL)
            1000 mL NS
            IV set 20 gtt/mL
            infusion pump
         Primary set:
            1000 mL LR
            IV set 20 gtt/mL

   Determine the following:

   a. Secondary IV:
      (1) Magnesium sulfate dosage.
      (2) Concentration of solution.
      (3) Volume of loading dose and infusion rate for pump.
      (4) Infusion rate per hour of magnesium sulfate.

   b. Primary IV: 75 mL/hr.

   c. Total fluid intake for 8 hours.

2. Oxytocin (Pitocin) for augmentation of labor.

    a. Give LR 500 mL over 30 minutes, then infuse at 75 mL/hr.

    b. Mix 15 units of oxytocin (Pitocin) in 250 mL NS.

        Start infusion at 2 milliunits/min, increase by 1 to 2 milliunits/min until labor pattern is established and contractions are 2 to 3 minutes apart. Notify physician before exceeding 40 milliunits/min.

        Available: Secondary set:
                oxytocin 10 units/mL
                250 mL NS
                IV set 20 gtt/mL
                infusion pump
            Primary set:
                1000 mL LR
                IV set 20 gtt/mL

For secondary IV line, the following calculations must be made:
    (1) Dose of oxytocin for IV.
    (2) Concentration of solution.
    (3) Infusion rate: Volume per minute and volume per hour.
    (4) Titration factor in milliunits per minute.

For primary IV line, the following calculation must be made:
    (1) Infusion rate for 500 mL over 30 minutes.

3. Preterm labor.

    a. Mix terbutaline 5 mg in 250 mL NS.

        Begin infusion at 15 mcg/min; increase by 2 mcg/min until contractions subside. Do not exceed 80 mcg/min.

    b. Start NS 1 L at 100 mL/hr.

        Available: Secondary set:
          terbutaline 1 mg/1 mL ampule
          250 mL NS
          IV set 20 gtt/mL
        Primary set:
          1000 mL NS
          IV set 20 gtt/mL

For secondary IV line, the following calculations must be made:
    (1) Dose of terbutaline for IV.
    (2) Concentration of solution.
    (3) Infusion rate: Volume per minute and volume per hour.
    (4) Titration factor in micrograms per minute and hour.

For primary IV line, the following calculation must be made:
    (1) Infusion rate for 100 mL/hr.

4. Oxytocin (Pitocin) for augmentation of labor.

    a. Mix 35 units of IV Oxytocin (Pitocin) in 1000 mL of LR.

        Start infusion at 5 milliunits/min; increase by 2 milliunits/min until regular contractions begin.

b. Give 1000 mL LR over 3 hours.

Available: Secondary set:
Oxytocin (Pitocin) 10 units/mL
1000 mL LR
IV set 20 gtt/mL
Primary set:
1000 mL LR
IV set 20 gtt/mL

For secondary IV line, the following calculations must be made:
(1) Dose of oxytocin (Pitocin) for IV.
(2) Concentration of solution.
(3) Infusion rate: Volume per minute and volume per hour.
(4) Titration factor in milliunits per minute.

For primary IV line, the following calculation must be made:
(1) Infusion rate for 1000 mL over 3 hours.

ANSWERS   SUMMARY PRACTICE PROBLEMS

1. a. Secondary IV:

(1) Magnesium sulfate dosage:

$$\frac{D}{H} \times V = \frac{20\,g}{5\,g} \times 10\,mL = 40\,mL \text{ or 4 ampules of magnesium sulfate}$$

(2) Concentration of solution:

$$20\,g = 20,000\,mg$$
$$20,000\,mg : 500\,mL :: X\,mg : 1\,mL$$
$$500\,X = 20,000$$
$$X = 40\,mg$$

The concentration of solution is 40 mg/mL.

(3) Volume of loading dose:

$$4\,g = 4000\,mg$$
$$40\,mg : 1\,mL :: 4000\,mg : X\,mL$$
$$40\,X = 4000$$
$$X = 100\,mL$$

Infusion rate for 30 minutes:

$$100\,mL \div \frac{30\,min}{60\,min/hr} = 100 \times \frac{\overset{2}{\cancel{60}}}{\underset{1}{\cancel{30}}} = 200\,mL/hr$$

(4) Infusion rate: volume per hour:

$$2\,g = 2000\,mg$$
$$\frac{2000\,mg/hr}{40\,mg/mL} = 50\,mL/hr$$

b. Primary IV:
After the loading dose: Set IV rate at 75 mL/hr.

c. Total IV intake over 8 hours:

Volume of loading dose		100 mL
Volume of secondary IV	50 mL × 8 =	400 mL
Volume of primary IV	75 mL × 8 =	+600 mL
		1100 mL

2. a. Secondary IV:

(1) Oxytocin dosage: $\dfrac{D}{H} \times V = \dfrac{15 \text{ units}}{10 \text{ units}} \times 1 \text{ mL} = 1.5 \text{ mL}$

Add 1.5 mL of oxytocin to 250 mL of NS.

(2) Concentration of solution

15 units = 15,000 milliunits

15,000 milliunits : 250 mL = X milliunits : 1 mL

$$250 \text{ X} = 15,000$$
$$\text{X} = 60 \text{ milliunits/mL}$$

(3) Infusion rate: $\dfrac{\text{Concentration/minute}}{\text{Concentration of solution}} = \dfrac{2 \text{ milliunits/min}}{60 \text{ milliunits/mL}}$

$$= 0.033 \text{ mL/min}$$
$$0.033 \text{ mL/min} \times 60 \text{ min/hr} = 1.98 \text{ mL/hr}$$

(4) Titration factor: $\dfrac{2 \text{ milliunits/min}}{60 \text{ milliunits/mL}} = 0.033 \text{ mL/min} \times 60 \text{ min/hr} = 1.9 \text{ mL/hr or } 2 \text{ mL/hr}$

$$\dfrac{3 \text{ milliunits/min}}{60 \text{ milliunits/mL}} = 0.05 \text{ mL/min} \times 60 \text{ min/hr} = 3 \text{ mL/hr}$$

$$\dfrac{4 \text{ milliunits/min}}{60 \text{ milliunits/mL}} = 0.06 \text{ mL/min} \times 60 \text{ min/hr} = 3.6 \text{ mL/hr or } 4 \text{ mL/hr}$$

$$\dfrac{5 \text{ milliunits/min}}{60 \text{ milliunits/mL}} = 0.08 \text{ mL/min} \times 60 \text{ min/hr} = 4.8 \text{ mL/hr or } 5 \text{ mL/hr}$$

NOTE

With this concentration of solution, there is a 1:1 relationship between milliunits/mL and mL/hr.

b. Primary IV: $500 \text{ mL LR} \div \dfrac{\text{Minutes to administer}}{60 \text{ min/hr}} = 500 \text{ mL} \div \dfrac{30 \text{ minutes}}{60 \text{ min/hr}}$

$$= 500 \times \dfrac{60}{30}$$

$$= 1000 \text{ mL in 30 min}$$

3. a. Secondary IV:

(1) Terbutaline dosage:

$$\dfrac{D}{H} \times V = \dfrac{5 \text{ mg}}{1 \text{ mg}} \times 1 \text{ mL} = 5 \text{ mL or 5 ampules of terbutaline}$$

Add 5 mL of terbutaline to 250 mL NS.

(2) Concentration of solution:

5 mg = 5000 mcg

5000 mcg : 250 mL :: X mcg : 1 mL

$$250 \text{ X} = 5000$$
$$\text{X} = 20 \text{ mcg/mL}$$

(3) Infusion rate:

$$\frac{\text{Concentration/minute}}{\text{Concentration of solution}} = \frac{15 \text{ mcg/min}}{20 \text{ mcg/mL}}$$

$$= 0.75 \text{ mL/min}$$

$$= 0.75 \times 60 = 45 \text{ mL/hr}$$

(4) Titration factor:

$$\frac{20 \text{ mcg/min}}{60 \text{ mcg/mL}} = 0.1 \text{ mL/min}$$

$$0.1 \text{mL/min} \times 60 \text{ min/h r} = 6 \text{ mL/hr}$$

b. Primary IV: Set infusion pump to deliver 100 mL/hr.

4. a. Secondary IV:

(1) Oxytocin (Pitocin) dosage:

$$\text{BF: } \frac{D}{H} \times V = \frac{35 \text{ units}}{10 \text{ units}} \times 1 \text{ mL} = 3.5 \text{ mL}$$

Add 3.5 mL of oxytocin (Pitocin) to 1000 mL of LR.

(2) Concentration of solution:

$$35 \text{ units} = 35,000 \text{ milliunits}$$

RP: D : V :: H : X

35,000 milliunits : 1000 mL :: X milliunits : 1 mL

$$1000 \, X = 35,000$$

$$X = 35 \text{ milliunits/mL}$$

(3) Infusion rate:

$$\frac{\text{Concentration/minute}}{\text{Concentration of solution}} = \frac{5 \text{ milliunits/min}}{35 \text{ milliunits/mL}}$$

$$= 0.14 \text{ mL/min}$$

$$= 0.14 \times 60 = 8.4 \text{ mL/hr}$$

(4) Titration factor:

$$\frac{7 \text{ milliunits/min}}{35 \text{ milliunits/mL}} = 0.2 \text{ mL/min}$$

$$\frac{9 \text{ milliunits/min}}{35 \text{ milliunits/mL}} = 0.25 \text{ mL/min}$$

$$\frac{11 \text{ milliunits/min}}{35 \text{ milliunits/mL}} = 0.31 \text{ mL/min}$$

b. Primary IV: 1000 mL LR $\div \dfrac{\text{Minutes to administer}}{60 \text{ min/hr}} = 1000 \text{ mL} \div \dfrac{180 \text{ minutes}}{60 \text{ min/hr}}$

$$= 1000 \times \frac{60}{180}$$

$$= 333 \text{ mL/hr}$$

NEXT-GENERATION NCLEX® EXAMINATION-STYLE QUESTIONS

A 30-year-old primigravida, who is 36 weeks pregnant, presents to the Labor and Delivery triage. The client appears very anxious and diaphoretic. She reports having a headache and dizziness. Upon assessment, the nurse notices that the patient is edematous with notable +2 pitting edema in her bilateral lower extremities. Vital signs: HR 100, BP 186/108, Resp 28, SpO2 97%, Temp 100 F (37.7 C). Her past medical history includes BMI 40, anxiety, and hypothyroidism. The patient has no known drug allergies and is taking daily prenatal vitamins and levothyroxine. The following labs were ordered: Complete blood count (CBC), Comprehensive metabolic panel (CMP), and Urine dipstick test.

Choose the most likely option for the information missing from the statements below by selecting from the lists of options provided.

The nurse recognizes that the patient's __A__ is elevated, which is concerning. If the patient's laboratory results show __B__ the nurse needs to monitor carefully for symptoms of __C__.

Option A	Option B	Option C
Temperate	Hypokalemia	Preeclampsia
Heart rate	Anemia	Preterm labor
Blood pressure	Leukocytosis	Placenta Previa
Respirations	Thrombocytosis	Eclampsia
Oxygen saturation	Proteinuria	HELLP syndrome

ANSWERS NEXT-GENERATION NCLEX® EXAMINATION-STYLE QUESTIONS

Option A	Option B	Option C
Temperate	Hypokalemia	**Preeclampsia**
Heart rate	Anemia	Preterm labor
Blood pressure	Leukocytosis	Placenta Previa
Respirations	Thrombocytosis	Eclampsia
Oxygen saturation	**Proteinuria**	HELLP syndrome

Rationale:

The patient is demonstrating symptoms of Preeclampsia as evidence by being over 20 weeks of gestation with elevated blood pressure and proteinuria. Preeclampsia is associated with an increased risk of maternal and fetal morbidity and/or mortality. The other listed choices do not correlate with the patient's presenting symptoms of preeclampsia.

For additional practice problems, refer to the Obstetric Dosages section of the Elsevier's Interactive Drug Calculation Application, Version 1 on evolve.

CHAPTER 17

Home Care and Community

Although the metric system is widespread in the clinical area, the home setting generally does not have the devices of metric measure. This becomes a problem when liquid medication is prescribed in metric measure for the home patient. Measuring spoons and syringes with metric measurements are available in pharmacies, and families should be encouraged to purchase them. All pediatric liquid medication must be measured using a metric measuring device. If metric devices are not available, the community nurse should be able to assist the adult patient in converting metric to household measure.

Preparation of solutions in the home setting may involve conversion between the metric and household systems. Solutions used in the home setting can be used for oral fluid replacement, topical application, irrigation, or disinfection. Although the majority of the solutions are available in stores, solutions that can be prepared in the home can be effective and less costly than the commercially premixed items.

When commercially prepared drugs are too concentrated for the patient's use and must be diluted, it is necessary to calculate the strength of the solution to meet the therapeutic need as prescribed by the physician. Knowledge of solution preparation and of metric-household conversion can be useful skills for the community nurse.

METRIC TO HOUSEHOLD CONVERSION

When changing from metric to household measure, use the ounce from the apothecary system as an intermediary, because there is no clear conversion between the two systems.

The conversion factors for volume are:

Ounces to milliliters: multiply ounces $\times$ 29.57 or 30

Milliliters to ounces: multiply milliliters $\times$ 0.034

The conversion factors for weight are:

Ounces to grams: multiply ounces $\times$ 28.35

Grams to ounces: multiply grams $\times$ 0.035

Note that weight and volume measures differ in the metric system. The properties of crystals, powders, and other solids account for the differences more so than the liquids. Also, as liquid measures increase in volume, there are greater discrepancies between metric and standard household measure. Table 17.1 shows the current approximate equivalents. Deciliters and liters are also included with the volume measurements. These terms will be seen more commonly as the use of the metric system increases. Although conversion charts are helpful guides, a metric measuring device would be optimal for drug administration. Standard household measuring devices should be used instead of tableware if a metric device is not available.

NOTE

When a measuring device comes from the manufacturer with a drug, it should be used. If a liquid drug has no measuring device, one should be purchased from the pharmacy, and the pharmacist can help choose the correct device. If a measuring device cannot be obtained, then standard household measuring devices can be used.

TABLE 17.1 Household to Metric Conversions (Approximate)

Standard Household Measure	Apothecary	Metric Volume	Metric Weight
$^1/_8$ teaspoon	7-8 gtt or $^1/_{48}$ oz	0.6 mL	0.6 g
$^1/_4$ teaspoon	15 gtt or $^1/_{24}$ oz	1.25 mL	1.25 g
$^1/_2$ teaspoon	30 gtt or $^1/_{12}$ oz	2.5 mL	2.5 g
1 teaspoon	60 gtt or $^1/_6$ oz	5 mL	5 g
1 tablespoon or 3 teaspoons	$^1/_2$ oz	15 mL	15 g
2 tablespoons or 6 teaspoons	1 oz	$^1/_4$ dL or 30 mL	30 g
$^1/_4$ cup or 4 tablespoons	2 oz	$^1/_2$ dL or 60 mL	60 g
$^1/_3$ cup or 5 tablespoons	$2^1/_2$ oz	$^3/_4$ dL or 75 mL	75 g
$^1/_2$ cup	4 oz	1 dL or 120 mL	120 g
1 cup	8 oz	$^1/_4$ L or 250 mL	230 g
1 pint	16 oz	$^1/_2$ L or 480-500 mL	
1 quart	32 oz	1 L or 1000 mL	
2 quarts or $^1/_2$ gallon	64 oz	2 L or 2000 mL	
1 gallon	128 oz	$3^3/_4$ L or 3840-4000 mL	

PRACTICE PROBLEMS ▶ I METRIC TO HOUSEHOLD CONVERSION

Answers can be found on page 384.

Use Table 17.1 to convert metric to household measure.

1. Bismuth subsalicylate 15 mL every hour up to 120 mL in 24 hr.

_____

2. Ceclor 5 mL four times per day.

_____

3. Tylenol elixir 1.25 mL every 6 hours as necessary for temperature greater than 102° F.

_____

4. Maalox 30 mL after meals and at bedtime.

_____

5. Neo-Calglucon 7.5 mL three times per day.

_____

6. Gani-Tuss NR liquid 10 mL, q6h, prn.

_____

7. Castor oil 60 mL at bedtime.

_____

Use Table 17.1 for conversions.

8. Metamucil 5 g in 1 glass of water every morning.

_____

9. Dilantin-30 pediatric suspension 10 mL twice per day.

_____

10. Homemade pediatric electrolyte solution:

H_2O 1 L, boiled _____

Sugar 30 g _____

Salt 1.25 g _____

Lite salt 2.5 g _____

Baking soda 2.5 g _____

11. A nonalcoholic mouthwash:

H_2O 500 mL boiled _____

Table salt 5 g _____

Baking soda 5 g _____

12. Magic mouthwash:

Benadryl 50 mg/10 mL _____

Maalox 10 mL _____

13. Gastrointestinal cocktail for gastric upset:

Belladonna/phenobarbital elixir, 10 mL _____

Maalox, 30 mL _____

Viscous lidocaine, 10 mL _____

PREPARING A SOLUTION OF A DESIRED CONCENTRATION

All solutions contain a solute (drug) and a solvent (liquid). Solutions can be mixed three different ways:

1. *Weight to weight:* Involves mixing the weight of a given solute with the weight of a given liquid.

EXAMPLE

5 g sugar with 100 g H_2O

This type of preparation is used in the pharmaceutical setting and is the *most accurate*. Scales for weight to weight preparation are not usually found in the home setting.

2. *Weight to volume:* Uses the weight of a given solute with the volume of an appropriate amount of solvent.

EXAMPLE

10 g of salt in 1 L of H_2O

or

$\frac{1}{3}$ oz of salt in 1 qt of H_2O

Again, a scale is needed for this preparation.

3. *Volume to volume:* Means that a given volume of solution is mixed with a given volume of solution.

EXAMPLE

30 mL of hydrogen peroxide 3% in 1 dL H_2O

or

2 T of hydrogen peroxide 3% in $\frac{1}{3}$ c H_2O

Preparation of solutions volume to volume is commonly used in both clinical and home settings. After a solution is prepared, the strength can be expressed numerically in three different ways:

1. A ratio—1:20 acetic acid
2. A fraction—5 g/100 mL acetic acid
3. A percentage—5% acetic acid

With a ratio, the first number is the solute and the second number is the solvent. In a fraction, the numerator is the solid and the denominator is the liquid. A solution labeled by percentage indicates the amount of solute in 100 mL of liquid. All pharmaceutically prepared solutions use the metric system, and the ratio, fraction, and percentages are interpreted in *grams per milliliter*.

Changing a Ratio to Fractions and Percentages

Change a ratio to a percentage or a fraction by setting up a proportion using the following variables:

Known drug : Known volume : : Desired drug : Desired volume

A proportion can also be set up like a fraction:

$$\frac{\text{Known drug}}{\text{Known volume}} = \frac{\text{Desired drug}}{\text{Desired volume}}$$

 YOU MUST REMEMBER

Any variable in this formula can be found if the other three variables are known.

EXAMPLE Change acetic acid 1: 20 to a percentage

$$1\,g : 20\,mL = X\,g : 100\,mL$$
$$20\,X = 100$$
$$X = 5\,g$$
$$1\,g : 20\,mL = 5\,g : 100\,mL$$

Note: In percentage, the volume of liquid is 100 mL.

The ratio can be expressed as a fraction, 5 g/100 mL, or as a percentage, 5%. Another method of changing a ratio to a percentage involves finding a multiple of 100 for volume (denominator), then multiplying both terms by that multiple.

PRACTICE PROBLEMS ▶ II PREPARING A SOLUTION OF A DESIRED CONCENTRATION

Answers can be found on pages 384 to 385.

Change the following ratios to fractions and percentages.

1. 4:1

2. 2:1

3. 1:50

4. 1:3

5. 1:1000

6. 1:10,000

7. 1:4

8. 1:5000

9. 1:200

10. 1:10

In the previous problems, grams per milliliter is the unit of measure used for preparing solutions. Scales for measuring grams are rarely found in the clinical area or the home environment. Volume (in milliliters) is the common measurement of drugs for administration. Drugs that are powders, crystals, or liquids are measured in graduated measuring cups with metric, apothecary, or household units. The milliliter, although a volume measure, can be substituted for a gram, a measure of mass, because at 4° C, 1 mL of water weighs 1 g. Mass and volume differ with the type of substance; thus grams and milliliters are not exact equivalents in all instances, but they can be accepted as approximate values for preparation of solutions.

Calculating a Solution From a Ratio

To obtain a solution from a ratio, use the proportion or fraction method.

EXAMPLES **PROBLEM 1:** Prepare 500 mL of a 1 : 100 vinegar-water solution for a vaginal douche.

$$Known\ drug : Known\ volume :: Desired\ drug : Desired\ volume$$
$$1\,mL \quad : \quad 100\,mL \quad :: \quad X\,mL \quad : \quad 500\,mL$$
$$100\,X = 500$$
$$X = 5\,mL$$

or

$$\frac{Known\ drug}{Known\ volume} = \frac{Desired\ drug}{Desired\ volume}$$

$$\frac{1\,mL}{100\,mL} = \frac{X}{500\,mL}$$

$$100\,X = 500$$

$$X = 5\,mL$$

Answer: 5 mL of vinegar added to 500 mL of water is a 1 : 100 vinegar-water solution.
Note: Five milliliters did not increase the volume of the solution by a large amount. When volume and volume solutions are mixed, the total amount of *desired volume* should not be exceeded. Therefore it is important to determine the volume of desired drug first, then remove that volume from the appropriate amount of solvent (solution). When mixing the solution, begin with the desired drug and add the premeasured solvent. This process ensures that the solution has an accurate concentration.

PROBLEM 2: Prepare 100 mL of a 1 : 4 hydrogen peroxide 3% and normal saline mouthwash.

$$\text{Known drug : Known volume :: Desired drug : Desired volume}$$
$$1 \text{ mL} \quad : \quad 4 \text{ mL} \quad :: \quad X \text{ mL} \quad : \quad 100 \text{ mL}$$
$$4X = 100 \text{ mL}$$
$$X = 25 \text{ mL}$$

25 mL of hydrogen peroxide 3% is the amount of desired drug. To calculate the amount of normal saline, use the following formula:

$$\text{Desired volume} - \text{Desired drug} = \text{Desired solvent}$$
$$100 \text{ mL} \quad - \quad 25 \text{ mL} \quad = \quad 75 \text{ mL}$$

Answer: 75 mL of saline and 25 mL of hydrogen peroxide 3% make 100 mL of a 1 : 4 mouthwash.

Calculating a Solution From a Percentage

To obtain a solution from a percentage, use the same formula with either the proportion or fraction method.

EXAMPLE   Prepare 1000 mL of a 0.9% NaCl solution.

$$\text{Known drug : Known volume :: Desired drug : Desired volume}$$
$$0.9 \text{ g} \quad : \quad 100 \text{ mL} \quad :: \quad X \text{ g} \quad : \quad 1000 \text{ mL}$$
$$100X = 900$$
$$X = 9 \text{ g or } 9 \text{ mL}$$

Answer: 9 g or 9 mL of NaCl in 1000 mL makes a 0.9% NaCl solution.

PREPARING A WEAKER SOLUTION FROM A STRONGER SOLUTION

When a situation requires the preparation of a weaker solution from a stronger solution, the amount of desired drug must be determined. The known variables are the desired solution, the available or on-hand solution, and the desired volume. The formula can be set up with the strength of the solutions expressed in either ratio or percentage. The proportion method or the fractional method can be used to solve the problem. The first ratio or fraction, the desired solution (weaker solution), is the numerator, and the available or on-hand solution (stronger solution) is the denominator.

Desired solution: Available solution :: Desired drug: Desired volume

or

$$\frac{\text{Desired solution}}{\text{Available solution}} = \frac{\text{Desired drug}}{\text{Desired volume}}$$

EXAMPLES Prepare 500 mL of a 2.5% aluminum acetate solution from a 5% aluminum acetate solution. Use water as the solvent.

$$2.5\% \; : \; 5\% \; :: X : 500 \text{ mL}$$

$$2.5 \text{ mL}: 5 \text{ mL}:: X : 500 \text{ mL}$$

$$5 X = 1250$$

$$X = 250 \text{ mL}$$

Answer: Use 250 mL of 5% aluminum acetate to make 500 mL of 2.5% aluminum acetate solution.

Determine the amount of water needed.

$$\text{Desired volume} - \text{Desired drug} = \text{Desired solvent}$$

$$500 \text{ mL} \quad - \quad 250 \text{ mL} \quad = \quad 250 \text{ mL}$$

or

Same problem using the fractional method:

$$\frac{2.5\%}{5\%} \times \frac{X}{500 \text{ mL}} =$$

$$5 X = 1250$$

$$X = 250 \text{ mL of 5\% aluminum acetate}$$

or

Same problem but stated as a ratio:

Prepare 500 mL of a 1: 40 aluminum acetate solution from a 1: 20 aluminum acetate solution with water as the solvent.

$$\frac{1}{40} : \frac{1}{20} :: X : 500 \text{ mL}$$

$$\frac{1}{20}X = \frac{500}{40}$$

$$X = \frac{500}{\underset{2}{\cancel{40}}} \times \frac{\overset{1}{\cancel{20}}}{1} = \frac{500}{2}$$

$$X = 250 \text{ mL of 5\% aluminum acetate solution}$$

Guidelines for Home Solutions

For solutions prepared by patients in the home, directions need to be very specific and in written form, if possible. People often think that more is better. Teach the patient that solutions can be dangerous if they are too concentrated. Higher concentrations of solutions can irritate tissues and prevent the desired effect. Recommend that standard measuring spoons and cups be used rather than tableware. Level measures rather than heaping measures of dry solutes should be used. Utensils and containers for solution preparation should be *clean or sterilized by boiling* if used for infants. Mixing acidic solutions in aluminum containers should be avoided, especially if the solution is for oral use. Although there is no evidence of toxicity, a metallic taste is noticeable. Glass, enamel, or plastic containers can be used. Solutions should be made fresh daily or just before use. Oral solutions, especially for infants, require refrigeration; topical solutions do not.

When preparing the solution, start with the desired drug and then add the solvent. This helps to disperse the drug and ensures that the desired volume of solution is not exceeded. If the volume of solvent is several liters, then it is not always practical to subtract a small volume of solute.

Solution problems are best calculated within the metric system. Fractional and percentage dosages are difficult to determine within the household system.

PRACTICE PROBLEMS ▶ III PREPARING A WEAKER SOLUTION FROM A STRONGER ONE

Answers can be found on pages 385 to 387.

Identify the known variables and choose the appropriate formula. Perform calculations needed to obtain the following solutions using the metric system. Use Table 17.1 to obtain the household equivalent.

1. Prepare 250 mL of a 0.9% NaCl and sterile water solution for nose drops.

2. Prepare 250 mL of a 5% glucose and sterile water solution for an infant feeding.

3. Prepare 1000 mL of a 25% Betadine solution with sterile saline for a foot soak.

4. Prepare 2 L of a 2% Lysol solution for cleaning a changing area.

5. Prepare 20 L of a 2% sodium bicarbonate solution for a bath.

6. Prepare 100 mL of a 50% hydrogen peroxide 3% and water solution for a mouthwash.

7. Prepare 500 mL of a modified Dakin's solution 0.5% from a 5% sodium hypochlorite solution with sterile water as the solvent.

8. Prepare 1500 mL of a 0.9% NaCl solution for an enema.

9. Prepare 2 L of a 1: 1000 Neosporin bladder irrigation with sterile saline. (Omit the household conversion.)

10. Determine how much alcohol is needed for a 3:1 alcohol and white vinegar solution for an external ear irrigation. Vinegar 30 mL is used. Solve using the proportion method.

11. Prepare 1000 mL of a 1: 10 sodium hypochlorite and water solution for cleaning.

12. Prepare 1000 mL of a 3% sodium hypochlorite and water solution.

13. Prepare 2000 L of a 1:9 Lysol solution to clean colorfast linens soiled with body fluids. (Omit the household conversion.)

14. Prepare 6 L of a 1: 1200 bleach bath solution, using household bleach and water, for eczema. Determine how much bleach is needed.

15. Prepare a 0.12% bleach bath solution, using household bleach and 20 gallons of water, to reduce methicillin-resistant *Staphylococcus aureus* (MRSA) colonization. Determine how much bleach is needed.

HYDRATION MANAGEMENT

Calculate Daily Fluid Intake for an Adult

Hydration problems normally increase with age as total body water is lost when muscle mass decreases. With aging, the sensation of thirst diminishes and the physiological response to dehydration is not sufficient to meet metabolic needs. Kidney function begins to decline in middle age, slowly decreasing the ability of the kidney to concentrate urine, resulting in increasing water loss. Add health care problems, such as dementia and diabetes, along with commonly used medication that increases fluid loss, such as diuretics and laxatives, and dehydration is a real risk.

Dehydration can exacerbate problems such as urinary tract and respiratory tract infections but can cause more subtle problems in the elderly, such as confusion, decreased cognitive function, incontinence, constipation, and falls. All elderly adults, especially those over 85 years old, should be assessed for dehydration on the basis of physical assessment, laboratory data, cognitive assessment, pattern of fluid intake, and medical condition. Once daily fluid intake is established, nursing measures can be taken to maintain an adequate hydration.

Standard Formula for Daily Fluid Intake*

100 mL/kg for the first 10 kg of weight

50 mL/kg for the next 10 kg of weight

15 mL/kg for the remaining kg

The standard formula includes fluid contained in foods. To determine how much liquid alone an adult needs to consume, multiply the daily fluid intake by 75%.

EXAMPLE Adult weight is 94 kg

$$\frac{-10 \text{ kg}}{84 \text{ kg}} \times 100 \text{ mL} = 1000 \text{ mL}$$

$$\frac{-10 \text{ kg}}{74 \text{ kg}} \times \frac{50 \text{ mL} = 500 \text{ mL}}{15 \text{ mL} = \underline{1110 \text{ mL}}}$$

$$2610 \text{ mL}$$

2610 mL × 75% = 2610 × 0.75 = **1957.5 or 1958 mL fluid/day**

---

*Adapted from Skipper, A. (Ed.) (1998). *Dietitians handbook of enteral and parenteral nutrition*. Rockville, Maryland: Aspen Publishers.

Calculate Daily Fluid Intake for a Febrile Adult

When an adult is febrile, the need for fluids increases by 6% for each degree over normal temperature. For example, a 94-kg adult with an oral temperature of 100.8° F, 2° above normal, needs a 12% increase in fluid. To find the increase, multiply the fluid/day, 1958 mL, by the percent increase, 12%, and add that to the total fluid/day.

$$1958 \text{ mL} \times 12\% = 1958 \times 0.12 = 234.9 \text{ or } 235 \text{ mL}$$
$$1958 \text{ mL} + 235 \text{ mL} = 2193 \text{ mL}$$

PRACTICE PROBLEMS ▶ IV HYDRATION MANAGEMENT

Answers can be found on pages 387 to 388.

1. Calculate the standard formula, then the fluid need of an adult weighing 84 kg.

2. Calculate the standard formula, then the fluid need of an adult weighing 63 kg.

3. Calculate the standard formula, then the fluid need of an adult weighing 70 kg.

4. Calculate the standard formula, then the fluid need of an adult weighing 100 kg.

5. Calculate the standard formula, then the fluid need of an adult weighing 69 kg with a fever of 101° F.

BODY MASS INDEX (BMI)

The importance of weight for the determination of overall health status and drug therapy must be emphasized. The current international standard is "body mass index" for adults and children as the criteria for healthy weight, overweight, and obese persons.

Body mass index (BMI) is a weight-for-height index that takes the place of previously used height and weight tables. BMI is a part of health assessments and is used as an indicator of risk factors for chronic diseases.

Calculate Body Mass Index Using Two Formulas

a. BMI pounds and inches formula:

$$\frac{\text{Weight in pounds}}{(\text{Height in inches})(\text{Height in inches})} \times 703$$

EXAMPLE   A person who weighs 165 pounds and is 6 ft 1 inch (73 inches) has a BMI of:

$$\frac{165}{73 \times 73} \times 703 = 21.8 \text{ BMI}$$

b. BMI metric formula:

$$\frac{\text{Weight in kg}}{(\text{Height in meters})(\text{Height in meters})}$$

EXAMPLE   A person who weighs 165 pounds and is 6 ft 1 inch (73 inches) has a BMI of:

$$73 \text{ inches} \times 0.0254 \text{ meters} = 1.854 \text{ meters}$$
$$165 \text{ lbs} \div 2.2 \text{ kg} = 75 \text{ kg}$$
$$\frac{75}{(1.854)(1.854)} = \frac{75}{3.437} = 21.8 \text{ BMI}$$

PRACTICE PROBLEMS ▶ V BODY MASS INDEX

Answers can be found on page 388.

1. What is the BMI for a female weighing 208 lbs and who is 5 ft 2?
2. What is the BMI for a male weighing 198 lbs and who is 5 ft 11?
3. What is the BMI for a female weighing 112 lbs and who is 5 ft 4 inches tall?
4. What is the BMI for a male weighing 165 lbs and who is 6 ft 1 inch tall?
5. What is the BMI for a male weighing 60 lbs with a height of 3 ft 10 inches?

ANSWERS

I Metric to Household Conversion

1. Bismuth subsalicylate 15 mL = 1 T; no more than 8 T in 24 hr
2. Ceclor 5 mL = 1 t
3. Tylenol elixir 1.25 mL = $\frac{1}{4}$ t
4. Maalox 30 mL = 2 T
5. Neo-Calglucon 7.5 mL = $1\frac{1}{2}$ t
6. Gani-Tuss NR 10 mL = 2 t
7. Castor oil 60 mL = 4 T or $\frac{1}{4}$ c
8. Metamucil 5 g = 1 t
9. Dilantin-30 pediatric suspension 10 mL = 2 t

10. H_2O 1 L = 1 qt
    Sugar 30 g = 2 T
    Salt 1.25 g = $\frac{1}{4}$ t
    Lite salt 2.5 g = $\frac{1}{2}$ t
    Baking soda 2.5 g = $\frac{1}{2}$ t
11. H_2O 500 mL = 1 pt
    Table salt 5 mL = 1 t
    Baking soda 5 mL = 1 t
12. Benadryl 50 mg/10 mL = 2 t
    Maalox 10 mL = 2 t
13. Belladonna/phenobarbital elixir, 10 mL = 2 t
    Maalox 30 mL = 2 T
    Viscous lidocaine 10 mL = 2 t

II Preparing a Solution Of a Desired Concentration

1. 4:1 = X:100
   X = 400
   $\frac{400}{100}$, 400%
2. 2:1 = X:100
   X = 200
   $\frac{200}{100}$, 200%
3. 1:50 = X:100
   50 X = 100
   X = 2
   $\frac{2}{100}$, 2%

4. 1:3 = X:100
   3 X = 100
   X = 33.3
   $\frac{33.3}{100}$, 33.3%
5. 1:1000 = X:100
   1000 X = 100
   X = 0.1
   $\frac{0.1}{100}$, 0.1%
6. 1:10,000 = X:100
   10,000 X = 100
   X = 0.01
   $\frac{1}{10,000}$, 0.01%

7. $1:4 = X:100$
   $4X = 100$
   $X = 25$
   $\dfrac{25}{100}, 25\%$

8. $1:5000 = X:100$
   $5000X = 100$
   $X = 0.02$
   $\dfrac{0.02}{100}, 0.02\%$

9. $1:200 = X:100$
   $200X = 100$
   $X = 0.5$
   $\dfrac{0.5}{100}, 0.5\%$

10. $1:10 = X:100$
   $10X = 100$
   $X = 10$
   $\dfrac{10}{100}, 10\%$

III Preparing a Weaker Solution From a Stronger One

1. Known drug: 0.9% NaCl
   Known volume: 100 mL
   Desired drug: X
   Desired volume: 250 mL

$0.9:100::X:250$
$100X = 225$
$X = 2.25$ mL

2.25 mL of NaCl in 250 mL of water yields a 0.9% NaCl solution. Household equivalents are approximately $^1/_2$ teaspoon salt and 1 cup sterile water.

2. Known drug: 5% glucose (sugar)
   Known volume: 100 mL
   Desired drug: X
   Desired volume: 250 mL

$5:100::X:250$
$100X = 1250$
$X = 12.5$ mL

12.5 mL of sugar in 250 mL of water yields a 5% glucose solution. Household equivalents are approximately 1 tablespoon in 1 cup of sterile water.

3. Known drug: 25% Betadine
   Known volume: 100 mL
   Desired drug: X
   Desired volume: 1000 mL

$25:100::X:1000$
$100X = 25,000$
$X = 250$ mL
1000 mL $- 250$ mL $= 750$ mL

250 mL of Betadine in 750 mL saline yields a 25% Betadine solution. Household equivalents are 1 cup Betadine in 3 cups sterile saline.

4. Known drug: 2% Lysol
   Known volume: 100 mL
   Desired drug: X
   Desired volume: 2 L = 2000 mL

$2:100::X:2000$ mL
$100X = 4000$
$X = 40$ mL

40 mL of Lysol in 2 L of water yields a 2% Lysol solution. Household equivalents are 2 tablespoons and 2 teaspoons (40 mL) of Lysol to 2 quarts or $^1/_2$ gallon of water.

5. Known drug: 2% sodium bicarbonate
   Known volume: 100 mL
   Desired drug: X
   Desired volume: 20,000 mL

$2:100::X:20,000$ mL
$100X = 40,000$
$X = 400$ mL or 400 g

400 mL or 400 g of sodium bicarbonate (baking soda) in 20,000 mL of water yields a 2% sodium bicarbonate solution. Household equivalents are $1^1/_2$ cups and 2 tablespoons baking soda in 5 gallons of water.

6. Known drug: 50% hydrogen peroxide   50:100::X:100
   Known volume: 100 mL   100 X = 5000
   Desired drug: X   X = 50 mL
   Desired volume: 100 mL   100 mL − 50 mL = 50 mL

50 mL of hydrogen peroxide 3% in 50 mL water yields a 50% solution. Household equivalents are approximately 3 tablespoons of hydrogen peroxide 3% in 3 tablespoons of water.

7. Known drug: 0.5%   0.5:5::X:500
   Available solution: 5%   5 X = 250
   Desired drug: X   X = 50 mL
   Desired volume: 500 mL   500 mL − 50 mL = 450 mL

50 mL of 5% sodium hypochlorite in 450 mL sterile water yields a 0.5% modified Dakin's solution. Household equivalents are 3 tablespoons and 1 teaspoon of Dakin's solution in 1 pint minus 3 tablespoons of water.

8. Known drug: 0.9%   0.9:100::X:1500
   Known volume: 100 mL   100 X = 1350
   Desired drug: X   X = 13.5 mL
   Desired volume: 1500 mL

13.5 mL of NaCl in 1500 mL water yields a 0.9% NaCl solution. Household equivalents are $2\frac{1}{2}$ teaspoons of salt in $1\frac{1}{2}$ quarts of water.

9. Known drug: 1 mL   1:1000::X:2000
   Known volume: 1000 mL   1000 X = 2000
   Desired drug: X   X = 2 mL
   Desired volume: 2000 mL

2 mL of Neosporin irrigant in 2000 mL of sterile saline yields a 1:1000 solution for continuous bladder irrigation. This treatment is done primarily in the clinical setting.

10. Use ratio and proportion to solve this problem.
   3:1::X:30 mL
     X = 90 mL

Add 90 mL of alcohol to 30 mL of vinegar to yield a 3:1 solution for an external ear wash. Household equivalents are 6 tablespoons of alcohol and 2 tablespoons of vinegar.

11. Known drug: 1 mL   1:10::X:1000
   Known volume: 10 mL   10 X = 1000
   Desired drug: X   X = 100 mL
   Desired volume: 1000 mL   1000 mL − 100 mL = 900 mL

100 mL of sodium hypochlorite (bleach) in 900 mL water yields a 1:10 sodium hypochlorite solution. Household equivalents are $\frac{1}{3}$ cup and 2 tablespoons sodium hypochlorite in approximately 1 quart minus $\frac{1}{3}$ cup and 2 tablespoons of water.

12. Known drug: 3 mL   3:100::X:1000
   Known volume: 100 mL   100 X = 3000
   Desired drug: X   X = 30 mL
   Desired volume: 1000 mL   1000 mL − 30 mL = 970 mL

30 mL of sodium hypochlorite (bleach) in 970 mL water yields a 3% sodium hypochlorite solution. Household equivalents are 2 tablespoons in 1 quart minus 2 tablespoons of water.

13. Use ratio and proportion to solve this problem.

$$1:9::X:2000 \text{ mL}$$
$$9 X = 2000 \text{ mL}$$
$$X = 222 \text{ mL}$$

Desired volume $-$ Desired drug $=$ Desired solvent
2000 mL $-$ 222 mL $= 1778$ mL

222 mL of Lysol in 1778 mL of water yields a 1:9 cleansing solution for colorfast linens soiled with body fluids.

14. Use ratio and proportion to solve this problem.

$$1:1200::X:6000 \text{ mL}$$
$$1200 X = 6000$$
$$X = 5 \text{ mL}$$

5 mL of household bleach in 6 L of water yields a 1:1200 bleach bath solution for eczema.

15. Convert gallons to liters.
1 gallon $= 4$ liters
20 gallons $\times$ 4 liters/gallon $= 80$ liters

Use ratio and proportion to solve this problem.

$$0.12 \text{ mL}:0.1 \text{ L}::X:80 \text{ L}$$
$$0.1 X = 9.6$$
$$X = 96 \text{ mL or } 3\frac{1}{4} \text{ ounces}$$

$3\frac{1}{4}$ ounces of bleach in 20 gallons of water yields a 0.12% bleach bath solution for MRSA decolonization.

IV Hydration Management

1. Adult weight is 84 kg

$$\underline{-10 \text{ kg}} \times 100 \text{ mL} = 1000 \text{ mL}$$
$$74 \text{ kg}$$
$$\underline{-10 \text{ kg}} \times 50 \text{ mL} = 500 \text{ mL}$$
$$64 \text{ kg} \times 15 \text{ mL} = \underline{960 \text{ mL}}$$
$$2460 \text{ mL}$$

2460 mL $\times$ 75% $=$ 2460 $\times$ 0.75 $=$ 1845 mL per day

2. Adult weight is 63 kg

$$\underline{-10 \text{ kg}} \times 100 \text{ mL} = 1000 \text{ mL}$$
$$53 \text{ kg}$$
$$\underline{-10 \text{ kg}} \times 50 \text{ mL} = 500 \text{ mL}$$
$$43 \text{ kg} \times 15 \text{ mL} = \underline{645 \text{ mL}}$$
$$2145 \text{ mL}$$

2145 mL $\times$ 75% $=$ 2145 $\times$ 0.75 $=$ 1608.75 or 1609 mL per day

3. Adult weight is 70 kg

$$\underline{-10 \text{ kg}} \times 100 \text{ mL} = 1000 \text{ mL}$$
$$60 \text{ kg}$$
$$\underline{-10 \text{ kg}} \times 50 \text{ mL} = 500 \text{ mL}$$
$$50 \text{ kg} \times 15 \text{ mL} = \underline{750 \text{ mL}}$$
$$2250 \text{ mL}$$

$$2250 \text{ mL} \times 75\% = 2250 \times 0.75 = 1687.5 \text{ or } 1688 \text{ mL per day}$$

4. Adult weight is 100 kg

$$\underline{-10 \text{ kg}} \times 100 \text{ mL} = 1000 \text{ mL}$$
$$90 \text{ kg}$$
$$\underline{-10 \text{ kg}} \times 50 \text{ mL} = 500 \text{ mL}$$
$$80 \text{ kg} \times 15 \text{ mL} = \underline{1200 \text{ mL}}$$
$$2700 \text{ mL}$$

$$2700 \text{ mL} \times 75\% = 2700 \times 0.75 = 2025 \text{ mL per day}$$

5. Adult weight is 69 kg

$$\underline{-10 \text{ kg}} \times 100 \text{ mL} = 1000 \text{ mL}$$
$$59 \text{ kg}$$
$$\underline{-10 \text{ kg}} \times 50 \text{ mL} = 500 \text{ mL}$$
$$49 \text{ kg} \times 15 \text{ mL} = \underline{735 \text{ mL}}$$
$$2235 \text{ mL}$$

$$2235 \text{ mL} \times 75\% = 2235 \times 0.75 = 1676 \text{ mL per day}$$

$6\% \times 3° = 18\%$ for increased temperature
$1676 \text{ mL} \times 18\% = 1676 \times 0.18 = 301.6 \text{ or } 302 \text{ mL}$
$1676 \text{ mL} + 302 \text{ mL} = 1978 \text{ mL per day}$

V Body Mass Index

1. 5 feet 2 inches = 62 inches ($12 \times 5 = 60$ inches $+ 2$ inches $= 62$ inches)

$$\frac{208}{(62)(62)} \times 703 = \frac{208}{3844} \times 703 = 0.054 \times 703 = 38 \text{ BMI}$$

2. 5 feet 11 inches = 71 inches

$$\frac{198}{(71)(71)} \times 703 = \frac{198}{5041} \times 703 = 0.039 \times 703 = 27.4 \text{ BMI}$$

3. 5 feet 4 inches = 64 inches

$$\frac{112}{(64)(64)} \times 703 = \frac{112}{4096} \times 703 = 0.027 \times 703 = 19 \text{ BMI}$$

4. 6 feet 1 inch = 73 inches

$$\frac{165}{(73)(73)} \times 703 = \frac{165}{5329} \times 703 = 0.031 \times 703 = 21.8 \text{ BMI}$$

5. 3 feet 10 inches = 46 inches

$$\frac{60}{(46)(46)} \times 703 = \frac{60}{2116} \times 703 = 0.028 \times 703 = 19.7 \text{ BMI}$$

NGN® PREP

1. A multi-generational family with a member, who has contracted a highly contagious virus, wants information regarding how to clean and disinfect their home to prevent the spread of the virus to the rest of the family. They all share one bathroom. It is known that a 2 : 100 household bleach solution from 5-9% household bleach and water will disinfect and kill the virus on hard surfaces such as toilet seat, sink, fixtures and doorknobs.

Choose the most likely option for the information missing from the statement below by selecting from the lists of options provided.

As the home health care nurse, you instruct the family to mix __A__ of household bleach or __B__ teaspoons, with __C__ of water or __D__, for cleaning.

Option A	Option B	Option C	Option D
20 mL	2 teaspoons	1000 mL	32 oz
30 mL	3 teaspoons	960 mL	64 oz
40 mL	4 teaspoons	2000 mL	48 oz
50 mL	5 teaspoons	500 mL	12 oz

2. As a home health care nurse, you are caring for a 52-year-old former homeless man with liver disease from alcoholism. He has severe onychomycosis and was instructed by his healthcare provider to soak his feet daily in a 1 : 2 white vinegar and water solution for 20 minutes. Preparation of this solution involves adding __A__ of white vinegar to 1000mL warm water. Household measure would be __B__ white vinegar to __C__ water.

Option A	Option B	Option C
250 mL	24 oz	64 oz
500 mL	16 oz	96 oz
300 mL	8 oz	32 oz
100 mL	120 z	128 oz

ANSWERS - NGN® PREP

1. **Option A:** Known Drug: Known Volume = Desired Drug: Desired volume

$$2mL : 100mL = X : 1000mL$$
$$100X = 2000$$
$$X = 20mL$$

Option B: 1 teaspoon = 5mL

$$20ml \div 5mL/teaspoon = 4 \text{ teaspoons}$$

Option C: 1000mL provides enough disinfecting solution for 24hours.

Option D: 1000mL ÷ 30mL/oz = 33oz, or 32oz or 1 quart

2. Option A: Known Drug: Known Volume :: Desired Drug: Desired Volume

$$1 \quad : \quad 2 \quad :: \quad X \quad : \quad 1000mL$$

$$2X = 1000mL$$

$$X = 500mL$$

Option B:

$$\frac{500mL}{30mL/oz} = 16.6 \text{ or } 16oz$$

Option C:

$$\frac{1000mL}{30mL/oz} = 33.3 \text{ or } 32oz$$

PART V

POST-TEST: ORAL PREPARATIONS, INJECTABLES, INTRAVENOUS, AND PEDIATRICS

The post-test is for testing the content of Part III, Oral Preparations, Injectables (subcutaneous and intramuscular), Insulin, Intravenous, and Chapter 15, Pediatric Critical Care. The test is divided into four sections. There are 65 drug problems, which should take 1 to 1½ hours to complete. You may use a conversion table as needed. The minimum passing score is 57 correct, or 88%. If you have more than two drug problems wrong in a section of the test, return to the chapter in the book for that test section and rework the practice problems.

ORAL PREPARATIONS

Answers can be found on pages 418 to 420.

1. Order: nifedipine (Adalat CC) 60 mg, po, daily for 1 week; then 90 mg, po, daily.
   Drug available:

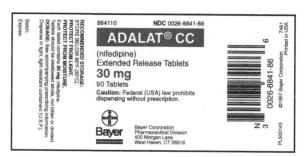 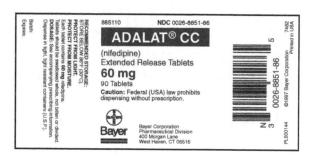

   a. Which Adalat CC container would you use for the first week?_____

   b. Explain how you would give 90 mg._____

2. Order: Crestor (rosuvastatin calcium)
   10 mg, po, daily at bedtime.
   Drug available:

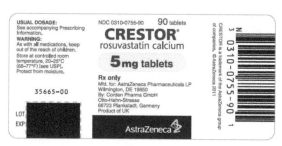

   a. How many tablet(s) would you give? _____

   b. When is/are the tablet(s) given? _____

3. Order: pravastatin sodium (Pravachol) 20 mg, po, at bedtime.

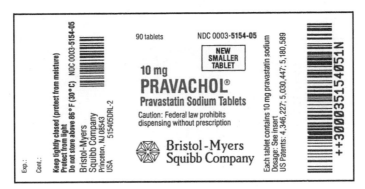

How many tablets of Pravachol should the patient receive? _____

4. Order: nitroglycerin (Nitrostat) gr 1/200, SL, STAT.
Drug available:

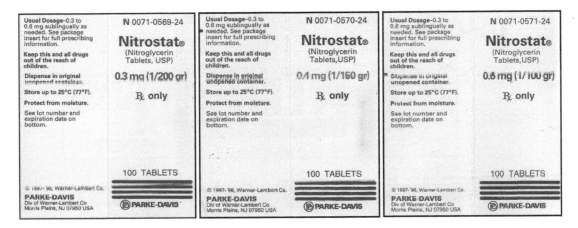

This drug dosage is ordered in the apothecary system, but the metric dosage is also on the drug label.

The drug is available in three different strengths. Which drug label would you select? Why?

_____

5. Order: clorazepate dipotassium (Tranxene) 7.5 mg in AM and 15 mg, po, at bedtime.
Drug available:

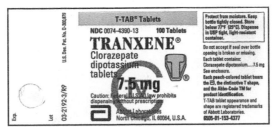

a. How many tablet(s) should the patient receive in the AM? _____

b. How many tablets should the patient receive at bedtime? _____

6. Order: clarithromycin (Biaxin) 0.5 g, bid × 10 days, po.
Drug available:

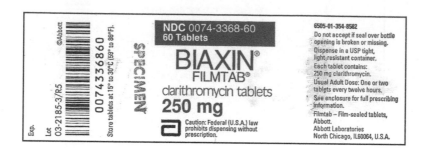

    a. 0.5 gram is equivalent to _____ milligrams.

    b. How many tablets would you give per dose? _____

7. Order: acetaminophen (Tylenol) 650 mg, po, prn, for headache.
Drug available:

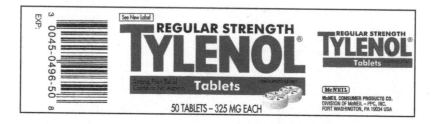

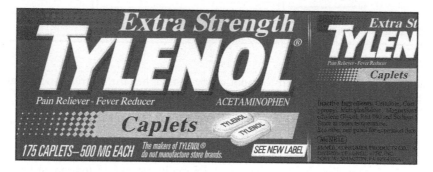

    a. Which Tylenol bottle would you select? _____

    b. How many tablets or caplets should the patient receive? _____

8. Order: allopurinol (Zyloprim) 0.2 g, po, bid.
   Drug available:

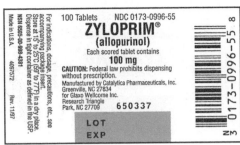

    a. 0.2 g is equivalent to_____milligrams.

    b. The patient should receive how many tablets of allopurinol per dose? _____

9. Order: prochlorperazine (Compazine) 10 mg, po, tid.
   Drug available:

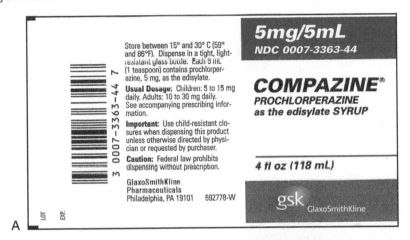

    a. Which Compazine bottle would you select? Why? _____

    b. How many milliliters would you give? _____

10. Order: olanzapine (Zyprexa) 10 mg, po, daily.
    Drug available:

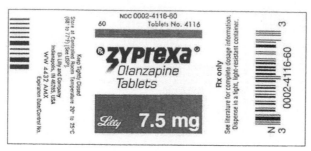

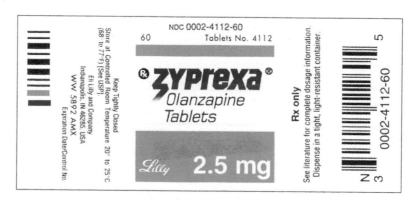

a. Which Zyprexa bottle would you select? Why? _____

b. How many tablet(s) would you give? _____

11. Order: Synthroid (levothyroxine) 0.0375 mg, po, daily.
    Drug available:

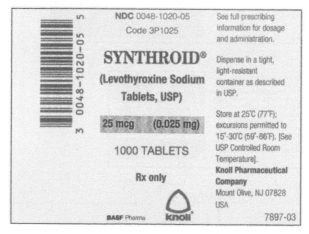 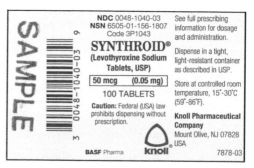

a. The micrograms for 0.0375 mg would be? _____

b. Which Synthroid bottle would you select? _____

c. How many tablet(s) would you give per day? _____

12. Order: cefuroxime axetil (Ceftin) 500 mg, po, q12h.
Drug available:

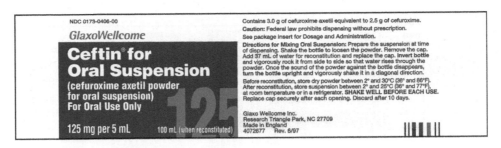

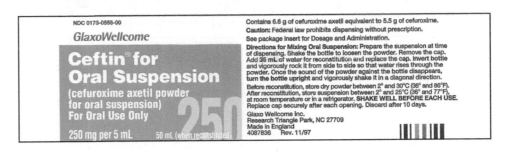

a. Which Ceftin bottle would you select? Explain _____

b. The patient would receive how many grams _____ or milligrams _____ of Ceftin per day?

c. How many milliliters should the patient receive per dose? _____

13. Order: cefaclor (Ceclor) 250 mg, po, q8h.
Drug available:

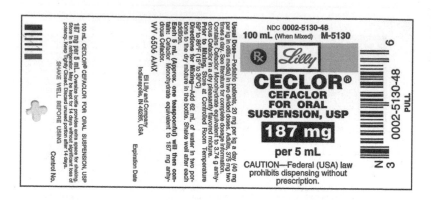

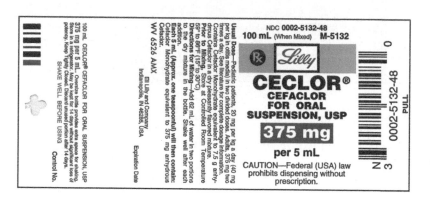

a. Which Ceclor bottle would you select? _____

b. How many milliliters should the patient receive per dose? _____

c. Is there another solution to this drug problem? _____

14. Order: simvastatin (Zocor) 40 mg, po, daily.
Drug available:

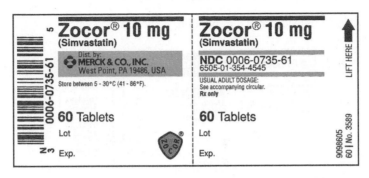

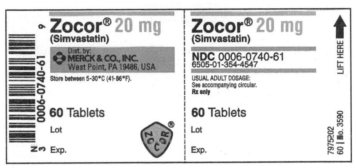

    a. Which Zocor bottle would you select? Why? _____

    b. How many tablets should the patient receive? _____

15. Order: ziprasidone (Geodon) 40 mg, po, bid.
After a week (7 days later) 60 mg, po, bid.
Drug available:

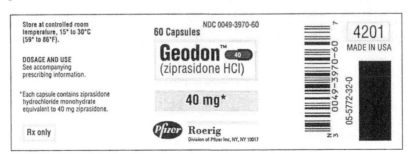

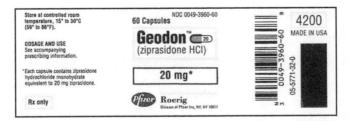

    a. Which Geodon bottle(s) would you select to give 40 mg? _____

    b. How many Geodon capsule(s) would you give for 40 mg per dose per day? _____

    c. Which Geodon bottle(s) would you select to give 60 mg per dose? _____

    d. How many Geodon capsule(s) from which bottle would you give per dose? _____

    Per day? _____

16. Order: Amoxil (amoxicillin) 0.4 g, po, q8h.
Drug available:

    a. Change grams into milligrams: 0.4 grams = _____milligrams.

    b. How many milligrams should the patient receive per dose? _____

    c. How many milliliters should the patient receive? _____

17. Order: lamivudine (Epivir) 150 mg, po, q12h.
Drug available:

    a. How many milligrams would you give per day? _____

    b. How many milliliters would you give per dose? _____

18. Order: etretinate (Tegison) 0.75 mg/kg/day, po, in two divided doses. Patient weighs 150 pounds.
Drug available: Tegison 10-mg and 25-mg capsules.

    a. How many kilograms does the patient weigh? _____

    b. How many milligrams of Tegison should the patient receive per day? _____

    c. Which bottle of Tegison would you select and how many capsules of Tegison per dose?

    _____

19. Order: theophylline 5 mg/kg/LD (loading dose), po. Patient weighs 70 kg.
Drug available: Oral solution 80 mg/15 mL and 150 mg/15 mL.

    a. How milligrams should the patient receive? _____

    b. Which oral solution bottle would you select? _____

    c. How many milliliters of theophylline should the patient receive as a loading dose?

    _____

20. Order: docusate sodium (Colace) 100 mg, po, bid per NG (nasogastric) tube.
Drug available: Colace 50 mg/5 mL. Osmolality of docusate sodium is 3900 mOsm. The desired osmolality is 500 mOsm.

    a. How many milliliters of Colace should the client receive? _____

    b. How much water dilution is needed to obtain the desired osmolality? _____

INJECTABLES

Answers can be found on pages 421 to 423.

21. Order: hydroxyzine (Vistaril) 25 mg, deep IM, STAT.
Drug available: (50 mg = 1 mL)

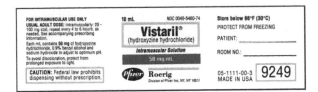

How many milliliters of Vistaril would you give? _____

22. Order: digoxin (Lanoxin) 0.25 mg, IM, daily.
Drug available:

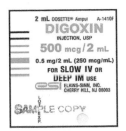

How many milliliters of digoxin would you give per dose? _____

23. Order: meperidine (Demerol) 40 mg and atropine sulfate 0.5 mg, IM, STAT.
Drug available:

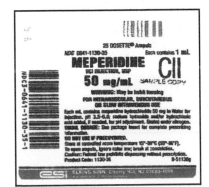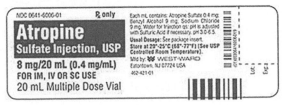

    a. How many milliliters of meperidine and how many milliliters of atropine would you administer?

_____

    b. Explain how the two drugs would be mixed. _____

24. Order: heparin 2500 units, subcut, q6h.
Drug available:

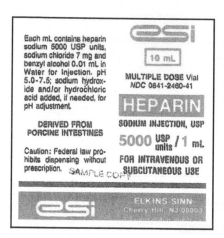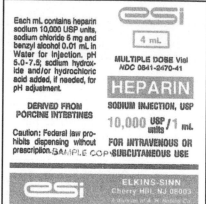

a. Which heparin would you use? _____

b. How many milliliters of heparin should the patient receive? _____

25. Order: Lovenox (enovaparin sodium) 20 mg, subcut, q12h.
Drug available:

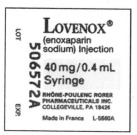

How many milliliters would you give? _____

26. Order: naloxone (Narcan) 0.5 mg, IM, STAT.
Drug available:

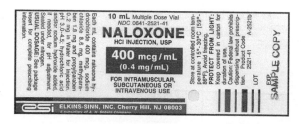

How many milliliters of naloxone should the patient receive? _____

27. Order: Humulin 70/30 insulin 35 units, subcut, in AM.
Drug available:

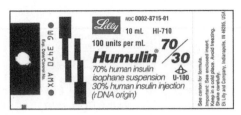

Indicate on the unit-100 insulin syringe how many units of 70/30 insulin should be given.

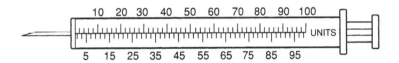

28. Order: Humulin N insulin 45 units and Humulin R (regular) 10 units.

a. Explain the method for mixing the two insulins.

_____

b. Mark on the unit-100 insulin syringe how much Humulin R insulin and Humulin N insulin should be withdrawn.

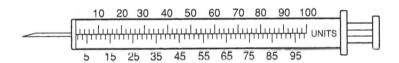

29. Order: vitamin B$_{12}$ 500 mcg, IM, 3 times a week.
Drug available:

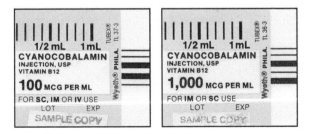

a. Which cyanocobalamin would you select? Why?

_____

b. How many milliliters would you give? _____

30. Order: morphine 8 mg IM, STAT.
Drug available:

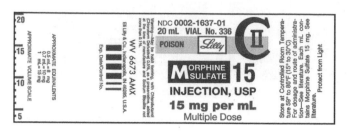

How many milliliters of morphine would you administer? _____

31. Order: phytonadione (AquaMEPHYTON) 5 mg, IM, STAT.
Drug available:

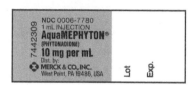

How many milliliters of AquaMEPHYTON would you administer? _____

32. Order: ranitidine HCl (Zantac) 35 mg, IM, q8h.
Drug available:

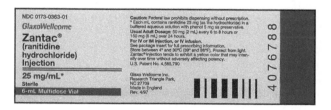

How many milliliters of Zantac should the patient receive per dose? _____

33. Order: tobramycin (Nebcin) 3 mg/kg/day, IM, in three divided doses.
Patient weighs 145 pounds.
Drug available: (80 mg = 2 mL)

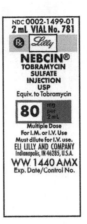

  a. How many kilograms does the patient weigh? _____

  b. How many milligrams of Nebcin should the patient receive per day? _____

  c. How many milligrams of Nebcin should the patient receive per dose? _____

  d. How many milliliters of Nebcin would you administer per dose? _____

34. Order: bethanechol chloride (Urecholine) 2.5 mg, subcut, STAT and may repeat in 1 hour.
Drug available: (Note: 5.15 mg = 5 mg or 5.15 mg = 5.2 mg [tenths])

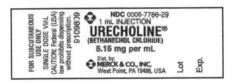

How many milliliters of Urecholine would you give? _____

35. Order: methotrexate 20 mg, IM, every other week.
Drug available:

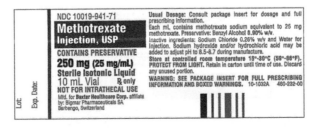

How many milliliters should the nurse administer? _____

36. Order: Tazidime (ceftazidime) 250 mg, IM, q8h.
Drug available:

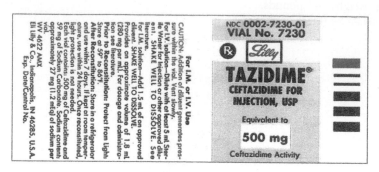

a. How much diluent would you add to the Tazidime vial? (See label.) _____

The diluent when mixed in the vial would equal _____

b. How many milligrams should the patient receive per day? _____

c. How many milliliters would you give IM per dose? _____

d. What type of syringe would you use? _____

37. Order: cefamandole (Mandol) 500 mg, IM, q12h.
Drug available:

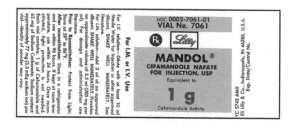

a. How much diluent would you mix with the Mandol powder? (See label for mixing.)

_____

b. How many milliliters should be given per dose? _____

38. Order: cefazolin (Ancef) 0.25 g, IM, q12h.
Mixing: Add 2.0 mL of diluent = 2.2 mL of drug solution.
Drug available:

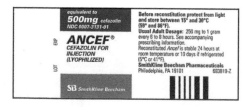

a. Change grams in order to milligrams; drug label is in milligrams. _____

b. How many milliliters of Ancef should the patient receive per dose? _____

39. Order: Rocephin (ceftriaxone) 500 mg, IM, q12h. Suggested dose: 1-2 g/day.
Drug available:

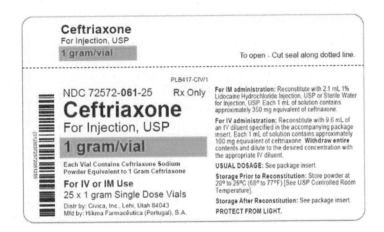

a. Is the dose per day within the suggested drug parameters? _____

Explain _____

b. How many milliliters of sterile water should be injected into the Rocephin 1-g vial? _____

c. After reconstitution, 1 mL of Rocephin solution would yield _____

d. How many mL of the Rocephin solution would you give per dose? _____

40. Order: ceftazidime (Fortaz) 750 mg, IM, q12h.
Add 2.5 mL of diluent = 3 mL of drug solution.
Drug available:

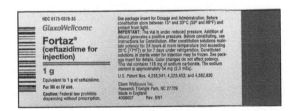

How many milliliters of ceftazidime would you administer per dose? _____

41. Order: gentamicin sulfate 4 mg/kg/day, IM, in three divided doses.
Patient weighs 165 pounds.
Drug available: gentamicin 10 mg/mL and 40 mg/mL.

a. How many kilograms does the patient weigh? _____

b. How many milligrams of gentamicin per day should the patient receive? _____

c. How many milligrams of gentamicin per dose? _____

d. Which gentamicin bottle would you select? Explain.

_____

e. How many milliliters of gentamicin per dose should the patient receive? _____

DIRECT IV ADMINISTRATION

Answers can be found on page 423.

42. Order: furosemide (Lasix) 30 mg, IV direct, STAT.
    Drug available:

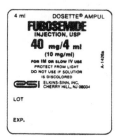

   Instruction: Direct IV infusion not to exceed 10 mg/min.

   How many milliliters should the patient receive? _____

43. Order: diltiazem (Cardizem) 15 mg, IV direct, STAT.
    Drug available:

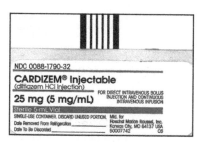

   Instruction: Direct IV infusion. Initial dose: 0.25 mg/kg over 2 minutes. Patient weighs 60 kg.

   a. How many milligrams should the patient receive? _____

   b. Is the Cardizem dose ordered within the drug parameter? _____

   c. Give the number of milliliters to administer.

   _____

INTRAVENOUS

Answers can be found on pages 424 to 425.

44. Order: 1000 mL of 5% dextrose/0.45% NaCl in 8 hours.
    Available: 1 liter of 5% D/½ NS; IV set labeled 10 gtt/mL.
    How many drops per minute should the patient receive?

   _____

45. Order: 500 mL of D₅W in 2 hours.
Available: 500 mL of D₅W; IV set labeled 15 gtt/mL.
How many drops per minute should the patient receive?

_____

46. Order: potassium chloride 20 mEq in 1000 mL in D₅W to run 8 hours.
Drug available:

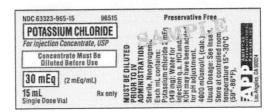

a. How many milliliters should be mixed in 1000 mL of 5% dextrose in water to be given IV over 8 hours? _____

b. How many drops per minute should the patient receive using a macrodrip IV set (10 gtt/mL)?

_____

47. Order: ticarcillin disodium (Ticar) 600 mg, IV, q6h.
Available: Calibrated cylinder (Buretrol) set with drop factor 60 gtt/mL; 500 mL D₅W.
Drug available: Add 2 mL of sterile water to yield 1 gm/2.6 mL.

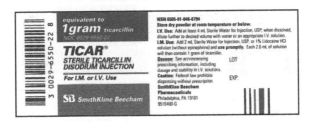

Instruction: Dilute drug in 60 mL of D₅W and infuse in 30 minutes.

a. _Drug calculation:_

_____

b. _Flow rate calculation:_

_____

48. Order: Infuse Eptifibatide 75 mg in 100 mL NS at 2 mcg/kg/min. Patient weighs 105 kg.
Available: Infusion pump.
The concentration of solution is 0.75 mg/mL.
Drug available:

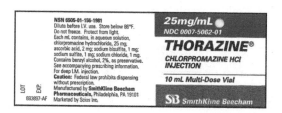

Determine the infusion rate for a specific body weight by calculating:

a. Concentration per minute_____

b. Concentration per hour_____

c. Volume per minute _____

d. Volume per hour_____

49. Order: chlorpromazine HCl (Thorazine) 50 mg, IV, to run for 4 hours.
Available: Secondary set: drop factor 15 gtt/mL; 500 mL of NS (normal saline solution)
Drug available:

Instruction: Dilute Thorazine 50 mg in 500 mL of 0.9% NaCl (NS) to run for 4 hours.

a. *Drug calculation:*

_____

b. *Flow rate calculation:*

_____

50. Order: cefoxitin (Mefoxin) 1 g, IV, q6h.
Drug available: ADD-Vantage vial

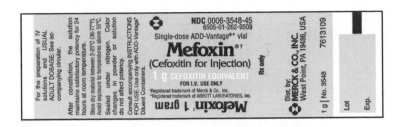

Set and solution: 50 mL of IV diluent bag for ADD-Vantage; Mefoxin 1-g vial for ADD-Vantage.
Instruction: Dilute Mefoxin in 50 mL of NaCl bag and infuse in 30 minutes.

a. How would you prepare Mefoxin 1-g powdered vial using the diluent bag? (See page 253.)

_____

b. Infusion pump rate (mL/hr): _____

For the following problems, add the drug solution to the volume of IV solution.

51. Order: cefepime HCl (Maxipime) 0.5 g, IV, q12h.
Available: Infusion pump.
Add 2.0 mL diluent — 2.5 mL.
Drug available:

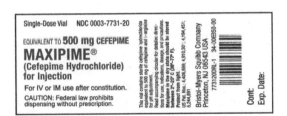

Instruction: Dilute in 50 mL of D$_5$W and infuse over 20 minutes.

a. _Drug calculation:_

_____

b. _Infusion pump rate:_

_____

52. Order: diltiazem (Cardizem) 10 mg/hr, IV for 5 hours.
Available: Infusion pump; 500 mL of D_5W.
Drug available:

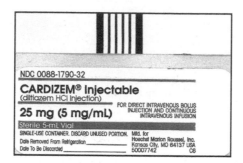

Instruction: Infuse diltiazem 10 mg/hr over 5 hours.
Drug parameter: 5-15 mg/hr for 24 hours.

a. *Drug calculation:* How many milligrams of Cardizem should the patient receive over 5 hours?

_____

b. How many milliliters of Cardizem should be mixed in the 500 mL of D_5W? _____

c. *Infusion pump rate:*

_____

53. Order: ciprofloxacin (Cipro) 100 mg, IV, q6h.
Drug available:

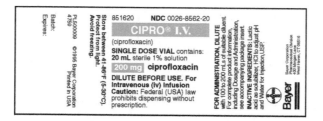

Set and solution: Secondary set with drop factor 15 gtt/mL; 100 mL of D_5W.
Instruction: Dilute drug in 100 mL of D_5W and infuse in 30 minutes; also calculate rate for infusion pump.

a. *Drug calculation:* _____

b. *Flow rate calculation* with secondary set (gtt/min): _____

c. *Infusion pump rate* (mL/hr): _____

54. Order: ifosfamide (Ifex) 1.2 g/m²/day for 5 consecutive days.
    Patient: Weight: 150 pounds; height: 70 inches = 1.98 m².
    Available: Infusion pump; 5% dextrose solution.
    Add 20 mL of diluent to 1 g of Ifex.
    Drug available:

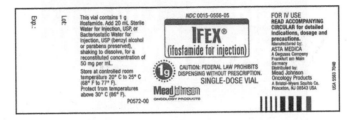

Instruction: Dilute Ifex in 50 mL of D₅W; infuse over 30 minutes.

  a. *Drug calculation:*

_____

    How many grams or milligrams of Ifex should the patient receive?

_____

  b. How much diluent would you add to 2.4 g of Ifex? _____

  c. *Infusion pump rate:*

_____

PEDIATRICS

Answers can be found on pages 425 to 427.

55. Child with heart failure.
    Order: Lanoxin (digoxin) pediatric elixir 0.4 mg, po, daily.
    Child's age and weight: 3 years, 12 kg.
    Pediatric dose range: 0.03–0.04 mg/kg.
    Drug available:

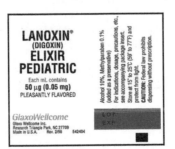

  a. Is this drug dose within the safe dosing range? _____

  b. How many milliliters would you administer? _____

56. Child with a high fever.

Order: ibuprofen (Motrin) 0.1 g, q6-8hrs, PRN for a temperature greater than 102° F.

Child's age and weight: 3 years, 15 kg.

Pediatric dose range: 100 mg, q6-8h, not to exceed 400 mg/day.

Drug available: (100 mg = 5 mL)

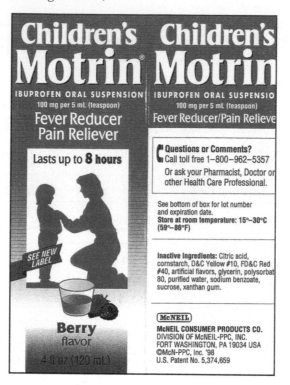

a. Is this drug dose within the safe dosing range? _____

b. How many milliliters should the child receive per dose? _____

57. Child with strep throat.

Order: penicillin V potassium (Veetids) 400,000 units, po, q6h.

Child's age and weight: 8 years, 53 pounds.

Pediatric dose range: 25,000–90,000 units/kg/day in three to six divided doses.

Drug available:

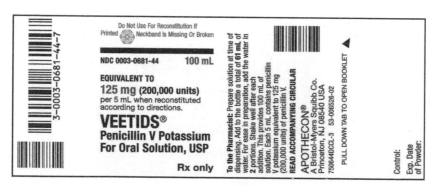

a. How many kilograms does this child weigh? _____

b. Is this drug dose within the safe dosing range? _____

c. How many milliliters of penicillin V (veetids) would you administer? _____

58. Child with otitis media.
Order: amoxicillin (Amoxil) 250 mg, po, q6h.
Child's age and weight: 5 years, 19 kg.
Pediatric dose range: 20-40 mg/kg/day in three divided doses.
Drug available:

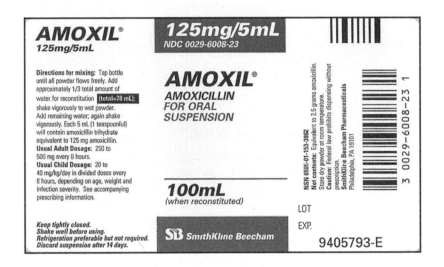

a. What are the dosing parameters for this child? _____

b. Is this drug dose within the safe dosing range? _____

c. How many milliliters would you administer? _____

59. Child with pruritus.
Order: diphenhydramine HCl (Benadryl) 25 mg, po, tid.
Child's age and weight: 2 years, 16 kg.
Pediatric dose: 5 mg/kg/day.
Drug available: Benadryl 12.5 mg/5 mL.

a. Is this drug dose within the safe dosing range? _____

b. How many milliliters would you administer? _____

60. Child with severe bacterial infection.
Order: clindamycin (Cleocin) 150 mg, po, q8h for 7 days.
Child's age and weight: 5 years, 45 pounds.
Pediatric dose range: 20-40 mg/kg/day in three divided doses.
Drug available:

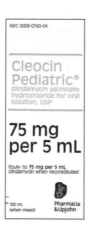

    a. How many kilograms does the child weigh? _____

    b. What are the dosage parameters for this child? _____

    c. Is this drug dose within the safe dosing range? _____

    d. How many milligrams should the child receive per day? _____

    e. How many milliliters should the child receive per dose? _____

61. Child with epilepsy.
Order: levetiracetam (Keppra) 150 mg IV q12h.
Child's age and weight: 3 years, 35 pounds.
Pediatric dose range: 20-60 mg/kg/day.
Drug available:

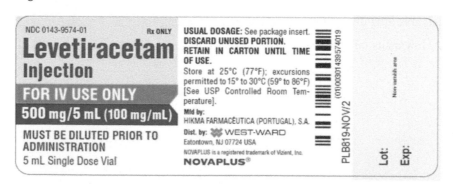

Instruction: Dilute drug in 100 mL NS and infuse over 15 minutes.

    a. How many kilograms does the child weigh? _____

    b. What are the dosing parameters for this child? _____

    c. Is this drug dose within the safe dosing range? _____

    d. How many milliliters should the child receive? _____

62. Child with severe systemic infection.
    Order: tobramycin (Nebcin) 15 mg, IV, q8h.
    Child's age and weight: 18 months, 10 kg.
    Pediatric dose range: 3-5 mg/kg/day in three divided doses.
    Drug available:

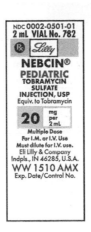

a. Is this drug dose within the safe dosing range? _____

b. How many milliliters of tobramycin would you give per dose? _____

63. Child with a severe central nervous system (CNS) infection.
    Order: ceftazidime (Fortaz) 250 mg, IV, q6h.
    Child's age and weight: 6 years, 27 kg.
    Pediatric dose range: 30-50 mg/kg/day in three divided doses.
    Add 2.0 mL of diluent = 2.4 mL of drug solution.
    Drug available:

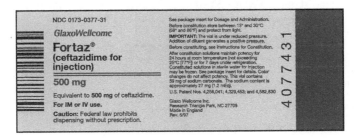

a. Is this drug dose within the safe dosing range? _____

b. How many milliliters of Fortaz would you administer? _____

64. Child with a severe urinary tract infection.
   Order: cefazolin (Ancef) 400 mg, IV, q8h.
   Child's age and weight: 5 years, 49 pounds.
   Pediatric dose range: 50-100 mg/kg/day in three divided doses.
   Drug available:

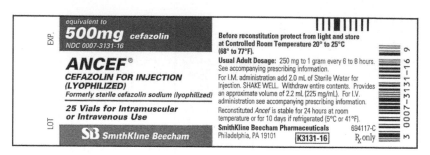

   Instruction: Mix Ancef with 1.8 mL to equal 2.0 mL = 500 mg. Buretrol: Dilute drug in 50 mL of IV diluent; infuse over 30 minutes.

   a. How many kilograms does the child weigh? _____

   b. Is this drug dose within the safe dosing range? _____

   c. How many milliliters of Ancef should be withdrawn from the vial? _____

   d. Flow rate calculation (gtt/min): _____

65. Child with a severe respiratory tract infection.
   Order: kanamycin (Kantrex) 60 mg, IV, q8h.
   Child's age and weight: 1 year, 26 pounds.
   Pediatric dose range: 15 mg/kg/day, q8-12h.
   Drug available:

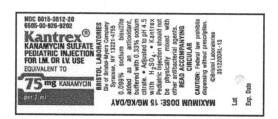

   a. How many kilograms does the child weigh? _____

   b. What are the dosage parameters for this child? _____

   c. Is this drug dose within the safe dosing range? _____

   d. How many milligrams should the child receive per day? Per dose? _____

   e. How many milliliters should the child receive per dose? _____

ANSWERS

Oral Preparations

1. **a.** The Adalat CC, 60-mg tablet container
   b. For 90 mg, remove 1 tablet from the 30-mg tablet container and 1 tablet from the 60-mg tablet container.
2. (a) 2 tablets; (b) bedtime
3. 2 tablets of Pravachol
4. Nitrostat 0.3 mg (use conversion table as needed). The strength in the order and on the drug label are the same.

5. **a.** 1 tablet in the AM
    b. 2 tablets at bedtime
6. **a.** 0.5 gram = 500 mg
    b. 2 tablets
7. **a.** 325-mg bottle
    b. 2 tablets from the 325-mg bottle
8. **a.** 0.2 g = 200 mg
    b. 2 tablets
9. **a.** Compazine 5 mg/5 mL; Compazine 5 mg/mL is for injection.
    b. 10 mL
10. **a.** Select Zyprexa 2.5-mg tablets. The nurse could give 1 tablet of Zyprexa 7.5 mg and 1 tablet of Zyprexa 2.5 mg = 10 mg. If the nurse does not have the two strengths of Zyprexa, then the nurse should use the 2.5-mg tablets.

    b. BF: $\dfrac{D}{H} \times V = \dfrac{10 \text{ mg}}{2.5 \text{ mg}} \times 1 \text{ tab} = 4 \text{ tablets}$

    or

    RP: $\quad$ H $\quad$: $\quad$ V $\quad$ :: $\quad$ D $\quad$:X
    $\quad\quad$ 2.5 mg:1 tab :: 10 mg:X
    $\quad\quad\quad\quad$ 2.5 X = 10
    $\quad\quad\quad\quad\quad$ X = 4 tablets

11. **a.** 37.5 mcg = 0.0375 mg
    b. 0.025-mg or 25-mcg bottle

    c. BF: $\dfrac{D}{H} \times V = \dfrac{0.0375}{0.025} \times 1 =$

    $\quad\quad\quad 1\frac{1}{2}$ tablets

    or

    RP: $\quad$ H $\quad$: $\quad$ V $\quad$ :: $\quad\quad$ D $\quad$: X
    $\quad\quad$ 0.025 mg:1 tab :: 0.0375 mg:X tab
    $\quad\quad\quad\quad$ 0.025 X = 0.0375
    $\quad\quad\quad\quad\quad\quad$ X = $\quad$ $1\frac{1}{2}$ tablets

    or

    FE: $\dfrac{H}{V} = \dfrac{D}{X} = \dfrac{25 \text{ mcg}}{1 \text{ tab}} = \dfrac{37.5 \text{ mcg}}{X} =$
    $\quad$ (Cross multiply) 25 X = 37.5
    $\quad\quad\quad\quad$ X = $1\frac{1}{2}$ tablets

    or

    DA: tab $= \dfrac{1 \text{ tab} \quad \times \; 0.0375 \text{ mg}}{0.025 \text{ mg} \; \times \quad\quad 1} = 1\frac{1}{2}$ tablets

12. **a.** Select 250-mg/5-mL bottle. However, either bottle could be used; 125 mg/5 mL = 20 mL.
    b. 1 gram; 1000 mg
    c. 500 mg = 10 mL of Ceftin 250 mg/5 mL
13. **a.** Either 187 mg/5 mL or 375 mg/5 mL.
    b. With (preferred) 187-mg/5-mL bottle:

    $\dfrac{250 \text{ mg}}{187 \text{ mg}} \times 5 \text{ mL} = \dfrac{1250}{187} = 6.68$ or 7 mL per dose

    c. With the 375 mg/5 mL, 3.3 mL per dose.
14. **a.** Zocor 20-mg bottle. Either bottle; however, with the 10-mg Zocor bottle, more tablets would be taken (Zocor 10-mg bottle = 4 tablets).
    b. 2 tablets (Zocor 20-mg bottle). If using the 10mg Zocor bottle, 4 tablets would be taken.
15. **a.** Select Geodon 40-mg bottle.
    b. 1 capsule of Geodon 40 mg per dose; 2 capsules per day.
    c. Select both Geodon 40 mg and Geodon 20 mg to equal 60 mg.
    d. Per dose, give 1 capsule from the 40-mg bottle and 1 capsule from the 20-mg bottle to equal 60 mg. You can NOT cut a capsule in half, so both bottles of Geodon would be needed. Per day, give 2 capsules from Geodon 40-mg bottle and 2 capsules from the Geodon 20-mg bottle.

16. a. Change 0.4 grams to milligrams = 400 mg
  b. 400 mg per dose.

  c. BF: $\dfrac{D}{H} \times V = \dfrac{400 \text{ mg}}{250 \text{ mg}} \times 5 \text{ mL} =$

  8 mL of amoxicillin

  or
  RP: H : V :: D : X
    250 mg:5 mL::400 mg:X mL
      250 X = 2000
        X = 8 mL

  or
  FE: $\dfrac{H}{V} = \dfrac{D}{X} = \dfrac{250}{5} = \dfrac{400}{X} =$

  (Cross multiply) 250 X = 2000
    X = 8 mL of amoxicillin

  or
  DA: mL $= \dfrac{5 \text{ mL} \times \overset{4}{\cancel{1000}} \text{ mg} \times 0.4 \cancel{g}}{\underset{1}{\cancel{250}} \cancel{mg} \times 1 \cancel{g} \times 1} = 8 \text{ mL}$

17. a. 300 mg per day

  b. BF: $\dfrac{D}{H} \times V = \dfrac{150 \text{ mg}}{10 \text{ mg}} \times 1 \text{ mL} =$

  $\dfrac{150}{10} = 15 \text{ mL}$

  or
  DA: mL $= \dfrac{1 \text{ mL} \times \overset{15}{\cancel{150}} \text{ mg}}{\cancel{10} \cancel{mg} \times 1} = 15 \text{ mL}$

18. a. 150 pounds = 68 kg
  b. 0.75 × 68 = 51 mg or 50 mg per day
  c. Select 25-mg capsule bottle. One capsule per dose or 2 capsules per day in divided doses.

19. a. 5 mg × 70 kg = 350-mg loading dose
  b. Select the 150-mg/15-mL bottle.

  c. BF: $\dfrac{D}{H} \times V = \dfrac{\overset{7}{\cancel{350}} \text{ mg}}{\underset{3}{\cancel{150}} \text{ mg}} \times 15 \text{ mL} = \dfrac{105}{3} = 35 \text{ mL}$ theophylline

  or
  DA: mL $= \dfrac{15 \text{ mL} \times \overset{7}{\cancel{350}} \text{ mg}}{\underset{3}{\cancel{150}} \text{ mg} \times 1} = \dfrac{105}{3} = 35 \text{ mL}$ theophylline

20. a. 10 mL = 100 mg Colace per dose.

  b. $\dfrac{\textit{Known mOsm} \ (3900) \times \text{Volume of drug (10 mL)}}{\text{desired mOsm (500)}} = \dfrac{39,000}{500} = 78 \text{ mL}$ drug solution and water

  78 mL of drug solution and water − 10 mL of drug solution = 68 mL of water to dilute the osmolality of the drug

Injectables

21. ½ mL or 0.5 mL

$$\mathbf{BF:} \frac{D}{H} \times V = \frac{\overset{1}{\cancel{25} \text{ mg}}}{\underset{2}{\cancel{50} \text{ mg}}} \times 1 \text{ mL} = \frac{1}{2} \text{ mL}$$

or

DA: no conversion factor needed

$$\text{mL} = \frac{1 \text{ mL} \times \overset{1}{\cancel{25} \text{ mg}}}{\underset{2}{\cancel{50} \text{ mg}} \times 1} = \frac{1}{2} \text{ mL or } 0.5 \text{ mL}$$

or

$$\mathbf{RP:} \quad H \; : \; V \; :: \; D \; : X$$
$$50 \text{ mg} : 1 \text{ mL} :: 25 \text{ mg} : X$$
$$50 X = 25$$
$$X = \frac{1}{2} \text{ mL or } 0.5 \text{ mL}$$

22. 1 mL

23. a. Meperidine 0.8 mL; atropine 1.25 mL or 1.3 mL

  b. (1) Draw 1.25 mL of air and insert into the atropine bottle.

  (2) Withdraw 1.25 mL of atropine and 0.8 mL of meperidine from the ampule.

24. a. Could use either vial, units 5000/mL or units 10,000/mL.

  b. 0.5 mL from the units 5000 vial or 0.25 mL from the units 10,000 vial.

25. 0.2 mL of Lovenox

26. 1.25 mL of Naloxone

27. Withdraw 35 units of Humulin 70/30.

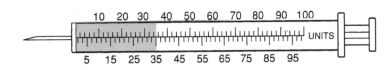

28. a. Withdraw the regular Humulin R insulin first and then the Humulin N insulin.

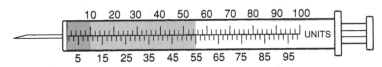

  b. Total of 55 units of Humulin R and Humulin N insulin (10 units regular, 45 units Humulin N).

29. a. Select 1000 mcg/mL. If you chose the 100-mcg/mL cartridge, you would need 5 cartridges to give 500 mcg.

  b. ½ mL or 0.5 mL

30. RP: $\quad$ H : V :: D :X

$\quad\quad\quad$ 15 mg : 1 mL :: 8 mg : X

$\quad\quad\quad\quad\quad$ 15 X = 8

$\quad\quad\quad\quad\quad\quad$ X = 0.533 or 0.5 mL of morphine (round off to tenths)

or

DA: $mL = \dfrac{1 \text{ mL} \times 8 \text{ mg}}{15 \text{ mg} \times 1} = \dfrac{8}{15} = 0.533$ or 0.5 mL of morphine (round off to tenths)

31. ½ mL or 0.5 mL

32. 1.4 mL

33. a. 145 ÷ 2.2 = 65.9 kg or 66 kg

$\quad$ **b.** 3 mg × 66 kg = 198 mg/day

$\quad$ **c.** 198 ÷ 3 = 66 mg per dose

$\quad$ **d. BF:** $\dfrac{66 \text{ mg}}{80} \times 2 \text{ mL} = \dfrac{132}{80} = 1.65$ or 1.7 mL per dose (round off to tenths)

$\quad\quad$ **or**

$\quad\quad$ **DA:** $mL = \dfrac{2 \text{ mL} \times 66 \text{ mg}}{80 \text{ mg} \times 1} = \dfrac{132}{80} = 1.7$ mL per dose

34. 0.5 mL or 0.48 mL = 0.5 mL (tenths)

35. RP: $\quad$ H : V :: D :X

$\quad\quad\quad$ 25 mg : 1 mL :: 20 mg : X

$\quad\quad\quad\quad$ 25 X = 20

$\quad\quad\quad\quad\quad$ X = 0.8 mL of methotrexate

$\quad$ Give 0.8 mL of methotrexate.

or

DA: $mL = \dfrac{1 \text{ mL} \times 20 \text{ mg}}{25 \text{ mg} \times 1} = \dfrac{20}{25} = 0.8$ mL

36. a. Add 1.5 mL of diluent: 1.8 mL total.

$\quad$ **b.** 750 mg per day

$\quad$ **c. BF:** $\dfrac{D}{H} \times V = \dfrac{250 \text{ mg}}{500 \text{ mg}} \times 1.8 \text{ mL} = 0.9$ mL of Tazidime

$\quad\quad$ **or**

$\quad\quad$ **RP:** $\quad$ H : V :: D : X

$\quad\quad\quad\quad$ 500 mg : 1.8 mL :: 250 mg : X mL

$\quad\quad\quad\quad\quad$ 500 X = 450

$\quad\quad\quad\quad\quad\quad$ X = 0.9 mL of Tazidime

$\quad$ **d.** 3-mL syringe for mixing and administering; unable to mix the drug and diluent with a tuberculin syringe.

37. a. Add 3 mL diluent = 3.5 mL of drug solution; 1 g = 1000 mg.

b. BF: $\dfrac{500 \text{ mg}}{1000 \text{ mg}} \times 3.5 \text{ mL} = \dfrac{1750}{1000} = 1.75$ mL or 1.8 mL per dose (round off to tenths)

38. a. 0.25 g = 250 mg

b. BF: $\dfrac{250 \text{ mg}}{500} \times 2.2 \text{ mL} = \dfrac{550}{500} = 1.1$ mL per dose **or** 1 mL

or

RP: H : V :: D :X
500 mg:2.2 = 250:X
500 X = 550

$$X = \dfrac{550}{500} = 1.1 \text{ mL or 1 mL}$$

or

DA: mL $= \dfrac{2.2 \text{ mL} \times 250 \text{ mg}}{500 \text{ mg} \times \quad 1} = 1.1$ mL or 1 mL of Ancef

39. a. Yes, the total dose is 1000 mg daily (1 g = 1000 mg).
   b. Inject 2.1 mL of sterile water into the vial.
   c. After reconstitution, 1 mL of Rocephin solution would yield 350 mg.

d. BF: $\dfrac{D}{H} \times V = \dfrac{500 \text{ mg}}{350 \text{ mg}} \times 1 \text{ mL} = 1.4$ mL of Rocephin

40. 2.25 mL Fortaz
41. a. 165 lbs ÷ 2.2 − 75 kg
   b. 4 mg × 75 kg = 300 mg/day
   c. 100 mg per dose
   d. Select 40-mg/mL bottle of gentamicin sulfate. (Normally less than 3 mL IM should be given at one site.)
   e. 2.5 mL of gentamicin per dose

Direct IV Administration

42. 3 mL
43. a. 0.25 mg × 60 kg = 15 mg according to drug parameters of Cardizem IV direct (bolus) over 2 minutes
   b. Yes, dose is within drug parameters.
   c. Administer 3 mL of IV Cardizem.

Intravenous

44. 125 mL per hour

$$\frac{125 \text{ mL} \times 10 \text{ gtt/min}}{60 \text{ min/hr}} = \frac{1250}{60} = 20.8 \text{ gtt/min or } 21 \text{ gtt/min}$$

45. $\dfrac{250 \text{ mL/hr} \times \overset{1}{\cancel{15}} \text{ gtt/mL}}{\underset{4}{\cancel{60}} \text{ min}} = \dfrac{250}{4} = 62.5 \text{ or } 63 \text{ gtt/min}$

46. a. BF: $\dfrac{D}{H} \times V = \dfrac{\overset{2}{\cancel{20}} \text{ mEq}}{\underset{3}{\cancel{30}} \text{ mEq}} \times 15 \text{ mL} = \dfrac{30}{3} = 10 \text{ mL of KCl}$

Inject 10 mL of potassium chloride in 1000 mL D$_5$W. The KCl should be injected into the IV bag and mixed well before the IV is hung.

b. $1000 \div 8 = 125 \text{ mL}$

$$\frac{125 \text{ mL} \times 10 \text{ gtt}}{60 \text{ min/hr}} = \frac{1250}{60} = 21 \text{ gtt/min}$$

47. Add 2.0 mL diluent = 2.6 mL of drug solution; 1 g = 1000 mg.

a. $\dfrac{\cancel{600} \text{ mg}}{\cancel{1000} \text{ mg}} \times 2.6 \text{ mL} = \dfrac{15.6}{10} = 1.56 \text{ mL or } 1.6 \text{ mL Ticar per dose (round off to tenths)}$

b. $\dfrac{\text{Amount of solution} \times \text{gtt/mL}}{\text{Minutes}} = \dfrac{60 \text{ mL} \times \overset{2}{\cancel{60}} \text{ gtt/mL}}{\underset{1}{\cancel{30}} \text{ min}} = 120 \text{ gtt/min}$

48. a. Concentration/min:
Body weight × Desired dose/kg/min
105 kg × 2 mcg/kg/min
   = 210 mcg/min

b. Concentration/hr:
210 mcg/min x 60 min/hr = 12,600 mcg/hr

c. Volume/min:

$$\frac{210 \text{ mcg/min}}{750 \text{ mcg/mL}} = 0.28 \text{ mL/min}$$

d. Volume/hr:
0.28 mL/min × 60 min/hr = 16.8 mL/hr

49. a. Add 2 mL Thorazine to 500 mL. For 4 hours: 500 mL ÷ 4 = 125 mL/hr.

b. $\dfrac{125 \text{ mL} \times \overset{1}{\cancel{15}} \text{ gtt/mL}}{\underset{4}{\cancel{60}} \text{ min/1 hr}} = \dfrac{125}{4} = 31 \text{ gtt/min for 4 hours}$

50. a. Use the Mefoxin 1-g vial for ADD-Vantage and mix drug in the 50 mL IV bag for ADD-Vantage.

b. Amount of sol $\div \dfrac{\text{Minutes to admin}}{60 \text{ min/hr}} = \text{mL/hr}$

$$50 \text{ mL} \div \frac{30 \text{ min}}{60 \text{ min}} = 50 \text{ mL} \times \frac{\overset{2}{\cancel{60}} \text{ min}}{\underset{1}{\cancel{30}} \text{ min}} = 100 \text{ mL/hr}$$

51. a. 0.5 g = 500 mg; add 2.0 mL of diluent = 2.5 mL of drug solution; 500 mg = 2.5 mL

b. Amount of solution $\div \dfrac{\text{Min to admin}}{60 \text{ min/hr}} = \text{mL/hr}$

$2.5 \text{ mL drug} + 50 \text{ mL} \div \dfrac{20 \text{ min}}{60 \text{ min/hr}} = 52.5 \text{ mL} \times \dfrac{\overset{3}{\cancel{60}}}{\underset{1}{\cancel{20}}} = 157.5 \text{ mL/hr or } 158 \text{ mL/hr}$

Set pump to deliver in 20 minutes.

52. a. 10 mg/hr × 5 hr = 50 mg Cardizem

b. $\dfrac{50 \text{ mg}}{5} \times 1 \text{ mL} = 10 \text{ mL Cardizem to add to } 500 \text{ mL}$

c. $10 \text{ mL drug solution} + 500 \text{ mL} \div \dfrac{300 \text{ min (5 hr)}}{60 \text{ min/hr}} = 510 \text{ mL} \times \dfrac{\overset{1}{\cancel{60}} \text{ min}}{\underset{5}{\cancel{300}} \text{ min (5 hr)}} = \dfrac{510}{5} = 102 \text{ mL/hr}$

53. a. *Drug calculation:*

$\text{BF:} \dfrac{D}{H} \times V = \dfrac{100 \text{ mg}}{200 \text{ mg}} \times 20 \text{ mL} = 10 \text{ mL}$ **or** $\text{RP:}\quad H : V :: D : X$
$200 \text{ mg} : 20 \text{ mL} :: 100 \text{ mg} : X \text{ mL}$
$200 X = 2000$
$X = 10 \text{ mL}$

or
$\text{FE:} \dfrac{H}{V} = \dfrac{D}{X} = \dfrac{200}{20} = \dfrac{100}{X} =$

(Cross multiply) $200X = 2000$
$X = 10 \text{ mL}$

or
$\text{DA: mL} = \dfrac{20 \text{ mL} \times \overset{1}{\cancel{100}} \text{ mg}}{\underset{2}{\cancel{200}} \text{ mg} \times 1} = 10 \text{ mL}$

b. *Flow rate calculation* (secondary set):

$\dfrac{110 \text{ mL } (100 + 10) \times \overset{1}{\cancel{15}} \text{ gtt/mL (set)}}{\underset{2}{\cancel{30}} \text{ min}} = 55 \text{ gtt/min}$

c. *Infusion pump rate:*

$110 \text{ mL} \div \dfrac{30 \text{ min to admin}}{60 \text{ min/hr}} = 110 \times \dfrac{\overset{2}{\cancel{60}}}{\underset{1}{\cancel{30}}} = 220 \text{ mL/hr}$

54. a. 1.2 g × 1.98 m² = 2.37 g or 2.4 g or 2400 mg

b. 2.4 g × 20 mL = 48 mL diluent added to Ifex vials

c. $(48 \text{ mL of drug solution} + 50 \text{ mL}) \div \dfrac{30 \text{ min}}{60 \text{ min}} = 98 \text{ mL} \times \dfrac{\overset{2}{\cancel{60}} \text{ min}}{\underset{1}{\cancel{30}} \text{ min}} = 196 \text{ mL/hr}$

Set pump to deliver in 30 minutes.

Pediatrics

55. a. Yes, the drug dose is within the safe dosing range.
0.03 mg × 12 kg = 0.36 mg
0.04 mg × 12 kg = 0.48 mg

b. $\text{BF:} \dfrac{D}{H} \times V = \dfrac{0.4 \text{ mg}}{0.05 \text{ mg}} \times 1 \text{ mL} = 8 \text{ mL of digoxin}$

$\text{DA: mL} = \dfrac{1 \text{ mL} \times 0.4 \text{ mg}}{0.05 \text{ mg} \times 1} = \dfrac{0.4 \text{ mg}}{0.05 \text{ mg}} = 8 \text{ mL of digoxin}$

56. **a.** Yes, the drug dose is within the safe dosing range.
   b. 5 mL
   0.1 gram = 100 mg
   Drug available: 100 mg: 5 mL
57. **a.** 53 lbs ÷ 2.2 = 24 kg
   b. Yes, the drug dose is within the safe dosing range.
   Dosing parameters: 25,000 units × 24 kg = 600,000 units and 90,000 units × 24 kg = 2,160,000 units/day.
   Child to receive 400,000 units × 4 daily doses (q6h) = 1,600,000 units/day.
   c. **RP:**   H   : V ::   D   :X
              200,000 units : 5 mL :: 400,000 units : X
                    200,000 X = 2,000,000
                          X = 10 mL of veetids

   400,000 units = 10 mL per dose
58. **a.** Dosing parameters: 20 mg × 19 kg = 380 mg/day and 40 mg × 19 kg = 760 mg/day.
   b. No, the drug dose is *NOT* within the safe dosing range. Do NOT administer. Notify the physician or responsible health care provider.
   Child ordered 250 mg × 4 daily doses (q6h) = 1000 mg/day. *This dose is not safe, it exceeds the dosing parameters for this child.*
   c. Do not administer medication.
59. **a.** Yes, the drug dose is within the safe dosing range.
   Dosing parameter: 5 mg × 16 kg = 80 mg.
   Child to receive 25 mg × 3 daily doses (tid) = 75 mg

   b. **BF:** $\dfrac{D}{H} \times V = \dfrac{\overset{2}{\cancel{25}}}{\underset{1}{\cancel{12.5}}\,mg} \times 5\,mL = 10\,mL$ of Benadryl

60. **a.** 45 lbs ÷ 2.2 = 20.45 or 20.5 kg.
   b. Dosage parameters:
   20 mg × 20.5 kg/day = 410 mg/day.
   40 mg × 20.5 kg/day = 820 mg/day.
   c. Yes, the drug dose is within the safe dosing range.
   d. 150 mg × 3 daily doses = 450 mg.
   The child should receive 450 mg of Cleocin per day.

   e. **BF:** $\dfrac{D}{H} \times V = \dfrac{\overset{2}{\cancel{150}}}{\underset{1}{\cancel{75}}} \times 5\,mL = 10\,mL$ per dose   **or**   **DA:** $mL = \dfrac{5\,mL \times \overset{2}{\cancel{150}\,mg}}{\underset{1}{\cancel{75}}\,mg \times 1} = 10\,mL$ per dose

61. **a.** 35 lbs ÷ 2.2 = 15.9 or 16 kg.
   b. Dosing parameters: 20 mg × 16 kg/day = 320 mg/day and 60 mg × 16 kg/day = 960 mg/day.
   c. No, the drug dose is *NOT* within the safe dosing range. Do NOT administer. Notify the physician or responsible health care provider.
   Child ordered 150 mg × 2 daily doses (q12h) = 300 mg/day. *This dose does not meet the dosing parameters for this child.*
   c. Do not administer medication.
62. **a.** Yes, the drug dose is within the safe dosing range.
   Dosing parameters: 3 mg × 10 kg = 30 mg/day and 5 mg × 10 kg = 50 mg/day.
   Child to receive 15 mg × 3 daily doses (q8h) = 45 mg/day.
   b. **RP:** H :   V   :: D   :   X
   20 mg : 2 mL :: 15 mg : X
            20 X = 30
              X = 1.5 mL of tobramycin

63. a. Yes, the drug dose is within the safe dosing range.
Dosing parameters: 30 mg × 27 kg = 810 mg/day; 50 mg × 27 kg = 1350 mg/day.
Child to receive 250 mg × 4 daily doses (q6h) = 1000 mg/day.

  b. DA: $\text{mL} = \dfrac{2.4 \text{ mL} \times \overset{1}{\cancel{250}} \text{ mg}}{\underset{2}{\cancel{500}} \text{ mg} \times 1} = 1.2 \text{ mL of Fortaz}$

64. a. 49 lbs ÷ 2.2 = 22.2 or 22 kg
  b. Yes, the drug dose is within the safe dosing range.
Dosing parameters: 50 mg × 22 kg = 1100 mg/day and 100 mg × 22 kg = 2200 mg/day.
Child to receive 400 mg × 3 daily doses (q8h) = 1200 mg/day

  c. BF: $\dfrac{D}{H} \times V = \dfrac{400 \text{ mg}}{500 \text{ mg}} \times 2 \text{ mL} = \dfrac{8}{5} = 1.6 \text{ mL of Ancef}$

  or

  DA: $\text{mL} = \dfrac{2 \text{ mL} \times \overset{4}{\cancel{400}} \text{ mg}}{\underset{5}{\cancel{500}} \text{ mg} \times 1} = \dfrac{8}{5} = 1.6 \text{ mL of Ancef}$

  d. *Flow rate calculation:* $\dfrac{50 \text{ mL} \times \overset{2}{\cancel{60}} \text{ gtt/mL}}{\underset{1}{\cancel{30}} \text{ min}} = 100 \text{ gtt/min}$

65. a. 26 lbs ÷ 2.2 = 11.8 or 12 kg
  b. Dosing parameter: 15 mg × 12 kg − 180 mg/day
  c. Yes, the drug dose is within the safe dosing range.
  d. Child to receive 180 mg/day or 60 mg per dose (180 mg ÷ 3 daily doses (q8h) = 60 mg)

  e. BF: $\dfrac{D}{H} \times V = \dfrac{60 \text{ mg}}{75 \text{ mg}} \times 2 \text{ mL} = \dfrac{120}{75} = 1.6 \text{ mL of Kantrex}$

  or

  FE: $\dfrac{H}{V} = \dfrac{D}{X} = \dfrac{75 \text{ mg}}{2 \text{ mL}} = \dfrac{60 \text{ mg}}{X}$

  (cross multiply) 75 X = 120
  X = 1.6 mL of Kantrex

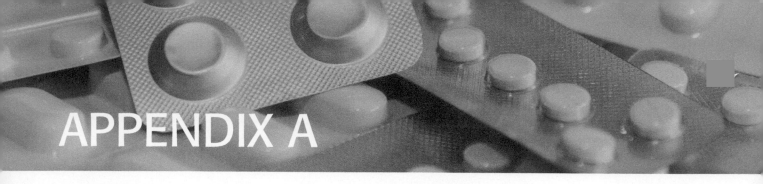

APPENDIX A

Guidelines for Administration of Medications

Outline **GENERAL DRUG ADMINISTRATION**
ORAL MEDICATIONS
INJECTABLE MEDICATIONS
INTRAVENOUS FLUID AND MEDICATIONS

GENERAL DRUG ADMINISTRATION

1. Wash hands and don gloves before preparing **all** medications.
2. All medication should be prepared in a clean, distraction-free environment.
3. Check medication order against physician's orders in the MAR (medication administration record) or eMAR (electronic medication administration record). Check for medication administration parameters, such as heart rate, respiration, and blood pressure.
4. Check label of drug container against medication order and physician's order. Verify 5 "rights": that you have the right patient, medication, dose, route of administration, and time of administration. If something is amiss, ask another nurse to verify the medication reconciliation with you.
5. Check all drug labels for an expiration date. Notify the pharmacy of outdated drugs, and return expired medication.
6. If a drug order is unclear, do not guess. Verify order with charge nurse, physician, and/or pharmacist.
7. Nurses are patient advocates and have the right to question and clarify drug orders. Physicians are responsible for medication orders. Nurses are responsible for administering medications correctly and safely.
8. Do not give medications that are poured or drawn up by someone else unless you witness the drug preparation. Dosages should be verified before administering them.
9. Do not leave medication sitting out unsupervised or out of your sight.
10. Identify patients by using their identification bracelets (ID bands) and by asking each patient to state his or her name and birth date.
11. Check if patient has any allergies to the drug or drug class. Patient should be wearing an allergy bracelet.
12. Explain to the patient what medication he or she is receiving and why.
13. Assist patient as necessary with taking medication (i.e., positioning or providing water). You must stay with the patient to make sure the medication is taken. Manage time by giving medications last to patients who need more assistance.

14. Promptly document in patient's MAR or eMAR that medication was given (especially STAT medications). If patient did not receive medication, document why in MAR or eMAR.
15. Record the amount of fluid taken orally or intravascularly with each medication if client's intake (I) and output (O) are being recorded.
16. Immediately report any medication errors to the physician and charge nurse. Document incident per your institution's policy. Evaluate the patient's condition immediately.
17. Nurses have a window of 30 minutes before and after the scheduled time to administer ordered medications. Check hospital policy because some facilities vary on time allowed before and after the scheduled administration time.
18. Patients have the right to refuse medications. Provide education for these patients. Notify physician of patient's refusal. Document refusal on patient's MAR or eMAR.

ORAL MEDICATIONS

1. Wash hands and don gloves before preparing oral medications.
2. Pour tablet or capsule into medicine cup (not your hand or into another medication container). Drugs prepared for unit dose can be opened at the time of administration in the patient's room. Discard drugs that are dropped on the floor and dispose of them per institutional policy.
3. Pour liquids into a container or cup placed on a flat surface and read measurement at eye level. Pour liquid medication from the opposite side of the bottle's label to avoid spilling on the label.
4. Do not mix liquid medications or tablets and liquid medications together. Ideally, medications should be given one at a time. Patient may take more than one tablet or capsule at a time (except oral narcotics, digoxin, and STAT medications) if they are comfortable doing so.
5. Evaluate patients' swallowing abilities by first having them take a sip of water. For a larger pill (e.g., potassium), ask patients if they feel comfortable swallowing it. Instant coughing after swallowing water may indicate that the patient is aspirating.
6. For the patient who has difficulty swallowing tablets and thin liquids, contact the physician and pharmacy to evaluate whether the medication can be crushed and given in applesauce.
7. Do not return poured medication to its container. Discard poured medication if unused.
8. Dilute liquid medication that irritates gastric mucosa (e.g., potassium products) or that could discolor or damage tooth enamel (e.g., saturated solution of potassium iodide). Evaluate whether these medications can be taken with meals.
9. Offer ice chips before administering bad-tasting medications to help numb patient's taste buds.
10. Assist patient into an upright position when administering oral medications. Stay with patient until medication is taken.
11. Give 50 to 100 mL of oral fluids with medications unless the patient has a fluid restriction.
12. Patients who have a nasogastric or gastric tube should receive their oral medications via this route. Tablets should be thoroughly crushed and diluted in sterile water or normal saline (NS). Medications should be given one at a time and flushed with sterile water or NS between each medication. Some medications cannot be crushed; therefore the form would need to be changed. Refer to your institution's policy. (See Chapter 8 for additional information.)
13. For drugs given by oral syringe, direct the syringe across the tongue and toward the side of the mouth.
14. If a patient spits out all of the liquid medication, repeat the dose. If the patient spits out half of the medication, repeat half of the dose. Notify the physician if there is a question regarding repeated doses. The physician may need to select another route of administration.

INJECTABLE MEDICATIONS

1. Wash hands and don gloves before preparing injectable medications.
2. Check medication order and medication label to determine method(s) for drug administration (e.g., intramuscular [IM] or subcutaneous [subcut]).
3. Check for drug compatibility before mixing drugs in the same syringe. Check institution's policy before mixing compatible drugs in a syringe to administer.
4. Do not give medications that are cloudy, discolored, or that have precipitated.
5. Select the proper syringe and needle size for the route and type of medication to be administered.
6. Select the injection site according to the drug, patient's age, and disease process.
7. Medication in ampules should be drawn up using a 15-micron filtered needle or filter straw. Once opened, the ampule cannot be used again and the unused solution should be discarded.
8. Do not reuse vials, needles, or syringes between patients.
9. Avoid the use of multiple-dose vials. If multiple-dose vials must be used, each patient should have his or her own vial, labeled with the date it was opened and stored according to manufacturer's directions.
10. Know alternative sites of administration. Do not administer injections into inflamed, edematous, or infected tissue. Lesions (moles, birthmarks, and scar tissue) and surgical sites should also be avoided.
11. When administering IM medications, aspirate the plunger before injecting the medication. If blood is aspirated, do not administer. Withdraw the needle and prepare a new solution. Check your institution's policy about aspirate when giving IM injections.
12. Do not massage the injection site when using the Z-track method, intradermal injections, or any anticoagulant solution.
13. Recognize that patients experiencing edema, shock, or poor circulation will have a slower tissue absorption rate with IM injections.
14. The site of injection on the patient's skin should be cleansed with an alcohol swab before injection.
15. Do not administer IM medications subcutaneously. Poor medication absorption and sloughing of the skin could occur.
16. Specific medications (e.g., narcotics) need to be discarded with a colleague and documented per your institution's policy.
17. Discard medication per your institution's policy. Discard needles into the proper sharps container.

INTRAVENOUS FLUID AND MEDICATIONS

1. Wash hands and don gloves before preparing and priming IV drugs or fluids.
2. Use aseptic technique when inserting IV catheters, administering medications, and changing IV tubing and fluids.
3. All products and medications for IV infusion should be clearly labeled with trade and generic names, along with the dosage and concentration of the drug or fluid, route of administration, expiration date, frequency, infusion rate, and sterility state.
4. Recognize signs of catheter-related infection, such as erythema, edema, induration or drainage at vascular access site, fever, and chills. These changes should be reported immediately to the charge nurse and physician.
5. Use peripheral access over central access when appropriate. Avoid placing an IV in areas of inflammation, bruises, breakdown, or infection; in the lower extremities; at surgical sites; or in extremities with neuromuscular or motor deficits.
6. IV tubing and fluid bags should be labeled with date, time, and initials of nurse. When multiple catheters or lumens are being used, all lines should be labeled (at the sites where they connect to the patient) with the name of the medication or fluid that is infusing.

7. Check patency of IV catheter before using by flushing the IV catheter with 2 mL of normal saline (NS). To clear IV tubing of a medication's solution, flush tubing with 15 mL of NS.
8. Do not forcefully irrigate IV catheters. The IV catheter could be kinked, infiltrated, or the force could dislodge a clot from the catheter site, leading to an embolus.
9. IV sites that are saline locked should be flushed at intervals that adhere to your institution's protocols.
10. Check for air bubbles in tubing. Remove air from tubing by repriming the tubing or by clamping below the air bubble and removing the air by aspirating with a syringe. Use the method that is indicated by unit policy.
11. Monitor all IV flow rates hourly or as needed. IV flow rates can be easily altered by the patient's position or by kinked tubing. Promptly address pump alarms.
12. Assess for signs of an allergic reaction to the IV drug. If signs of a reaction are noted, stop the administration of the drug and notify the prescriber immediately.
13. Use an infusion pump for any high-risk medications with a narrow therapeutic range to prevent medication errors. Every precaution should be taken to prevent "free flow" incidence of IV fluids. Check that the pump is infusing accurately.
14. Check compatibility of IV medications before infusing them together. Stop infusion immediately if precipitation is noted in the tubing.
15. Assess IV sites for signs of infiltration: swelling, coolness, leakage, and pain at insertion site. If these symptoms are found, remove IV and elevate arm. Use an infiltration scale to grade severity of the infiltration when documenting (see following page).
16. Monitor IV sites for signs of phlebitis, which is an inflammation of the vein, causing erythema and pain along the vessel. Remove the IV catheter if signs are present. A phlebitis scale should be used when documenting this site (see following page).
17. IV sites should be secured with tape or stat lock and stabilized to prevent the loss of IV access.
18. Change IV site dressing when soiled and per institution's policy. Ensure that IV sites are labeled with date and time of insertion, gauge size, and initials.
19. Change IV tubing every 24 to 48 hours. This includes all add-on devices, such as filters, extensions, ports, stopcocks, access caps, and needleless systems. Change IV fluid every 24 hours. Follow institution's policy.
20. Vascular access sites should be flushed at intervals according to institutional policies and procedures and manufacturer's recommendations.
21. Choose the flow-control device that best meets the clinical application for patients. Base this choice on factors such as severity of illness, type of therapy, clinical setting, age, and mobility.

Infiltration Scale

Grade	Clinical Criteria
0	No symptoms
1	Skin blanched
	Edema less than 1 inch in any direction
	Cool to touch
	With or without pain
2	Skin blanched
	Edema 1–6 inches in any direction
	Cool to touch
	With or without pain
3	Skin blanched, translucent
	Gross edema greater than 6 inches in any direction
	Cool to touch
	Mild to moderate pain
	Possible numbness
4	Skin blanched, translucent
	Skin tight, leaking
	Skin discolored, bruised, swollen
	Gross edema greater than 6 inches in any direction
	Deep pitting tissue edema
	Circulatory impairment
	Moderate to severe pain
	Infiltration of any amount of blood product, irritant, or vesicant

From *Infusion Nursing Standards of Practice.* (2006). New York: Infusion Nurses Society, p. S60.

Phlebitis Scale

Grade	Clinical Criteria
0	No symptoms
1	Erythema at access site with or without pain
2	Pain at access site with erythema and/or edema
3	Pain at access site with erythema and/or edema
	Streak formation
	Palpable venous cord
4	Pain at access site with erythema and/or edema
	Streak formation
	Palpable venous cord greater than 1 inch in length
	Purulent drainage

From *Infusion Nursing Standards of Practice.* (2006). New York: Infusion Nurses Society, p. S59.

REFERENCES

Adachi, W., & Lodolce, A. E. (2005). Use of failure mode and effects analysis in improving the safety of I.V. drug administration [electronic version]. *American Journal of Health-Systems Pharmacy, 62*(9):917-920.

ALARIS Medical Systems. (1999). *Volumetric infusion pump manual.*

Beckwith, C. M., Feddema, S. S., Barton, R. G., & Graves, C. (2004). A guide to drug therapy in patients with enteral feedingtubes: dosage form selection and administration methods. *Hospital Pharmacy, 39*:231.

Briars, G. L., & Bailey, B. J. (1994). Surface area estimation: pocket calculator vs. nomogram. *Archives of Disease in Childhood, 70*: 246-247.

Brunton L., & Chabner, B. (2011). *Goodman & Gilman's the pharmacological basis of therapeutics* (12th ed.). New York: McGraw-Hill.

Bryn Mawr Hospital. (2005). Perinatal units: policy and procedural manual. Bryn Mawr, Pa: Auhor.

Burz, S. (2006). *Smart pumps get smarter.* Retrieved from www.nursezone. com/job/technologyreport.asp?article ID_15520.

Carayon, P., Wetterneck, T. B., Schoofs Hundt, A., et al. (2008). Observing nurse interaction with infusion pump technologies [electronic version]. *Advances in Patient Safety: From Research to Implementation, 2*:349-364.

Casu, G., & Merella, P. (2015). *Diuretic Therapy in Heart Failure-Current Approaches.* European Cardiology Review. Retrieved from https://www.ecrjournal.com/articles/diuretic-therapy-heart-failure-current-approaches.

CNA Medical. (n.d.). *Refurbished infusion pumps.* Retrieved from www.cnamedical.com/infusionpumps.htm.

Conklin, S. (2004). *UW Hospital and clinics install "smart" intravenous pumps.* Retrieved from www.wistechnology.com/article. php?id_1186.

Cowan, D. (2009). *"Mission zero" with smart pumps* [electronic version]. *Pharmacy Solutions*, a supplement of *Nursing Management, 40*(11): 1-2.

Crass, R. (2001). *Improving intravenous (IV) medication safety at the point of care.* Boston: ALARIS.

Dennison, R. D. (2006). High alert drugs: Strategies for safe I.V. infusions. *American Nurse Today, 1*(2).

Department of Veterans Affairs, Veterans Health Administration. (2002). *Bar code medication administration, version 2, training manual.* Washington, D.C.: Authors.

Food and Drug Administration. (n.d.). *Dailymed.* Retrieved from http://dailymed.nlm.nih.gov/dailymed/.

Foster, J. (2006). *Intravenous in-line filters for preventing morbidity and mortality in neonates.* Retrieved from www.nichd.nih.gov/cochrane/foster2FOSTER.HTM.

Gahart, B., & Nazarento, A. (2015). *Intravenous medications* (31st ed.). St. Louis: Mosby.

Gardner, S. L., & Carter, B. S. (2011). *Merenstein & Gardner's handbook of neonatal intensive care* (7th ed). St. Louis: Mosby.

Gin, T., Chan, M. T., Chan, K. L., & Yen, P. M. (2002). Prolonged neuro- muscular block after rocuronium in postpartum patient. *Anesthesia- Analgesia, 94*(3):686-689.

Green, B. (2004). *What is the best size descriptor to use for pharmacokinetic studies in the obese?* Retrieved from www.ncbi.nlm.nih.gov/entrez/query.fegi?cmd.

Gurney, H. (1996). Dose calculation of anticancer drugs: a review of current practice and introduction of an alternative. *Journal of Clinical Oncology, 14*(9):590-611.

Gurney, H. P., Ackland, S., Gebski, V., & Farrell, G. (1998). Factors affecting epirubicin pharmacokinetics and toxicity: evidence against using body-surface areas for dose calculation. *Journal of Clinical Oncology, 16*:2299-2304.

Han, P.Y., Coombes, I.D., & Green, B. (October 4, 2004). *Factors predictive of intravenous fluid administration errors in Australian surgical care wards.* Retrieved from www.qhc.bmjjournals.com/cgi/content/full/14/3/179.

Hasler, R. A. (2004). *Administration of blood products.* ALARIS. Retrieved from www.cardinalhealth.com/alaris/support/clinical/pdfs/wp836.asp.

Hegenbarth, M. A., & American Academy of Pediatarics Committee on Drugs. (2008). Preparing for pediatric emergencies: Drugs to consider. *Pediatrics, 121*(2):433-443.

Hockenberry, M. J., & Wilson, D. (2011). *Wong's Nursing care of infants* (9th ed). St: Louis: Elsevier/Mosby.

Hodgson, B., & Kizior, R. (2006). *Mosby's 2006 drug consult for nurses.* St. Louis: Elsevier.

Husch, M., Sullivan, C., & Rooney, D. (2005). Insights from the sharp end of intravenous medication errors: Implications for infusion pump technology. *Quality & Safety in Health Care, 14*(2):80-86.

Infusion Nurses Society. (2011). *Infusion nursing: Standards of practice,* vol. 34. Philadelphia: Lippincott Williams & Wilkins.

Institute for Safe Medication Practices. (2005). *Preventing magnesium toxicity in obstetrics.* Retrieved from www.ismp.org/newsletters/acutecare/articles/20051020.asp.

Institute for Safe Medication Practices. (2010). *ISMP's guidelines for standard order sets.* Retrieved from http://www.ismp.org/Tools/guidelines/StandardOrderSets.asp.

Institute for Safe Medication Practices. (2013). *ISMP's list of error-prone abbreviations, symbols, and dose designations.* Retrieved from www.ismp.org.

Joanna Briggs Institute. (2001). *Maintaining oral hydration in older people* vol 5. Retrieved from www.joannabriggs.edu.au/best_practice/BPIShyd.php.

Johnson, N. L., Huang, J. T., & Chang, T. (1996). Control of a multichannel drug infusion pump using a pharmacokinetic model. United States. Abbott Laboratories (Abbott Park, IL). Retrieved from http://www.freepatentsonline.com/5522798.html.

Joppa, S. A., et al. A Practical Review of the Emerging Direct Anticoagulants, Laboratory Monitoring, and Reversal Agents. *Journal of Clinical Medicine.* vol. 7, no. 29, Feb. 2018, pp. 1-15.

The Joint Commission. (2000). *Infusion pumps: Preventing future adverse effects* (15th ed.). Retrieved from www.jointcommission.org/SentinelEvents/SentinelEventAlert/sea_15.htm.

The Joint Commission. (2001). *Sentinel event alert: Medication errors related to potentially dangerous abbreviations.* Retrieved from www.jointcommission.org.

Kaboli, P. J., Glasgow, J. M., Jaipaul, C. K., et al. (2010). Identifying medication misadventures: Poor agreement among medical record, physician, nurse, and patient reports [electronic version]. *Pharmacotherapy, 30*(5):529-538.

Kalyn, A., Blatz, S., & Pinelli, M. (2000). A comparison of continuous infusion and intermittent flushing methods in peripheral intravenous catheters in neonates. *Journal of Intravenous Nursing, 23*(3):146-153.

Kazemi, A., Fors, U. G. F., Tofighi, S., et al. (2010). Physician order entry or nurse order entry? Comparison of two implementation strategies for a computerized order entry system aimed at reducing dosing mediation errors. *Journal of Medical Internet Research, 12*(1):e5.

Kee, J. L., Hayes, E. R., & McCuistion, L. (2012). *Pharmacology: A nursing process approach* (7th ed.). Philadelphia: Saunders.

Kee, J. L., Paulanka, J. B., & Polek, C. (2010). *Fluids and electrolytes with clinical applications* (8th ed.). Albany, NY: Delmar Publishers.

Krupp, K., & Heximer, B. (1998). The flow. *Nursing, '98*(4):54-55.

Kuczmarski, R. J., & Flegal, K. M. (2000). Criteria for definition of overweight in transition: Background and recommendations for the United States. *American Society for Clinical Nutrition, 72*:1074-1081.

Kuschel, C. (2004). *Newborn services drug protocol.* Retrieved from http://www.adhb.govt.nz/newborn/DrugProtocols/Default.htm.

Lack, J. A., & Stuart-Taylor, M. E. (1997). Calculation of drug dosage and body surface area of children. *British Journal of Anaesthesia, 78*: 601-605.

Lacy, C. (1990-2000). *Drug information handbook* (7th ed.). Cleveland: Lexi-Corp, Inc.

Leahy-Patano, M. (2008). Safety at the pump [electronic version]. *Acuity Care Technology.*

Leidel, B. A., Kirchhoff, C., Bogner, V., et al. (2012). Comparison of intraosseous versus central venous vascular access in adults under resuscitation in the emergency department with in accessible peripheral veins. *Resuscitation, 83*(1):40-45.

Lilley, L. L., & Guanci, R. (1994). Getting back to basics. *American Journal of Nursing, 9*:15-16.

Lu, M., & Okeke, C. (2005). *Requirements for compounding sterile preparations: Evolution of USP's chapter.* Retrieved from http://www.usp.org/hqi/practitioner-Programs/newsletters/capsLink/.

Macklin, D., Chernecky, C., & Infortuna, M. H. (2011). *Math for clinical practice* (2nd ed.). St. Louis: Elsevier/Mosby.

Maddox, R. R., Danello, S., Williams, C. K., & Fields, M. (2008). Intravenous infusion safety initiative: Collaboration, evidence-based best practices, and "smart" technology help avert high-risk adverse drug events and improve patient outcomes [electronic version]. *Advances in Patient Safety: New Directions and Alternative Approaches, 1*(4):1-14.

Magnuson, V., Clifford, T. M., Hoskins, L. A., & Bernard, A. C. (2005). Enteral nutrition and drug administration, interactions, and complications. *Nutrition in Clinical Practice, 20*(6):618-624. Retrieved from www.ncp.aspenjournals.org/cgi/content/full/20/6/618.

McKinley Medical. (2001). *Ambulatory infusion pump.* Retrieved from www.mckinleymed.com.

McKinley Medical. (2001). *High tech IVs raise issues—intravenous infusion systems.* Retrieved from www.mckinleymed.com.

McKinley Medical. (n.d.). *Intravenous therapy.* Retrieved from www.mckinleymed.com/intravenous-therapy.shtml.

McKinley Medical. (n.d.). *Infusion pumps.* Retrieved from www.mckinleymed.com/infusion-pump-systems.shtml.

Medscape. (2006). *ASHP National Survey of pharmacy practice.* Retrieved from www.medscape.com/viewarticle/523005.

Mentes, J. C. (2004). *Hydration management evidence based-practice guidelines.* Iowa City: University of Iowa.

Mentes, J. C. (2006). Oral hydration in older adults. *American Journal of Nursing, 106*(6):40-48.

MMWR. (2005). *Immunization management issues.* CDC. Retrieved from www.cdc.gov/mmwr/preview/mmwrhtml/rr5416a3.htm.

Morris, D. G. (2010). Calculate with confidence (5th ed) St. Louis: Elsevier/Mosby.

Mulholland, J. M. (2011). *The nurse, the math, the meds* (2nd ed). St. Louis: Elsevier/Mosby.

Murray, M.D. (n.d.). *Unit-dose drug distribution systems.* Retrieved from www.ahrq.gov/clinic/ptsafety/chap10.htm.

National Coordinating Council for Medication Error Reporting and Prevention. (2005). *Council recommendation.* Retrieved from www.nccmerp.org/council/council1996-09-04.html.

National Institute of Health (NIH). (1998). *First federal obesity clinical guidelines released.* Retrieved from www.nhlbi.nih.gov/new/press/ober14f.htm.

Neville, K., Galinkin, J. I., Green, T. P., et al. (2015). Metric units and the preferred dosing of orally administered liquid medications. [electronic Version]. *Pediatrics, 1359*(4):784-787.

Niemi, K., Geary, S., Larrabee, M., & Brown, K. R. (2005). Standardized vasoactive medications: a unified system for every patient, everywhere. *Hospital Pharmacy, 40*(11):984-993.

Ogden, S. J. (2012). Calculation of drug dosages (9th ed.). St. Louis: Elsevier/Mosby.

Okeke, C. (2005). Pharmaceutical calculations in prescription compounding [electronic version]. *Pharmacopeial Forum, 31*(3):846.

Owen, D., Jew, R., Kaufman, D., & Balmer, D. (1997). Osmolality of commonly used medications and formulas in the neonatal intensive care unit. *Nutrition Clinics, 12*(4).

Oyama, A. (2000). Intravenous line management and prevention of catheter-related infections in America. *Journal of Intravenous Nursing, 23*(3):170-175.

PALL Medical. (n.d.). *Posidyne ELD intravenous filter set.* Retrieved from www.pall.com.

Partners Healthcare System, Inc. (2003). *Project 4: safe intravenous infusion systems.* Retrieved from www.coesafety.bwh.harvard.edu/linkPages/projectsPages/project4.htm.

PatientPlus. (n.d.). *Prescribing in children.* Retrieved from www.patient.co/uk/showdoc/40024942.

Physicians' Desk Reference. (69th ed.). Montvale, NJ: PDR Network, LLC.

Pinkney, S., Trbovich, P., Rothwell, S., et al. (2009). Smart medication delivery system: Infusion pumps. *Healthcare Human Factors Group.* Retrieved from http://www.ehealthinnovation.org/?q_smartpumps.

Praxbind. https://www.praxbind.com.

Ratain, M. J. (1998). Body-surface area as a basis for dosing of anticancer agents: science, myth, or habit? *Journal of Clinical Oncology, 16*(7): 2297-2298.

Rothschild, J. M. (2003). *Intelligent intravenous infusion pumps to improve medical administration safety.* AMIA Annual Symposium Process. Retrieved from www.pubmedcentral.nih.gov.articlerender.fegi?artid_1480207.

Savinetti-Rose, B., & Bolmer, L. (1997). Understanding continuous subcutaneous insulin infusion therapy. *American Journal of Nursing, 97*:42-49.

Skokal, W. (1997). Infusion pump update. *RN, 60*:35-38.

Spratto, G., & Woods, A. (2003). *PDR Nurse's drug handbook.* Albany, NY: Delmar Publishers.

Taxis, K. (2005). *Safety infusion devices.* Grogingen: BMJ Publishing-Group. Retrieved from www.qhc.bmjjournals.com/cgi/content/ ful/14/2/76.

Terry, J., Baranowski, L., Lonsway, R., & Hedrick, C. (1995). *Intravenous therapy: Clinical principles and practice.* Philadelphia: W.B. Saunders.

Tessella Support Services. (2005). *Software that saves your life.* ALARIS. Retrieved from www.tessella.com/literature/articles/tessarchive/alaris.htm.

Thimbleby, H., & Williams, D. (2013). Using nomograms to reduce harm from clinical calculations. *Proceedings of IEEE International Conference on Healthcare Informatics, 461-470.*

Toedter Williams, N. (2009). Medical administration through enteral feeding tubes [electronic version]. *American Journal of Health-Systems Pharmacy, 65*(24):2347-2357.

Truax Group (The). (2010). *Infusion pump safety.* Retrieved from http://www.patientsafetysolutions.com/docs/April_27_2010_Infusion_ Pump_Safety.htm.

Vanderveen, T. (2002). *Impact of intravenous (IV) infusion medication errors.* Retrieved from www.cardinalhealth.com/alaris/support/clinical/pdfs/wpguardrails.asp.

Vanderveen, T. (2005). *Medication safety: averting high-risk errors is first priority.* Patient Safety & Quality Healthcare. Retrieved from www.psqh.com/mayjun05/averting.html.

Wideman, M.V., Whittler, M.E., & Anderson, T.M. (n.d.). *Barcode medication administration: lessons learned from an intensive card unit implementation.* Columbia, Mo: Agency for Healthcare Research and Quality.

Wyeth, Laboratories (1988). *Intramuscular injections.* Philadelphia: Wyeth Laboratories.

Youngberg Webb, P., & Chilamkurti, R. (2009). *Formulations: RTU drug products, the keys to RTU parenterals* [electronic version]. *Pharmaceutical Formulation & Quality.*

INDEX

Page references with f indicate figures; those with t, tables.